Clinical Ophthalmology Companion

Anthony Zaborowski

Colin Cook

JUTA

Clinical Ophthalmology Companion
First published 2010

Juta and Company Ltd
PO Box 14373, Lansdowne, 7779, Cape Town, South Africa

ISBN 978-0-7021-8033-0

Project Manager: Johanna Breakey
Editor and proofreader: Lorraine Johnstone
Typesetter: Lebone Publishing Services
Indexer: Cecily van Gend
Cover designer: Genevieve Simpson
Printed in South Africa by ABC Press

Contents

Foreword viii

Acknowledgements ix

Abbreviations x

Chapter 1 Examination technique

General ophthalmic examination 1
Eyelids 2
Ptosis 3
Watering eye 4
Cornea 5
Glaucoma 6
Pupil 8
Lens and cataracts 9
Cataract surgery – pre-operative examination 9
Retina 10
Macula 11
Strabismus 11
Proptosis 12
Thyroid eye disease 13
Neuro-ophthalmology 14
Refractive surgery – pre-operative examination 18
Functional visual loss 19

Chapter 2 Eyelids and lacrimal system

Disorders of lid position 20
Blepharophimosis syndrome 20
Benign eyelid nodules and cysts 22
Allergic lid disorders 23
Eyelid infections 23
Disorders of the eyelashes 23
Miscellaneous acquired eyelid disorders 24
Miscellaneous congenital eyelid disorders 24
Eyelid tumours 25
Lacrimal disorders 26

Chapter 3 Conjunctiva

Dry eye syndrome 29
Xerophthalmia 30
Conjunctival degenerations 31
Miscellaneous inflammations 35
Chronic progressive conjunctival cicatrisation 37
Tumours of the conjunctiva 39

Chapter 4 Cornea and sclera

Congenital abnormalities 42
Anterior chamber cleavage syndromes 44
Iridocorneal endothelial syndrome .. 46
Corneal dystrophies 46
Herpes zoster ophtalmicus 51
Keratitis 52
Ocular microbiology 59
Peripheral ulcerative keratitis 60
Phlyctenular disease 63
Keratoconus 65
Climate droplet keratopathy 68
Metabolic keratopathies 69
Miscellaneous keratopathies 73
Involutional diseases 77
Pterygium 79
Chemical burns 80
Contact lens 82
Keratoplasty 82
Limbal stem cell 85
Amniotic membrane 86
Scleritis 86
Episcleritis 88

Chapter 5 Glaucoma

Classification 90
Intraocular pressure 93
Disc changes in glaucoma 95
Gonioscopy 97

Primary chronic open angle glaucoma 97
Normal tension glaucoma 100
Ocular hypertension 101
Primary angle closure glaucoma 102
Congenital glaucoma 104
Secondary glaucomas 106
Neovascular glaucoma 108
Pigment dispersion 111
Pseudocapsular exfoliation 112
Inflammatory glaucoma 113
Lens-related glaucoma 114
Post-cataract surgery glaucoma 115
Ciliary block glaucoma 116
Iridocorneal dysgenesis 117
Iridocorneal endothelial syndrome 117
Tumours 117
Vitreoretinal surgery and corneal grafts 118
Glaucoma post-VR surgery 118
Genetics 118
Perimetery 119
Glaucoma drugs 122
Antifibrotic agents 124
Neuroprotection 124
Glaucoma imaging 124
Glaucoma in pregnancy 125
Studies in glaucoma 126

Chapter 6 Lens

Classification of cataracts 128
Congenital lens defects 128
Ectopia lentis 129
Senile cataracts 131
Secondary cataracts 131
Pre-operative evaluation 132
Biometery 133
Intraocular lenses 134
Viscoelastics 135
Surgical complications 136
Endophthalmitis 138
Post-operative astigmatism 139
Developmental cataracts 139
Cataract surgery in special situations 141
Cataract surgery in uveitis 142
Lens-induced uveitis and glaucoma 144

Chapter 7 The uvea

Aniridia 145
Iridocorneal endothelial (ICE) syndrome 146
Iris degenerations and atrophies 146
Uveitis classification 147
Clinical features of uveitis 148
Anterior uveitis – causes 148
Arthritis and uveitis 149
Gastrointestinal (GIT) diseases associated with uveitis 150
Renal diseases associated with uveitis 150
Behçet's disease 150
Sarcoidosis 152
Pars planitis 155
Vogt-Koyanagi-Harada (VKH) syndrome 155
Sympathetic uveitis 156
Fuchs' heterochromic iridocyclitis 157
Toxoplasmosis 158
Childhood uveitis 159
Juvenile idiopathic arthritis 162
Bacterial endophthalmitis 164
Fungal endophthalmitis 166
Ocular tuberculosis 167
Syphilis 168
Fungal uveitis 168
Viral uveitis 169
Parasitic uveitis 170
Ocular Leprosy 171
Uveitis masquerade syndromes 172
Uveal tumours 173
Choroidal melanoma 174
Ideopathic multifocal White Dot syndromes 177
Steroids 178
Cataract surgery in uveitis 182
Cilio choroidal detachment 184

Chapter 8 Retina and vitreous

Congenital retinal pigment epithelium and vascular abnormalities 185
Retinopathy of prematurity 186
Retinoblastoma 190
Retinitis pigmentosa 196
Angioid streaks 199
Albanism 200
Phacomatoses 200
Age-related macular degeneration .. 203
Choroidal neovascularisation 207
Retinal vein occlusions 208
Retinal arterial occlusive disease 211
Macular disease 214
Epiretinal membrane 214
Cystoid macular oedema 216
Central serous chorioretinopathy 217
Drug-induced maculopathies 218
Miscellaneous maculopathies 219
Hereditary fundal dystrophies 220
Vitreoretinal interface abnormalities .. 225
Diabetic retinopathy 227
Proliferative retinopathies 232
Eale's disease 233
Telangiectasias 234
Sickle cell retinopathy 235
Hypertensive retinopathy 236
Macroaneurysm 237
Vasculitis 237
Retinal detachment 238
Proliferative vitreoretinopathy 243
Peripheral retinal degenerations 244
Tears 245
Retinal pigment epithelium detachment 247
Retinoschisis 247
Myopia 248
Choroidal dystrophies 249
Choroidal folds 251
Vitreous disorders 251
Vitreous haemorrhage 253
Optic disc tumours 253
Fluorescein and ICG angiography 254
Optical coherence tomography 256
Electrodiagnostics 256
The electro-oculogram 257
Trauma 258

Chapter 9 The orbit

Anophthalmos 260
Craniosynostoses 260
Cystic lesions of the orbit 261
Dysthyroid eye disease 262
Idiopathic orbital inflammatory disease (orbital pseudotumour) .. 265
Lacrimal gland 267
Orbital lymphoma 269
Orbital infections 269
Orbitotomy 271
Other orbital tumours 272
Causes of proptosis 274
Orbital radiology 275
Rhabdomyosarcoma 276
Orbital trauma 276
Vascular lesions of the orbit 279

Chapter 10 Strabismus

Prevalence classification 282
Versions and vergences 283
Congenital esotropia 285
Accomodative esotropia 287
Other esotropias 288
Exotropia 290
Vertical deviations 292
Obliques 293
Paralytic and restrictive strabismus 295
Syndromes 296
Miscellaneous strabismus 298
Amblyopia 298
Monofixation syndrome 300
Motor adaptations (abnormal postures) 301
Sensory adaptations 301
Surgery 303
Surgical complications 305
Botulinum toxin (Botox) 306

Chapter 11 Neuro-ophthalmology

Congenital disc anomalies 307
Swollen disc 309
Optic atrophy 311
Anterior ischaemic optic neuropathy 313
Optic neuritis 315
Multiple sclerosis 317
Traumatic optic neuropathy 319
Nutritional and toxic optic neuropathies 320
Optic nerve tumours 321
Neuro-ophthalmic associations of diabetes mellitus 323
Cerebral aneurysms 323
Brain lesions 324
Cortical blindness 325
Headache and migraine 326
Myopathies 328
Nystagmus and spontaneous eye movement disorders 329
Optic chiasm syndrome 335
Diplopia 336
Third (oculomotor) nerve 338
Fourth (trochlear) nerve 340
Sixth (abducens) nerve 342
Seventh (facial) nerve 344
Combined ocular motor nerve palsies 346
Supranuclear and internuclear gaze palsies 348
Vascular malformations 352
Pupil 353
Visual fields 356
Neuroimaging 360

Chapter 12 Trauma

Chemical burns 361
Blunt trauma 363
Penetrating eye injuries 363
Stabbed orbit 365
Orbital fractures 365
Intraocular foreign bodies 367
Uveal trauma 369
Traumatic retinopathy 371

Chapter 13 Refractive error and refractive surgery

Refractive error 372
Anisometropia 376
Abnormalities of accommodation 377
Optical aberrations 378
Asthenopia 379
Astigmatism of oblique incidence 379
Aphakia 380
Spectacles 381
Power and notation of lenses 383
Toric lenses 383
Prisms 384
Contact lenses 385
Basic principles of refractive surgery 387
Classification of corneal refractive surgery 389
Intraocular surgery 389
Photoablation 390
Thermokeratoplasty 392
Incisional and inlay corneal surgery 392
IOL power calculation after refractive surgery 393
Presbyopia 393
Refractive surgery in ocular and systemic disease 395

Chapter 14 Systemic diseases

Acquired immune deficiency syndrome (AIDS) 397
Albinism 399
Chromosomal disorders 399
Haematological disorders and the eye 400
Leprosy 401
Liver disease 402
Metabolic disorders and the eye 402
Microphthalmos 403
Musculoskeletal disease and the eye 404
Myasthenia gravis 405
Phacomatoses 406
Rheumatoid arthritis 409

Skin diseases 410
Rubella 410
Syphilis 411

Chapter 15 Community eye health

Principles of prevention of blindness 412
Cataract 416
Refractive error 417
Childhood blindness 419
Glaucoma 422
Diabetic retinopathy 423

Foreword

From 1987 until 2004 Colin Cook was responsible for the development and provision of clinical and surgical ophthalmology services at Edendale Hospital in Pietermaritzburg. This included the training of both ophthalmic medical officers and nurses. During the training sessions Professor Cook provided handouts that proved to be especially popular, concise and user friendly.

In 2007 Anthony Zaborowski, who had passed through the programme, decided to produce an ophthalmology text that could be available as a "companion" to the busy ophthalmologist. He persuaded Colin Cook to join him in this endeavour, which would be based predominantly on the updated handouts.

The first edition of the *Clinical Ophthalmology Companion* has now come to fruition.

The Clinical Ophthalmology Companion has been written to complement rather than replace the many existing excellent referral texts. It is intentionally small enough to be carried by the ophthalmologist or optometrist in training, and is intended to serve as a readily available reference for utilisation in the everyday clinical setting.

The book has been compiled in an abbreviated and list-driven format, thereby presenting basic clinical information that is easy to access and to understand. The Companion concentrates on management, but includes aetiology, pathology, and pathophysiology where these are relevant for clinical reasons.

The book has fulfilled the authors' goals and should prove to be a real companion to both those in training and to the well established practitioner.

Anthony Murray
Emeritus Professor
University of Cape Town

Acknowledgements

Alcon Laboratories have made a generous donation towards the production of this book. We thank Alcon for their commitment to education in ophthalmology and their unfailing support for academic projects.

My sincere thanks to my co-author and mentor Professor Cook. Your organised and practical approach to ophthalmology is the inspiration behind this book. Thank you for your wisdom and guidance which has been the foundation of my career.

Anthony Zaborowski

Abbreviations

AACG acute angle closure glaucoma
AC anterior chamber
AC PIOL anterior chamber phakic intraocular lens
AC/A accommodative convergence / accommodation
ACC anterior corneal curvature
AGIS Advanced Glaucoma Intervention Study
AHP anomalous head posture
AIDS acquired immune deficiency syndrome
AION anterior ischaemic optic neuropathy
AK arcuate keratototomy
ALT argon laser trabeculoplasty
AMD age-related macular degeneration
AMPP acute multifocal placoid pigmented epitheliopathy
AN aniridia
ANA antinuclear antibody
ANCA antineutrophilic cytoplasmic antibody
APD afferent papillary defect
ARC anomalous retinal correspondence
ARMD age related macular degeneration
ARN acute retinal necrosis
ASAP as soon as possible
ATP adenosine triphosphate
AV arteriovenous

BAB blood aqueous barrier
BD twice daily
BHL bilateral hilar lymphadenopathy
BP blood pressure
BPES blepharophimosis ptosis epicanthus inversus syndrome
BRAO branch retinal artery occlusion
BRVO branch retinal vein occlusion
BSS balanced salt solution

CACG chronic angle closure glaucoma
c-ANCA classical anti-neutrophil cytoplasmic antibody
CHRPE congenital hypertrophy of the retinal pigment epithelium
CIGTS Collaborative Initial Glaucoma Treatment Study
CK conductive keratoplasty
CMO cystoid macular oedema
CMV cytomegalovirus
CNS central nervous system
CNTGS Collaborative Normal Tension Glaucoma Study
CNV choroidal neovascularisation
COAG chronic open angle glaucoma
COWS cold opposite, warm same
CRAO central retinal artery occlusion
CRF chronic renal failure
CRP c-reactive protein
CRVO central retinal vein occlusion
CSA cyclosporin A
CSCR central serous chorioretinopathy
CSF cerebrospinal fluid
CSMO clinically significant macular oedema
CSR cataract surgery rate
CT computerised tomography
CUWD cold up, warm down
CVA cerebrovascular accident
CXR chest X-ray

D-ACE drain air cryopexy explant
dB decibels
DBR diabetic retinopathy
DCCT Diabetes Control and Complications Trial
DD disc diameters
DHD dissociated horizontal deviation
DIDMOAD diabetes insipidus, diabetes mellitus, optic atrophy, deafness
DNA deoxyribonucleic acid
DR diabetic retinopathy
DRS Diabetic Retinopathy Study
DRVS Diabetic Retinopathy Vitrectomy Study
DVD dissociated vertical deviation
EBV Epstein-Barr virus
ECCE extracapsular cataract extraction
ECLE extracapsular lens extraction
EDTA ethylenediaminetetraacetic acid

EEP electrically-evoked potential
ELISA enzyme-linked immunosorbent assay
EMGT Early Manifest Glaucoma Trials
ENT ear nose and throat
EOG electrooculogram
EOM extraocular muscles
ERG electroretinogram
ERM epiretinal membrame
ERP early receptor potential
ESR erythrocyte sedimentation rate
ETDRS Early Treatment Diabetic Retinopathy Study
EUA examination under anaesthetic

FAZ foveal avascular zone
FB foreign body
FBC full blood count
FDA Food and Drug Administration
FDT Frequency Doubling Technology perimetry
FEM fast eye movements
FTA fluorescent treponemal antibody

GDx Glaucoma Diagnosis machine
GIT gastro-intestinal tract
Gy gray

hb haemoglobin
HIV human immunovirus
HLA human leukocyte antigen
HRT Heidelberg retinal tomography
HZO herpes zoster ophthalmicus

ICE syndrome iridocorneal endothelial syndrome
ICG indocyanine green
ICL implantable contact lens
ICLE intracapsular lens extraction
ICP intracranial pressure
IgA immunoglobulin A
IgG immunoglobulin G
IMI intramuscular injection
Intacs intrastromal corneal ring segments
IO inferior oblique
IOFB intraocular foreign body
PAN polyarteritis nodosa
IOL intraocular lens
IOOA inferior oblique overaction
IOP intraocular pressure
IR inferior rectus
IRMA intraretinal microvascular anomalies
ISNT inferior superior nasal temporal
IVI intravenous injection
IVI MP intravenous methylprednisolone
IVT intravitreal

JIA juvenile idiopathic arthritis

KP keratic precipitates

LASEK laser subepithelial keratomileusis
LASIK laser-assisted in situ keratomileusis
LDH lactate dehydrogenase
LFT liver function test
LOCS Lens Opacification Classification System
LR lateral rectus
LTK laser thermokeratoplasty

MD mean deviation
MEWDS (Multiple Evanescent White Dot Syndrome)
MI myocardial infarction
MMC mitomycin C
MP methylprednisolone
MR medial rectus
MRA magnetic resonance angiogram
MRI magnetic resonance imaging
MS multiple sclerosis

NB nota bene
NFL nerve fibre layer
NMDA N-methyl-D-aspartate
NPDBR non-proliferative diabetic retinopathy
NPL no perception of light
NS nuclear sclerosis
NSAID non-steroidal anti-inflammatory drug
NVD new vessels at the disc
NVE new vessels elsewhere
OCT optical coherence tomography
OKN optokinetic nystagmus
ON optic nerve

PAS peripheral anterior synechiae
PC posterior capsule
PCC posterior corneal curvature
PCIOL posterior chamber intraocular lens
PCO posterior capsular opacification
PCOAG primary chronic open angle glaucoma
PCR polymerase chain reaction
PDR proliferative diabetic retinopathy
PDT photodynamic therapy
PED pigment epithelial detachment
PHPV persistent hyperplastic primary vitreous
PHTC Phenylthiocarbamide
PIOL phakic intraocular lens
PMMA polymethylmethacrylate
PO orally
POAG primary open angle glaucoma
PORN progressive outer retinal necrosis
PPV pars plana vitrectomy
PRK photorefractive keratectomy
PRN when required
PRP pan retinal photocoagulation
PS posterior synechiae
PSCLO posterior subcapsular lens opacity
PSD pattern standard deviation
PTB pulmonary tuberculosis
PVD posterior vitreous detachment

RA rheumatoid arthritis
RAO retinal artery occlusion
RB retinoblastoma
RD retinal detachment
RK radial keratototomy
RNA ribonucleic acid
ROP retinopathy of prematurity
RP retinitis pigmentosa
RPE retinal pigment epithelium
RRD rhegmatogenous retinal detachment
RT radiotherapy

SACE serum angiotensin converting enzyme
SBV single binocular vision
SEM slow eye movements
SITA Swedish Interactive Threshold Algorithm
SLE systemic lupus erythematosis
SO superior oblique
SOOA superior oblique overaction
SOUA superior oblique underaction
SR superior rectus
SRF subretinal fluid
SRK Sanders-Retzlaff-Kraft
SRNV subretinal neovascularisation
STD sexually transmitted disease
STIR short tau inversion recovery
SWAP Short Wavelength Automated Perimetry

TB tuberculosis
TED thyroid eye disease
TINU tubulointerstitial nephritis and uveitis
TORCH Toxoplasmosis Other viruses Rubella Cytomegalovirus Herpes
TPHA Treponema Pallidum Haemagglutination
TRD tractional retinal detachment
TSH thyroid stimulating hormone
TTT transpupillary diode thermotherapy

U+E urea and electrolytes
UC ulcerative colitis
UGH uveitis glaucoma hyphaema
US ultrasound
UV ultraviolet

VA visual acuity
Va ophthalmic branch of the trigeminal nerve
Vb maxillary branch of the trigeminal nerve
Vc mandibular branch of the trigeminal nerve
VEC Vincristine, Etoposide and Carboplatin
VEGF vasoendothelial growth factor
VER visual evoked response
VKH Vogt-Koyanagi-Harada syndrome
VR vitreoretinal

WCC white cell count
WEBINO wall-eyed bilateral internuclear ophthalmoplegia
WHO World Health Organisation
WR widal reaction (syphilis)

XL X-linked

YAG yttrium aluminium garnet

1

Examination technique

General ophthalmic examination 1
Eyelids 2
Ptosis 3
Watering eye 4
Cornea 5
Glaucoma 6
Pupil 8
Lens and cataracts 9
Cataract surgery – pre-operative examination 9
Retina 10
Macula 11
Strabismus 11
Proptosis 12
Thyroid eye disease 13
Neuro-ophthalmology 14
Refractive surgery – pre-operative examination 18
Functional visual loss 19

General ophthalmic examination

History

General

- Name
- Age
- Gender
- Race/ethnicity
- Occupation

Present ophthalmic

- Poor vision
- Double vision
- Pain
- Discharge
- Change in appearance

Past ophthalmic

- Medical
- Surgical
- Spectacles

General medical and surgical

- Diabetes
- Hypertension
- Arthritis
- Tuberculosis
- Allergies

Medication

Systemic enquiry

- Neurological
- Cardiovascular
- Respiratory
- Gastrointestinal
- Ear-nose-throat
- Musculoskeletal
- Dermatology

Family history

Social history

Examination

Vision

- Visual acuity – without correction, with pinhole, with correction

1

- Refraction – objective, subjective, near add
- Visual field – red confrontation
- Colour vision – Ishihara plates

Pupils

- Direct
- Consensual
- Near reflex
- Light-near dissociation

Ocular motility

- Proptosis, orbits, regional lymphadenopathy
- Stereopsis
- Versions
- Vergences
- Cover-uncover
- Alternate cover
- Prism fusional amplitudes

Slit lamp

- Adnexae – lids, lashes, brows, punctae, tear sac
- Tear film, tear meniscus, fluorescein, tear break-up time
- Conjunctiva, episclera, sclera, fornices
- Cornea, corneal sensation
- Anterior chamber
  - Iris
  - Pupil
  - Lens
  - Anterior vitreous
- Intraocular pressure

Ophthalmoscopy

- Direct, red-free
- Indirect
- Slit lamp lens
- Disc, vessels, posterior pole, macula, periphery

Special examinations

- Amsler grid examination
- Perimetry
- Arden grating acuity
- Corneal topography
- Exophthalmometry
- Farnsworth-Munsell colour test
- Gonioscopy
- Indentation fundal examination
- Keratometry
- Pachymetry
- Schirmer test

Eyelids

Lid position

- Ptosis (see separate exam format), retraction

Opening and closing

- Lagophthalmos

Margin and glands

- Cysts, blepharitis – anterior, posterior, mixed

Lashes

- Trichiasis, dystichiasis, madarosis, poliosis

Lymphatics

- Pre-auricular → upper lid + lateral canthus
- Submandibular → lower lid + medial canthus

Involutional ectropion

- Horizontal laxity – central part of lid can be pulled ≥ 8 mm from globe + does not snap back into normal position without blinking
- Medial canthal tendon laxity – pull lower lid laterally + observe punctum; abnormal → displacement of > 1–2 mm; mild laxity → punctum reaches limbus; severe laxity → punctum reaches pupil
- Lateral canthal tendon laxity – ability to pull the lower lid > 2 mm medially

Involutional entropion

- Horizontal lid laxity

Ptosis

History

- Age of onset
- Duration
- Predisposing factors
- Associated symptoms – diplopia, pain, variability, systemic diseases
- Family history

Examination

Pseudoptosis

- Lack of lid support e.g. enophthalmos, contralateral lid retraction, ipsilateral hypotropia (lid follows globe downwards), brow ptosis, dermatochalasis

Degree of ptosis

- Margin-reflex distance – normal is 4–4.5 mm
- Vertical fissure height – males = 7–10 mm, females = 8–12 mm
- Unilateral ptosis – compare with contralateral side; mild ≤ 2 mm; moderate – 3 mm; severe ≥ 4 mm
- Margin position – upper normally 2 mm below upper limbus and 1 mm above lower limbus

Levator function

- Negate frontalis with thumb
- Measure upper lid excursion from downgaze to upgaze
  - Normal: ≥ 15 mm
  - Good: 12–14 mm
  - Fair: 5–11 mm
  - Poor: < 4 mm

Skin crease position

- Used to guide initial incision
  - High crease → aponeurotic defect
  - Absent crease → congenital ptosis
- Measure – distance between upper lid margin + crease in downgaze: males = 8 mm, females = 10 mm

General

- Chin-lift, mechanical causes, lid lag on down gaze, Bell's phenomenon, Marcus Gunn jaw winking phenomenon, blepharophimosis, features of III palsy, features of Horner's syndrome corneal sensation, tear film, amblyopia in children

Pharmacological testing

- Tensilon, cocaine, hydro-xyamphetamine, adrenaline 1:1 000

Causes of Ptosis

- Congenital
  - Dystrophic
  - Blepharophimosis syndrome
  - Marcus-Gunn jaw winking
- Acquired
  - Involutional/senile
  - Myogenic – Myasthenia gravis, chronic progressive external ophthalmoplegia, myotonic dystrophy
  - Neurogenic – III palsy, Horner's syndrome
  - Traumatic + post-operative
  - Mechanical – tumours, scarring, oedema, anterior orbital lesions

Causes of lid retraction

- Thyroid eye disease
- Neurogenic
  - Contralateral unilateral ptosis
  - VII palsy
  - III misdirection
  - Marcus Gunn jaw winking
  - Parinaud's dorsal midbrain syndrome
- Mechanical – cicatrisation, surgical overcorrection
- Congenital – isolated, Duane's syndrome, Down's syndrome
- Miscellaneous – uraemia

Watering eye

History

- Use of topical medications
- Trauma, surgery
- Previous dacryocystitis
- Blood-tinged tears, pain

Examination

- Signs of ocular surface irritation with secondary hypersecretion
- Signs of outflow obstruction

External examination

- Tear overflow
- Corneal + conjunctival epithelium – fluorescein + rose bengal
- Marginal tear strip – especially if unilateral; precipitates; tear film break-up time
- Eyelids – ectropion; lagophthalmos → lacrimal pump malfunction; blepharitis, cysts, infections
- Dynamics of eyelid closure – one lid overriding the other
- Puncta – malposition, inflammation, stenosis, obstruction, material expression; reflux → canalicular system patent, nasolacrimal duct obstructed
- Lacrimal sac – palpate; mucous, stone, tumour
- Fluorescein disappearance test – normally little or no dye lasts > 3 mins; especially useful if unilateral abnormality
- Nasal examination – tumour, polyp, allergic rhinitis

Probing + irrigation

- Hard stop → canalicular system patent; irrigate for patency, sac will distend, ± fluid into nose
- Soft stop → canalicular obstruction, sac will not distend

Jones dye testing

- Only for suspected partial obstruction
- Primary – differentiates partial obstruction from primary hypersecretion
  - Fluorescein into conjuctival sac, 5 mins later → cotton bud into nose
  - Positive test – fluorescein recovered → primary hypersecretion
  - Negative test – no dye → partial obstruction, site unknown
- Secondary – if primary test negative, to identify site of obstruction
  - Done immediately after primary test
  - Irrigate system with normal saline with cotton bud in nose
  - Positive test – dye in nose → partial obstruction of nasolacrimal duct
  - Negative – no dye → canalicular or punctal obstruction

Contrast dacryocystography

- Lipiodol contrast injected into lacrimal sac

Lacrimal scintillography

- Technetium labelled tears in conjunctival sac

Computerised tomography scan

- Post-traumatic epiphora

Cornea

General

- Periocular skin, position + action of the eyelids, pre-auricular lymph nodes, globe placement, eyelid eversion → palpebral conjunctiva

Size

- Average 11.5 mm vertical, 12 mm horizontal
- Megalocornea ≥ 13 mm; microcornea ≤ 10 mm

Thickness

- Central cornea 490–560 μm, limbus 700–900 μm

Curvature

- Normal ± 44D

Epithelium

- Diffuse illumination, direct slit illumination, retro-illumination
- Punctate epithelial erosions – non-specific; stain with fluorescein but not rose bengal
- Punctate epithelial keratitis – viral; stain well with rose bengal, poorly with fluorescein
- Epithelial oedema ± bullae
- Filaments – stain well with rose bengal but not fluorescein
- Pannus

Stroma

- Slit illumination
- Scleral scatter (total internal reflection in cornea) – light incident on limbus, microscope central
- Infiltrates, oedema, vascularisation, scar

Endothelium

- Retro-illumination – fine endothelial changes, keratic precipitates
- Specular reflection – endothelial mosaic + guttata

Descemet's membrane

- Breaks (Haab's striae, birth trauma, keratoconus)
- Folds (striate keratopathy)

Nerves

Vessels

Perilimbal area

Corneal sensation

- Aesthesiometry – for evaluating neurotrophic keratopathy

Special examinations

- Keratometry – central 2–3 mm of cornea
- Corneal topography – colour-coded map
- Pachymetry
- Specular microscopy
  - Normal endothelial cell a regular hexagon
  - Normal cell density – 3 000/mm^2;
  - < 1 000 → high risk of endothelial decompensation from cataract surgery
  - Polymegathism – increase in variation of cell size
  - Pleomorphism – increase in variation in cell shape
- Anterior segment photography
- Confocal microscopy
- Schirmer test

Stains

- Fluorescein
  - Positive staining – punctate + ulcerative epithelial defects
  - Negative staining – highlights non-staining lesions, projecting through the tear film
  - Seidel test, dye disappearance test

- Rose bengal – stains devitalised cells
- Lissamine green

Glaucoma

History

- Symptoms – pain, redness, halos, blurring, trauma
- Ophthalmic history – surgery, previous diagnosis of glaucoma, other ocular diseases
- Past medical history – diabetes, cardiac, pulmonary, hypertension, migraine, neurological disease, renal stones
- Medication – steroids

Examination

Refraction

- Important for accurate perimetry
- Hyperopia → risk for angle closure
- Myopia → ? risk for open angle glaucoma

Pupils

- Compliance in miotic therapy
- Afferent pupil defect

Conjunctiva

- Injection in acute IOP elevation
- Allergic reactions from topical drop use
- Old surgery

Episclera and sclera

- Vessel dilation or angiomas in Sturge-Weber syndrome
- Old surgery

Cornea

- Haab's stria
- Enlarged cornea – buphthalmos
- Anterior segment anomalies in irido-corneal dysgenesis
- Krukenberg spindle
- Anterior Schwalbe's line
- Corneal oedema
- Signs of trauma – scars

Anterior chamber

- Depth
- Activity, pigment dispersion

Iris

- Heterochromia
- Atrophy
- Peripheral iridectomy
- Transillumination
- Ectropion uveae
- Corectopia
- Naevi
- Nodules
- Pseudocapsular exfoliation
- Rubeosis
- Signs of trauma – sphincter rupture, iridodenesis, vitreous in anterior chamber

Lens

- Pseudoexfoliative material on capsule
- Phacodenesis
- Size, shape, clarity
- IOL type + position
- Status of posterior capsule

Tonometry

- Goldmann
- Schiotz
- Perkins
- Air puff
- Tonopen

Gonioscopy

- + Indentation
- Corneal wedge
- Schwalbe's line
- Trabeculum
- Schlemm's canal
- Scleral spur
- Ciliary body
- Iris processes/root
- Blood vessels

Shaffer grading angle width	
■ Grade 4 (35–45°)	□ **Ciliary body** visible with ease □ Seen in myopia and aphakia □ Incapable of closure
■ Grade 3 (25–35°)	□ **Scleral spur** visible □ Incapable of closure
■ Grade 2 (20°)	□ **Trabeculum** identifiable □ Moderately narrow □ Angle closure possible but unlikely
■ Grade 1 (10°)	□ **Schwalbe's line** + top of trabecular meshwork visible □ Very narrow □ Risk of closure high
■ Slit angle	□ **No angle structures** visible but no iridocorneal touch □ Danger of imminent closure
■ Grade 0	□ **Closed angle** □ Iridocorneal touch

Optic nerve head

- Cup
- Disc size/height
- Cup-disc ratio
- Neuroretinal rim
    - ISNT rule (the neuroretinal rim is normally thickest inferiorly, followed by superiorly, nasally and is thinnest temporally)
    - Notching
- Blood vessels – nasalisation, bayoneting
- Nerve fibre layer – red-free light
- Peripapillary atrophy – alpha + beta zone

Clinically important disc signs	
■ Weak	□ Alpha and beta zone □ Peripapillary zone □ Cup > pallor □ Narrowing of retinal arteries
■ Moderate	□ ISNT rule not obeyed
■ Strong	□ Notch □ Nasal cupping □ Large cup for small disc □ Localised retinal nerve fibre layer loss □ Diffuse retinal nerve fibre layer loss □ Generalised retinal nerve fibre layer loss □ Acquired optic disc pit □ Optic disc haemorrhage □ Cup-disc ratio asymmetry ≥ 0.2

Imaging

- Stereoscopic disc photographs
- Heidelberg retinal tomography (HRT)
- Optical coherence tomography (OCT)
- Scanning laser polarimetry (GDx)

Perimetry

- Humphrey
- SITA
- SWAP
- Frequency doubling

Pupil

- Old photographs
- Size, shape, position, anisocoria
- Anisocoria – examine in light and dark
- Direct light reflex – patient fixates on a distant object
- Consensual light reflex
- Swinging flashlight test – remain 3–5 secs on each eye to allow pupillary stabilisation
- Near reflex
- Iris exam with lights on – heterochromia, atrophy
- Slit lamp exam – posterior synechiae, sphincter tears, iris atrophy, vermiform movements, gonioscopy

Specific pupil disorders

■ Afferent pupil defect (Marcus Gunn pupil)	□ 3–4+: Immediate pupil dilation □ 1–2+: No change in pupil size initially, followed by dilation □ Trace: Initial constriction, then escape to larger size than the same exercise on the other pupil
■ Amaurotic pupil	□ Maximum Marcus Gunn pupil
■ Adie's tonic pupil	□ Viral parasympathetic post-ganglionic denervation with regeneration from parasympathetic nerves serving the ciliary muscle □ Dilated pupil; poor or absent light reflex □ Slow constriction to near; slow redilation □ Accommodative paresis □ Segmental palsy of sphincter muscles □ Cholinergic sensitivity to weak pilocarpine solutions □ Holmes-Adie syndrome – Adie's pupil plus diminished deep tendon reflexes
■ Horner's syndrome	□ Sympathetic paralysis □ Miosis, ptosis ± anhidrosis □ Inferior lid higher (upside down ptosis) □ Iris heterochromia if congenital □ ± Dilated conjunctival + facial vessels, decreased IOP, increased accommodation □ Cocaine 4% – Horner's pupil does not dilate, normal pupil does (blocks re-uptake of adrenaline at the myoneural junction) □ Hydroxyamphetamine 1%: Pre-ganglionic – dilation, post-ganglionic – no dilation (causes release of adrenaline from nerve endings) □ Adrenaline 1:000: Pre-ganglionic – no dilation, pre-ganglionic – dilation (a normal nerve breaks adrenaline down quickly by monoamine oxidase)

- Argyll-Robertson pupils
  - Miotic + irregular
  - Light-near dissociation
  - Dilates poorly; poor response to light; brisk response to near
  - Usually bilateral, may be unilateral

Lens and cataracts

History

- Decreased visual acuity
- Glare
- Myopic shift
- Monocular diplopia

Examination

Morphology

- Subcapsular – anterior + posterior
- Nuclear
- Cortical
- Christmas tree

Maturity

- Immature
- Mature
- Hypermature
- Morgagnian

Lens Opacification Classification System (LOCS) score

- Posterior subcapsular (P0.1–P5.9)
- Cortical (C0.1–C5.9)
- Nuclear sclerosis (N0.1–N6.9)

Cataract surgery – pre-operative examination

History

- General health and medication
- Ocular history
  - Factors that could affect the surgical approach or prognosis e.g. trauma, inflammation, amblyopia, glaucoma
  - Outcome of previous surgery e.g. vitreous loss, endophthalmitis, cystoid macular oedema
- Social – need for surgery, post-op care and visual needs

Examination

Visual acuity

- ± Light projection ± pinhole ± best correction – in light + dark conditions
- Brightness acuity – visual acuity in bright room to assess effect of glare

Visual fields

- Confrontation, Humphrey

General

- Body habitus – tremor, bull neck, obesity, kyphosis

Adnexae

- Prominent brow, enophthalmos, blepharitis, tear film

Motility

- A significant phoria may break down post-op → diplopia
- Exclude pre-existing strabismus + amblyopia

Pupils

- Exclude afferent pupil defect

Conjunctiva

- Scarring, vascularisation can dictate surgical approach

Cornea

- Corneal thickness, opacities
- Guttata
  - Thickness > 600μ → poor prognosis for corneal clarity

1

Anterior chamber

- Depth – intumescent lens, posterior pathology
- Gonioscopy – peripheral anterior synechiae, angle neovascularisation especially if anterior chamber IOL anticipated

Iris

- Pupil size post-dilation
- Posterior synechiae

Lens

- Pseudocapsular exfoliation, phacodenesis, intumescence, subluxation, lenticular contribution to visual defect (assess with direct opthalmoscope red reflex)

Fundus

- Direct and indirect ophthalmoscopy
- Macula, optic nerve, retinal vessels, periphery

Potential acuity estimation

- To assess the lenticular contribution to visual loss; better for moderate lens opacities than dense lens opacities
- Laser inferometry – twin sources of monochromatic helium-neon laser light create a diffraction fringe pattern on the retinal surface. Transmission of this pattern is largely independent of lens opacity
- Potential acuity meter – a numerical or letter chart is projected through the lenticular opacities

Tests of macular function

- Maddox rod – loss of the red line caused by a large scotoma → macular disease
- Photostress test – get baseline visual acuity, then shine a light into the eye for 10 secs, then measure the time taken to read any 3 letters of the pre-stress acuity line
  - Best for checking one abnormal eye + comparing with good eye
  - Normal recovery time 27 secs; 99% of normal eyes recover within 50 secs
- Blue-light entoptoscopy – patient views an intense, blue, homogenous background; will see white blood corpuscles if macula functioning
- Purkinje's entoptic phenomenon – rapidly oscillating point source of light shone through closed eyelids; will see shadows of the retinal vasculature
- Electroretinogram, visual evoked potential

Pre-op measures

- Refraction
- Biometry
- Corneal pachymetry
- Specular microscopy
- B-scan ultrasound

Retina

External examination

- Tyres + sponges from previous surgery
- Conjunctiva + sclera for old ports, sutures, scarring

Fundus examination

- Disc, peripapillary area, blood vessels, posterior pole + macula, periphery

Indirect fundoscopy

- Indentation – to enhance visualisation of the peripheral retina + allows a dynamic exam; enhances contrast between choroid + sensory retina

Fundus drawing

- Detached retina → blue
- Flat retina → red
- Retinal veins → blue (arteries not drawn)
- Breaks → red with blue outline
- Flap of a retinal tear → blue

- Lattice → blue hatching
- Retinal pigment → black
- Exudates → yellow
- Vitreous opacities (including blood) → green

Three-mirror

- Central – 30 degree view of posterior pole
- Equatorial mirror (largest) – 30 degrees to equator
- Peripheral mirror (intermediate size) – equator to ora serrata
- Gonio mirror (smallest) – peripheral retina + pars plana

Linkoff's rules

- Shallow inferior detachment → inferior hole (hole on side where subretinal fluid slightly higher)
- Bullous inferior detachment → superior hole

B-scan

- Opaque media
- Dynamic ultrasonography with lateral eye movements

Macula

History

- Positive + negative scotomas
- Metamorphopsia, micropsia, macropsia

Amsler grid

- Evaluates central 10 degrees of field
- 10 cm square with 5 mm squares therein, 7 charts
- View at 30 cm

Photostress test

Fluorescein angiography

Dark adaptometry

- Useful in evaluating night blindness
- Goldman-Weekes adaptometry
- Expose to intense light, bleaching photoreceptors
- Then place in dark
- A series of flashing lights, gradually increasing in intensity
- Threshold when the patient first sees the light is plotted

Colour vision

- Ishihara, City Universal, Harvey-Rand-Rittler, Farnsworth-Munsell 100-hue, Farnsworth D15

Strabismus

History

- Present ophthalmic – age of onset, variability
- Past ophthalmic – glasses, previous surgery, previous eye problems; old photographs (strabismus or abnormal head position)
- Birth history
- Past medical history + systemic history – cerebral palsy, Down's syndrome, etc.
- Family

Examination

Visual acuity

- With + without correction (cycloplegic refraction)
- Occlusion, Volk's fixation, rotation test, preferential looking, optokinetic nystagmus, hundreds and thousands
- Near acuity

Appearance

- Abnormal head posture – head turn, tilt, chin-lift
- Gross abnormality

Stereopsis

- Titmus test
  - Fly tests gross stereopsis (3 000 secs of arc)
  - Circles test fine stereopsis (800–40 secs of arc)

- ◻ Animals test fine stereopsis (400–100 secs of arc)
- TNO random dot test, Lang test, Frisby test, base out prism test – 16D base out prism in front of one eye → corrective saccade to refixate if there is binocular single vision; useful in children who cannot do any of the above tests

Movements

- Ductions, versions, convergence
- Nystagmus
- Record diagrammatically as 1–4 + or – for each of the six directions of gaze for each of the eyes
- A or V pattern present
- Over- or underaction of any muscle (1–4 + or –)

Cover tests

- With + without correction
- Near and distance
- Primary position, 30 degrees left + right, 30 degrees up + down
- Hirschberg test (1 mm = 7 degrees = 15 dioptres)
- Krimsky test
- Prism cover
  - ◻ Cover → tropia
  - ◻ Cover-uncover → phoria
  - ◻ Alternate cover → phoria + tropia
  - ◻ Alternate prism cover → phoria + tropia
  - ◻ Simultaneous prism cover → tropia
- Type + size of deviation
- Signs of pseudosquint
- Parks 3-step test

Slit lamp exam + fundoscopy

- Including pupils

Special tests

- Dissimilar images
  - ◻ Maddox rod
  - ◻ Double Maddox rod (for bilateral IV palsy)
  - ◻ Maddox wing
- Sensory assessment
  - ◻ Synoptophore
  - ◻ Worth 4-dot
  - ◻ 4D base out prism
  - ◻ Bagolini striated lenses
  - ◻ After image
- Forced duction, forced generation
- Single binocular field
- Hess chart
- Maddox double prism
- Diplopia chart
- Tensilon test
- Electro-oculogram
- Optokinetic nystagmus
- Visual evoked response
- Bielschowsky phenomenon
- Neutral density filter

Proptosis

History

- Onset
- Duration
- Associated symptoms (pain)
- Variability

Examination

- True or pseudoproptosis – facial asymmetry, severe ipsilateral globe enlargement, ipsilateral lid retraction, contralateral enophthalmos
- Measurement of proptosis – Hertel exophthalmometer or ruler
  - ◻ 20 mm or difference > 2 mm → proptosis
  - ◻ Mild proptosis – 21–23 mm
  - ◻ Moderate – 24–27 mm
  - ◻ Severe – ≥ 28 mm
- Palpable masses
- Direction of proptosis – axial or non-axial
- Dystopia – displacement of the globe in the coronal plane
  - ◻ May co-exist with proptosis or enopthalmos
  - ◻ Measure from midline (nose) to nasal limbus

- Reducibility
- Variation with posture + valsalva
- Auscultation for bruit
- Corneal sensation/trigeminal nerve
- Extraocular motility III IV VI
- Forced duction
- Exposure keratopathy
- Pupil
- Disc – swelling, pallor, optociliary shunt vessels
- Choroidal folds
- Retinal vascular dilation + tortuosity
- Nasopharynx
- Regional lymphadenopathy
- Differential intraocular pressure test
- Systemic evidence of thyroid disease

Proptosis differential diagnosis

- Pseudoproptosis
    - Buphthalmos
    - Myopia
    - Contralateral enophthalmos
- Congenital
    - Craniosyntoses
    - Dermoid
    - Meningocoele
    - Encephalocoele
- Traumatic
    - Orbital + subperiosteal haemorrhage
    - Carotid-cavernous fistula
- Inflammatory
    - Idiopathic orbital inflammatory disease
    - Myositis
    - Posterior scleritis
    - Mucocoele
    - Dacryoadenitis
    - Tolosa Hunt syndrome
    - Cavernous sinus thrombosis
    - Wegeners granulomatosis
- Neoplastic
    - Benign – haemangioma, lymphangioma, neurofibroma
    - Malignant – rhabdomyosarcoma, glioma, meningioma, metastases, lymphoma, leukaemia, retinoblastoma, teratoma, sinus tumours, schwannoma, squamous cell carcinoma
- Metabolic
    - Dysthyroid eye disease
- Vascular
    - Varices, carotid-cavernous fistula
- Infective
    - Post-septal cellulitis, hydatid cyst

Thyroid eye disease

Systemic signs of thyrotoxicosis

Thyroid gland examination

Soft tissues

- Periorbital + lid swelling
- Conjunctival and episcleral hyperaemia
- Chemosis
- Superior limbic keratoconjunctivitis
- Keratoconjunctivitis sicca

Eyelids

- Dalrymple's sign
- Von Graefe's sign
- Kocher's sign

Proptosis

- Exposure keratopathy
- Hertel exophthalmometer or ruler

1

Ocular motility

- Extraocular muscle movements
- IOP in upgaze (fibrotic inferior rectus)

Optic nerve

- Disc hyperaemia, swelling

Mourits score

- Pain
  - At rest
  - With eye movement
- Swelling
  - Lids
  - Caruncle
  - Chemosis
  - Increasing proptosis
- Redness
  - Lids
  - Conjunctiva
- Decreasing function
  - Decreasing visual acuity
  - Decreasing eye movement

Neuro-ophthalmology

History

- Main complaint
- Minor complaints
- Past ophthalmic ± spectacles
- Neurological history – e.g. headaches, weakness, endocrine
- Past medical history
- Family

Examination

General

- Thyroid scars, habitus, wasting, facies, handshake, etc.

Higher function

- Minimental exam

Ocular

- Visual acuity + pinhole ± refraction
- Colour vision (Ishihara)
- Fields – red confrontation, perimetry
- Pupils – direct, consensual, near, light near dissociation
- Other optic nerve function tests – red desaturation, light brightness, contrast sensitivity
- Ocular motility – nystagmus, optokinetic drum
- Eye movements
  - Supranuclear – saccadic, smooth pursuit, vergence, vestibular
  - Infranuclear – III, IV, VI
  - Internuclear
- Slit lamp – anterior to posterior
- Fundoscopy

Cranial nerves

- I – Enquire only
- II – VA + pinhole, pupils, disc, fields, colour, brightness, red desaturation
- III, IV, VI – Ductions, versions, vergences, Parks 3-step test
- V – Dermatome + corneal sensation, open jaw against resistance
- VII – Close eyes, blow cheeks
- VIII – Rinne, Weber tests
- IX + X – Open mouth, uvula displacement; gag reflex (IX sensory, X motor)
- XI – Shrug shoulders against resistance
- XII – Tongue wasting + deviation

Motor

- Inspection – wasting, fasciculations, abnormal posture
- Tone – spasticity, rigidity
- Power
  - 0 – no movement
  - 1 – flicker of movement
  - 2 – movement when gravity eliminated
  - 3 – movement against gravity
  - 4 – movement against resistance
  - 5 – full muscle power
- Abnormal movements

Reflexes

- Upper and lower limbs, abdominal and cremasteric

Cerebellar

- Finger nose, past pointing, intention tremor, dysdiadokokinesis, heel-shin

Sensory

- Anterior columns (pain), posterior columns (proprioception, vibration)

Differential diagnosis: The swollen disc

Congenital	Drusen, hyaloid remnants, myelinated fibres, hypermetropia
Metabolic	Thyroid eye disease, diabetic papillopathy
Inflammatory	Papillitis, neuroretinitis, posterior scleritis, uveitis, sarcoidosis, TB
Neoplastic	Orbit or disc tumours – lymphoma, leukaemia, haemangioma, glioma, metastatic
Vascular	Hypertensive retinopathy grade IV, CRVO, proliferative retinopathy, AION – arteritic, non-arteritic
Systemic	Anaemia, hypoxia
Raised intra-cranial pressure	Papilloedema, benign intracranial hypertension
Hereditary	Leber's hereditary optic neuropathy
Mechanical	Papilloedema, ocular hypotony, retrobulbar mass

Causes of neuroretinitis

- Viral – Leber's idiopathic stellate neuroretinitis)
- Bartonella henselae (cat scratch disease)
- Toxoplasmosis
- Toxocara
- Histoplasmosis
- Syphilis
- Lyme disease

Causes of optic neuritis

- Idiopathic
- Demyelinating – isolated, multiple sclerosis, Devic's disease, Schilder's disease
- Parainfectious – viral infection, post-immunisation
- Infectious (TB, syphilis, sarcoidosis, cat scratch, cryptococcal, meningitis, zoster)
- Contiguous inflammation (sinuses, orbit, meninges)
- Post-viral syndrome
- Intraocular inflammation
- Autoimmune

1

Causes of anisocoria

- Physiological
- Horner's syndrome
- Adie's syndrome
- Posterior synechiae
- Iris atophy – acute angle closure glaucoma, herpes, anterior segment ischaemia
- Traumatic mydriasis – sphincter tears, ciliary nerve damage
- Pharmacological mydriasis or miosis
- III palsy
- Migrainous 'springing pupil'
- Pupil coloboma

Causes of diplopia

- Pseudodiplopia – patient actually means blur
- Physiological
- Pathological – binocular
  - Refractive – prismatic effect from spectacle correction
  - Neurogenic – III, IV, VI palsy, internuclear ophthalmoplegia, skew deviations
  - Myogenic – neuromuscular junction – myasthenia gravis, myotonic dystrophy; restrictive – thyroid eye disease, myositis, entrapment
  - Decompensated phoria
  - Cortical (rare)
  - Orbital pathology (dystopia)
- – monocular
  - Beam splitting opacities – cataract, corneal scars, etc.
  - Macular pathology
  - Astigmatism

Causes of vertical diplopia

- Myasthenia gravis
- Thyroid eye disease
- Orbital (trauma, tumour, inflammation, blowout fracture)
- III palsy
- Brown's syndrome
- Skew deviation
- IV palsy
  - Decompensated congenital
  - Acquired

Causes of light-near dissociation

Unilateral	Afferent pupil defect
	Adie's pupil
	Herpes zoster
	Aberrant regeneration of the III nerve
Bilateral	Optic neuropathy or severe retinopathy
	Neurosyphilis (Argyll-Robertson pupils)
	Diabetes Type 1
	Myotonic dystrophy
	Paranaud's dorsal midbrain syndrome
	Familial amyloidosis
	Encephalitis
	Chronic alcoholism

Causes of an abduction deficit

- VI palsy
- Duane's syndrome
- Muscle trauma, entrapment
- Thyroid eye disease
- Myasthenia gravis
- Esotropia with cross-fixation

Causes of chiasmal disease

Tumours	Pituitary adenoma, meningioma, craniopharyngioma, gliomas, metastases, etc.
Non-neoplastic masses	Aneurysms, sphenoidal sinus mucocoele, arachnoid cysts
Miscellaneous	Demyelination, inflammation, trauma, irradiation, vasculitis

Causes of Horner's syndrome

First order	Brain stem disease (tumours, vascular, demyelination)
	Spinal cord lesions (tumours, syringomyelia)
Second order	Chest lesions – carcinoma lung (Pancoast's tumour)
	Neck lesions – trauma, abscess, thyroid neoplasm, nodes
	Surgery – thyroid, neck dissection, carotid angiography
Third order	Cluster headaches/migraine
	Internal carotid artery dissection
	Carotid-cavernous fistula
	Nasopharyngeal carcinoma
	Cavernous sinus mass
	Otitis media

1

Conditions associated with benign intracranial hypertension

- 95% idiopathic
- Drugs – oral contraceptives, steroids, naladixic acid, tetracyclines, vitamin A, amiodarone
- Endocrine + metabolic – obesity, pregnancy, Addison's disease, eclampsia, menarche
- Obstruction of intracranial venous drainage – neck surgery, respiratory insufficiency, mediastinal mass
- Systemic illness – uraemia, meningitis, leukaemia, anaemia, idiopathic thrombocytic purpura, sarcoid, SLE

Causes of III palsy

- Nuclear (very rare)
- Fascicle – Nothnagel, Benedikt, Weber, Claude's syndrome
- Uncal herniation
- Posterior communicating artery aneurysm
- Tumour
- Cavernous sinus – aneurysm, Tolosa-Hunt, pituitary apoplexy, meningioma
- Orbital
- Ischaemic/vascular – vasculopaths (hypertension, diabetes), vasculitis (syphilis, autoimmune), ophthalmic migraine
- Trauma – subdural haematoma, uncal herniation
- Idiopathic (25%)

Causes of IV palsy

- Nuclear + fascicular – cerebrovascular accident, demyelination, trauma
- Subarachnoid – trauma, tumour
- Cavernous sinus
- Orbital – trauma, inflammation, tumour
- Isolated
    - Congenital
    - Acquired – 10% neoplasm aneurysm, 20% ischaemic, 30% idiopathic, 40% trauma

Refractive surgery – pre-operative examination

Exclude

- Nervous + anxious
- Psychiatric disease
- Narrow palpebral fissures
- Small orbit

Pre-visit

- Come without contact lenses (hard – not for 30 days, soft – not for 1 week)
- Be accompanied by someone – cycloplegic refraction required
- Bring old glasses + scripts

Early evaluation

- Autorefraction (with + without cycloplegia)

- Glasses – present + past
- Manifest refraction (red best duochrome for myopes + green best for hyperopes)
- Note any discrepancies between refractive cylinders + topographic astigmatism
- Pupil diameter – > 7 mm may need a wavefront analysis → might be higher order aberrations under scotopic conditions

Corneal topography + pachymetry

- For anterior + posterior surface profile
- Power profile
- Thickness map
- Detect anomalies e.g. keratoconus
- < 470 μm pachymetry → LASIK unlikely
- Difference of > 100 μm from thinnest zone to thickest zone → no LASIK
- Bow tie appearance on power map → no LASIK – may indicate keratoconus
- Structural weakness of the cornea is indicated by the highest point on the posterior profile coinciding with the highest point on the anterior profile, the point of maximum curvature, and the thinnest point on the pachymetry

Minimal stromal bed

- Must leave a minimum of 250–300 μm stromal bed post ablation

Rest of visit

- Family history (especially of keratoconus)
- Systemic medication
- Complete ophthalmic exam
- Pregnancy → undercorrection because water retention in the cornea
- Does the patient want monovision?

Functional visual loss

Special tests to detect malingering

Tests using lenses

- Fog with + 5.00, then add -5.00
- Polarising lenses + polarised Snellen letters
- Coloured lenses + letters (same principle)
- Paired cylinders 6D+ and 6D– placed parallel, then rotated transiently
- Strong plus lens, move reading print away

Tests using prisms

- Prism shift test – 4D base out prism placed in front of one eye while fixating the 6/12 letter, then look for movement
- 6D base down prism in front of the good eye with the 'blind' eye covered; sees double; move up while uncovering the 'blind' eye; sees double

Tests using fields

- Vary distance of testing to demonstrate a barrel constriction rather than a cone constriction
- Repeat on the tangent screen with the fixation point varied to demonstrate inconsistency
- Binocular visual field
- Colour fields

Other miscellaneous tests

- Size consistency – use different size letters at different distances, demonstrate inconsistent Snellen acuity
- Reading bar – at 15 cm, reading card at 30 cm
- Optokinetic nystagmus tape
- Stereoscopic tests – 40" stereoacuity = 6/6 in both eyes

Special tests

- Electroretinogram
- Visual evoked response

2

Eyelids and lacrimal system

Disorders of lid position 20
Blepharophimosis syndrome 20
Benign eyelid nodules and cysts . 22
Allergic lid disorders 23
Eyelid infections 23
Disorders of the eyelashes 23
Miscellaneous acquired eyelid disorders 24
Miscellaneous congenital eyelid disorders 24
Eyelid tumours 25
Lacrimal disorders 26

Disorders of lid position

Ectropion

- Congenital
- Acquired – involutional, paralytic, mechanical, cicatricial

Entropion

- Congenital
- Acquired – involutional, spastic, cicatricial

Ptosis

- Congenital
  - Dystrophic
  - Blepharophimosis epicanthus inversus ptosis syndrome
  - Marcus Gunn jaw winking
- Acquired
  - Involutional
  - Myogenic – myasthenia gravis, ocular dystrophy, progressive external ophthalmoplegia
  - Neurogenic – III palsy, Horner's syndrome
  - Traumatic
  - Mechanical – tumours, scarring

Blepharophimosis syndrome

Definitions

- Blepharophimosis syndrome
  - A rare congenital eyelid and orbit syndrome consisting of blepharophimosis, ptosis, epicanthus inversus and telecanthus
  - Also known as blepharophimosis ptosis epicanthus inversus syndrome (BPES)
- Telecanthus
  - Widened intercanthal distance with a normal interpupillary distance, caused by lengthening of the medial canthal ligament
- Hypertelorism
  - Increased separation between the bony orbits

Genetics

- Autosomal dominantly inherited or sporadic (positive family history in 75%)
- Mutation in gene FoxL2 on chromosome 3q23

Clinical features

- Blepharophimosis
  - Abnormal narrowness of the palpebral fissures, shortened horizontally and vertically

- Epicanthus inversus
  - A crescent shaped skin fold extending vertically from the lower lid to the upper lid and overlying the medial canthus
  - A prominent epicanthic fold is normal in Orientals
  - Three kinds of epicanthus: e. tarsalis – fold more prominent in the upper eyelid; e. inversus – fold more prominent in the lower eyelid; e. palpebralis – fold equally distributed between the upper and lower eyelids
- Ptosis
  - Due to hypoplasia or aplasia of levator palpebrae superiorus
  - Levator function is usually very poor
  - Three distinctive patterns: severe, bilateral ptosis (> 4 mm); moderate, bilateral ptosis (2 to 4 mm); asymmetrical ptosis
- Upper lid crease almost always absent
- Associated with a typical chin-tilt posture

Other ocular findings

- Upper lids rigid and tightly stretched over globes
- Lower lid ectropion
- Nasolacrimal drainage problems (18%)
- Flattened and widened nasal bridge
- Hypoplasia of the superior orbital rims
- Hypertelorism
- Hypermetropia (43%)
- Significant astigmatism
- Optic nerve hypoplasia
- Anterior chamber angle dysgenesis
- Strabismus
- Hypoplasia of the caruncle and semilunar fold
- Face may be flat and expressionless with stiff skin

Systemic associations

- Type 1: Associated with ovarian failure (premature menopause and female infertility)
- Type 2: Not associated with ovarian failure
- Mental retardation – more common in the sporadic form

Management

- Amblyopia
- Refraction
- Genetic/family counselling
- Paediatrics referral
- Surgery

Amblyopia

- 39% to 56%
- Higher with co-existent strabismus
- Early surgery in severe ptosis; patching and penalisation

Refraction

- Hypermetropia and astigmatism

Genetic/family counselling

- Autosomal dominant inheritance pattern
- Significant chance of female infertility

Paediatrics referral

- Developmental delay and concurrent neurological problems not uncommon, especially in sporadic form
- Other syndromes may present with blepharophimosis e.g. branchio-oto-renal syndrome
- A large number of patients with BPES have other unrecognised malformation syndromes with systemic abnormalities

Surgery

- The degree of blepharophimosis varies and not all cases require surgery
- Important for cosmesis and to prevent amblyopia
- Optimal age for surgery
  - With severe ptosis – before the age of 3

  - Mild to moderate ptosis – before the age of 5
- Telecanthus and epicanthus tend to improve with age
- Epicanthus inversus does not improve as much with age as e. palpebralis and e. tarsalis
- Mustarde 'jumping man' double Z-plasty or Y-V-plasty, followed a few months later by a ptosis repair

Correction of telecanthus and epicanthus inversus

- Six months prior to ptosis surgery
- Sometimes combined with shortening of elongated medial canthal tendons by transnasal wiring
- Epicanthic Z-plasty, double Z-plasty, Y-V-plasty, double Z-plasty (Mustarde) 'jumping man'

Correction of ptosis

- Usually bilateral frontalis sling procedures
- Rarely there may be enough levator function to allow ptosis correction by levator aponeurosis advancement

Prognosis

- Excellent cosmetic outcome in 80%

Benign eyelid nodules and cysts

Chalazion (meibomian cyst)

Pathology

- Chronic lipogranulomatous inflammatory cyst of meibomian gland
- Caused by blockage of gland orifice and stagnation of sebaceous secretions

Clinical features

- Painless nodule in tarsal plate
- May be associated with posterior blepharitis

Treatment

- May resolve spontaneously
- Incision and curettage
- Steroid injection – 80% success
- Systemic tetracycline if chalazia are recurrent

Hordeolum

Internal

- Pathology
  - Staphylococcal abscess of meibomian gland
- Clinical features
  - Painful nodule in tarsal plate
- Treatment
  - Systemic antibiotic
  - Incision and curettage

External

- Pathology
  - Staphylococcal abscess of lash follicle
- Clinical features
  - Painful nodule in lid margin
- Treatment
  - Nil, hot compresses, epilation of lash, topical antibiotic, systemic antibiotic

Molluscum contagiosum

- Pox virus
- Single or multiple, pale, waxy, umbilicated nodules
- Treat by curettage

Xanthelesma

- Yellowish subcutaneous plaque of cholesterol and lipid at the medial aspects of the eyelids
- Treat for cosmesis by excision or laser

Miscellaneous cysts

- Cyst of Moll – small translucent cyst on anterior lid margin
- Eccrine sweat gland hidrocystoma – less common, similar, not confined to lid margin
- Cyst of Zeis – small opaque cyst on anterior lid margin
- Sebaceous cyst

- Milia – tiny, white, round, occur in crops, derived from hair follicles or sebaceous glands

Allergic lid disorders

Acute allergic oedema

- May be due to insect bites, angiooedema, urticaria, drugs
- Painless pitting periorbital lid oedema
- May treat with topical steroids and systemic antihistamines

Contact dermatitis

- May be due to sensitivity to topical medication
- Localised erythema and crusting
- Treat with topical steroids

Atopic dermatitis (eczema)

- Common idiopathic skin condition, frequently associated with asthma and hay fever
- Thickening, crusting, fissuring of upper eyelids
- Treat with emolients to hydrate skin + topical steroids
- Ocular associations of atopic dermatitis include – staph blepharitis, vernal keratoconjunctivitis, cataract

Eyelid infections

- Herpes zoster
- Herpes simplex
- Impetigo (Staph aureus + β haemolytic Strep)
- Erysipelas (Strep pyogenes)
- Necrotising fasciitis (Strep pyogenes)

Chronic marginal blepharitis

Ulcerative (staphylococcal) anterior blepharitis

- Poliosis, trichiasis, broken lashes, loss of lashes, collarettes, hordeola, angular blepharitis, tear film instability
- May result in corneal infiltrates, phlyctenulosis, lower one third superficial punctate keratopathy, pannus
- Treat with lid hygiene, antibiotic/ steroid ointment

Seborrhoeic anterior blepharitis

- Excess sebaceous secretions, associated with seborrhoeic dermatitis
- Excess sebaceous secretions broken down to irritating fatty acids
- Treat with lid hygiene, antibiotic/ steroid ointment

Meibomian seborrhoea

- Excessive meibomian gland secretions
- Oil globules are visible capping the meibomian gland orifices
- Pressure on tarsus → expression of meibomian oil
- Tear film excessively oily and foamy
- Treat with systemic tetracycline x 6–12 weeks, lid hygiene, tear substitutes, topical steroids

Meibomianitis

- Inflammation and obstruction of meibomian glands
- Posterior lid margin shows diffuse or localised inflammation around the meibomian gland orifices
- Expressed meibomian gland secretions are turbid or inspissated
- Blockage of meibomina ducts → secondary cystic dilatation and formation of meibomian cysts
- Tear film instability may occur
- Treat with systemic tetracycline × 6–12 weeks, lid hygiene, tear substitutes, topical steroids

Disorders of the eyelashes

Trichiasis and distichiasis

Causes

- Distichiasis

2

- Abnormal extra lashes directed posteriorly, second row of lashes in the position of the meibomian gland orifices
- Congenital
- Acquired – metaplastic (Stevens-Johnson syndrome, trachoma)

- Trichiasis
  - Normal lashes directed posteriorly
  - With entropion
  - Misdirected lashes

Treatment

- Epilation, electrolysis, cryotherapy, argon laser ablation

Madarosis

- Decrease/loss of lashes

Causes

- Local – chronic blepharitis, burns
- Skin disorders – generalised alopecia, psoriasis
- Systemic disorders – myxoedema, systemic lupus erythematosis, syphilis, leprosy

Poliosis

- Premature localised whitening of hair, which may involve lashes and eyebrows
- Ocular associations – chronic blepharitis, sympathetic uveitis
- Systemic associations – Vogt-Koyanagi-Harada syndrome, Waardenburg syndrome

Miscellaneous acquired eyelid disorders

Dermatochalasis

- Redundant upper eyelid skin
- Treat by blepharoplasty

Blepharochalasis

- Recurrent episodes of painless non-pitting oedema of upper eyelids

Floppy eyelid syndrome

- Typically affects obese men
- Treat by horizontal lid shortening

Eyelid retraction

Causes

- Central nervous system – dorsal midbrain syndrome
- Peripheral nerve – aberrant III regeneration, Marcus Gunn phenomenon
- Neuromuscular junction – phenylephrine, unilateral ptosis with contralateral levator overaction
- Muscle – dysthyroid eye disease, hyperkalaemic periodic paralysis, systemic steroids, congenital levator fibrosis
- Congenital

Essential blepharospasm

- Idiopathic, progressive involuntary spasms of orbicularis oculi and upper facial muscles
- May occur in isolation, may occur as part of spectrum of dystonic movements
- Females > males

Treatment

- Botulinum toxin – subcutaneous injections into upper and lower lid and brow, repeat after 3–4 months if necessary
- Surgery – if becomes refractory to botulinum toxin
- Selective facial nerve avulsion and orbicularis myectomy

Miscellaneous congenital eyelid disorders

Epicanthic folds

- May cause pseudoesotropia

Telecanthus

- Increased distance between medial canthi as a result of long medial canthal tendons

- May have a number of systemic associations

Epiblepharon

- Extra horizontal row of skin that stretches across the lid margin

Coloboma

- May affect upper lid or lower lid
- Lower lid coloboma may have systemic associations

Eyelid tumours

Benign tumours

Viral wart (squamous cell papilloma)

- Pedunculated or sessile
- Raspberry like surface
- Treat by excision

Seborrhoeic keratosis (basal cell papilloma)

- Discrete, greasy brown lesion
- Treat by curettage or excision

Cutaneous horn

- May be associated with actinic keratosis or squamous cell carcinoma

Keratoacanthoma

- Central crater filled with keratin, surrounded by atypical epithelium

Solar keratosis

- Acanthosis, hyperkeratosis, parakeratosis and underlying chronic inflammatory cell infiltrate
- May become squamous cell carcinoma
- Treat by cryotherapy or excision

Epithelial cyst

- Developmental
  - Dermoid – contains sebum, hair, keratin
  - Epidermoid – no hair follicle contents
- Traumatic
  - Implantation

Juvenile xanthogranuloma

- Part of histiocytosis X group, seen in children > 1 year
- Orange skin lesions, iris lesions → spontaneous recurrent hyphaema
- Consists of diffuse granulomatous inflammatory reaction with histiocytes and Touton giant cells, variable vascularity

Naevus

- Junctional, compound, intradermal

Capillary haemangioma

- Females > males
- Predilection for upper lid
- Grows during first year, then starts to involute
- Complete resolution in 40% by 4 years, 70% by 7 years
- Systemic associations – high output heart failure, Kassabach-Merritt syndrome (thrombocytopaenia, anaemia), Maffuci's syndrome
- Amblyopia may occur from ptosis strabismus
- May require treatment to prevent amblyopia
- Treatment – conservative, steroid injection, surgical resection

Port wine stain (naevus flammeus)

- Rare, congenital
- Subcutaneous lesion composed of thin walled vessels and capillaries
- Usually unilateral and segmental, may be bilateral
- With age, darkens to red or purple, overlying skin becomes hypertrophied, coarse, nodular, friable
- May be associated with glaucoma in 45% of cases

- May be associated with Sturge-Weber syndrome in 5% of cases

Malignant tumours

Basal cell carcinoma

- Most common malignant eyelid tumour (90% of malignant lid tumours)
- Aetiology – actinic radiation
- Sites – lower lid > inner canthus > upper lid > lateral canthus
- Clinical types – nodular, ulcerative, cystic, fibrosing
- Behaviour – locally invasive, 'almost never' metastasises, medial canthus tumours particularly invasive
- Histology – arise from basal cells
- Variable melanin content
- Five histological types – solid, cystic, reticulate, keratotic, cicatrising
- Nests of basal cells show peripheral palisading and central pleomorphism
- Treatment – local excision or local radiotherapy
- Prognosis – 4% recurrence

Squamous cell carcinoma

- Less common (5–10% of malignant lid tumours)
- Aetiology – actinic radiation
- Usually preceded by solar keratosis
- Sites – lower lid > upper lid
- Clinical types – plaque like, nodular, ulcerating
- Behaviour – metastasise to regional lymph nodes
- Caruncle tumours are more aggressive
- Histology – arise from prickle cell layer
- Varies from well differentiated keratinising (dyskeratosis, cell nests, keratin pearls) to anaplastic spindle cell carcinoma
- Treatment – local excision and radiotherapy

Sebaceous gland carcinoma

- Rare
- May present as chalazion or chronic blepharoconjunctivitis
- Often diagnosed late
- 10% mortality
- Torre's syndrome – sebaceous gland tumour and visceral malignancy (usually carcinoma colon); more usual with benign tumours of the sebaceous gland

Melanoma

- Three types – superficial spreading, nodular, lentigo maligna
- Eyelid melanomas are often non-pigmented

Kaposi's sarcoma

- Vascular tumour
- Affects patients with AIDS
- Treat with radiotherapy

Lacrimal disorders

Causes of epiphora in neonates

- Distichiasis
- Congenital entropion
- Failure of canalisation – valve of Hasner
- Imperforate puncta
- Ectopic puncta
- Congenital nasolacrimal duct occlusion

Congenital nasolacrimal duct obstruction

- Most common congenital abnormality, present in up to 30% of neonates, 90% resolve by 6 months, 95% resolve by 1 year
- Occlusion occurs at entrance to nose beneath inferior turbinate, due to incomplete canalisation (valve of Hasner)
- Results in epiphora, mucocoele → pyocoele → acute dacryocystitis → chronic dacryocystitis + osteitis
- Treatment by massage and antibiotic drops, to prevent dacryocystitis
- Probing and syringing at 1 year if persistent
- If fails, balloon dacryoplasty, nasolacrimal duct intubation, dacrycystorhinostomy

Other congenital lid anomalies

- Imperforate puncta
- Failure of canalisation
- Absent valves
- Diverticula
- Fistula
- Duplication
- Atresia
- Congenital dacryocoele

Causes of epiphora in adults

- Adequate tear drainage
  - Hypersecretion – conjunctivitis, keratitis, sinusitis, hay fever, V irritation
  - Pseudoepiphora – tear secretion deficiency, lagophthalmos
  - Gustatory lacrimation/crocodile tears – aberrant VII regeneration
- Inadequate tear drainage
  - Obstruction to tear film movement – conjunctival chalasis
  - Deficiency in lacrimal pump – VII palsy, atonic eyelid
  - Punctum malposition – ectropion, congenital displacement
  - Punctal occlusion – congenital, post-irradiation, burns, trauma, neoplasm, cicatrising infection, drugs (phosphaline iodide), allergy (rubbing)
  - Lacrimal sac and nasolacrimal duct obstruction – congenital, fracture, tumour, infection, idiopathic, nasal polyp

Primary punctual stenosis

- Idiopathic, irradiation, herpes simplex lid infection, trachoma, cicatrising conjunctivitis
- Treat by dilatation, one-snip ampullotomy, two-snip ampullotomy, laser punctoplasty

Secondary punctual stenosis

Aetiology

- Punctal eversion

Treatment

- Ziegler cautery, medial conjunctivoplasty

2

Canalicular obstruction

Aetiology

- Idiopathic fibrosis, chronic dacryocystitis, herpes simplex infection, cicatrising conjunctivitis

Treatment

- Partial obstruction – intubation
- Complete obstruction – canaliculodacryocystorhinostomy

Acquired nasolacrimal duct obstruction

Aetiology

- Idiopathic, naso-orbital trauma, irradiation, Wegeners granulomatosis

Treatment

- Incomplete obstruction – intubation
- Complete obstruction – dacryocystorhinostomy

Chronic canaliculitis

- Actinomyces, streptomyces, candida, aspergillus
- Low grade infection with concretion formation
- Concretions contain gram-positive branching filaments

Treatment

- Probing and syringing, curettage, dacryocystorhinostomy

Acute dacryocycstitis

- Pneumococcus; also Staph, Strep, Diphtheroids
- Usually secondary to nasolacrimal duct obstruction
- X-ray sinuses to exclude sinus pathology

Treatment

- Aspirate pus with needle (avoid incision and drainage), systemic antibiotics, topical antibiotic
- Dacryocystorhinostomy when infection has resolved

Chronic dacryocystitis

- Following on acute dacryocystitis
- May be associated with osteitis
- Treat by dacrocystorhinostomy

Lacrimal sac tumours

- Benign
    - Papillomas – squamous cell, transitional cell, mixed
- Malignant
    - Papillary carcinoma – squamous cell, transitional cell
    - Lymphoma
    - Pseudotumour

3

Conjunctiva

Dry eye syndrome 29
Xerophthalmia 30
Conjunctival degenerations 31
Miscellaneous inflammations 35
Chronic progressive conjunctival cicatrisation 37
Tumours of the conjunctiva 39

Dry eye syndrome

Keratoconjunctivitis sicca

Incidence

- 10–15% of adults

Pathogenesis

- Decreased tear production
- Excessive tear evaporation
- Aqueous tear deficiency
- Mucin tear deficiency
- Lipid tear deficiency

Staining

- Rose bengal – stains dead/devitalised cells, mucous and cells inadequately protected by a mucin tear coating
- Lissamine green – does not stain healthy conjunctival epithelium, far less irritating; does not inhibit viral growth

Aetiology

- Aqueous deficiency
  - Congenital – congenital alacrima, hypoplasia, Riley-Day syndrome (familial dysautonomia)
  - Traumatic – chemical burns, irradiation, V cranial nerve paresis
  - Inflammatory – Sjögren's syndrome, dacryoadenitis, sarcoid, mumps, Stevens-Johnson syndrome, pemphigoid, HIV
  - Neoplastic – lymphoma, leukemia
  - Drugs – anticholinergics, antihistamines, phenothiazines, oral contraceptives, pregnancy
  - Other – idiopathic autoimmune dysfunction (Shy-Drager syndrome), Adie's syndrome, contact lens wear (decreased corneal senation), post-LASIK/PRK (decreased corneal sensation)
- Mucin deficiency
  - Conjunctival cicatricial diseases
  - Xerophthalmia (severe vitamin A deficiency)
- Lipid deficiency
  - Conjunctival cicatricial diseases
  - Chronic blepharitis and acne rosacea – bacteria → increase in free fatty acid in lipid secretions (and isotretinoin used in treatment of rosacea)
- Lid abnormalities
  - Exophthalmos
  - Ectropion
  - VII cranial nerve paresis, lagophthalmos
- Corneal surface abnormalities
  - Epitheliopathy with loss of villi
  - Scarring
  - Anaesthetic cornea

Sjögren's syndrome

Definition

- Triad of dry eyes, dry mouth, rheumatoid arthritis or other autoimmune disease

Associations

- Rheumatoid arthritis (incidence 15–30%), psoriatic arthiritis, polyarteritis nodosa, systemic sclerosis, systemic lupus erythematosis, Hashimoto's thyroiditis, chronic hepatobiliary disease, uveitis, HIV

Clinical features

- Common in menopausal women, insidious onset, cyclical course
- Multiple organ involvement in gut, liver, kidney, spleen, lung, thyroid, adrenals
- Also have dry tracheobronchial tree, dry vagina, dry stomach

Pathology

- Salivary gland biopsy – lymphocyte and plasma cell infiltration, with destruction of glandular elements

Symptoms

- Foreign body sensation, burning, photophobia, injection

Signs

- Decreased tear meniscus (< 1 mm)
- Decreased conjunctival lustre
- Debris in precorneal tear film
- Punctate epitheliopathy
- Filamentary keratitis
- ± Secondary staphylococcal infection

Investigations

- Schirmer 1 – without topical anaesthetic – tests total aqueous production basal and reflex
- Schirmer 2 – with topical anaesthetic – tests only basal production (normal 10–15 mm in 5 mins)
- Rose bengal stain – vital stain, taken up by damaged cells
- Tear break-up time – normal 15–45 secs, <10 secs = unstable tear film; may be decreased if there is decreased aqueous, mucin or lipid deficiency
- Lysozyme assay – enzyme decreased in dry eye; normally makes up 30% of protein content of tears; a measure of tear production by the main lacrimal gland
- Conjunctival impression cytology – gives information on quantity and morphology of goblet cells
- Infrared thermography of tear film – increased temperature + greater variation in temperature over a dry cornea

Management

- Artificial tears
  - Methylcellulose
  - Polyvinylalcohol
  - Mucormimetic
  - Petrolaclin, mineral oil, lanolin
  - Sodium hyaluronate
- Topical vitamin A → increased goblet cell count
- Topical cyclosporin A
- Topical steroids/nonsteroidal antiinflammatories
- Acetylcysteine → mucolytic effect
- Closure of puncta – temporary collagen, silicone or permanent with cautery
- Moist chamber – goggles, spectacles with cling wrap
- Lateral tarsorrhaphy
- Autologous nasal mucosal transplant
- Oral pilocarpine

Xerophthalmia

Definition

- The ocular diseases caused by severe vitamin A deficiency

Epidemiology

- A leading cause of blindness
- Responsible for 1% of blindness worldwide

- Prevalence is decreasing
- Pure xerophthalmia more common in Asia
- In Africa, combination of xerophthalmia, protein calorie malnutrition and measles occurs
- In some areas in South Africa, up to 50% of children have serological vitamin A deficiency
- May occur in unusual dietary practices, chronic alcoholism, lipid malabsorption (cystic fibrosis, biliary cirrhosis, bowel resection)

Sources of Vitamin A

- Prenatal – via placenta; maternal night blindness may develop in pregnancy
- Neonatal – breast milk
- Childhood – eggs, fish, liver

Classification (WHO)

- XN – Night blindness
- X1A – Conjunctival xerosis without Bitot's spots
- X1B – Conjunctival xerosis with Bitot's spots
- X2 – Corneal xerosis
- X3A – Corneal ulcer keratomalacia (< one third corneal surface)
- X3B – Corneal ulcer keratomalacia (> one third corneal surface)
- XS – Corneal scar
- XF – Xerophthalmic fundus

Clinical features

- Nyctalopia – night blindness – decreased vitamin A → decreased rhodopsin
- Conjunctival xerosis – interpalpebral region
- Bitot's spots – metaplastic keratinisation of areas of the conjunctiva
- Corneal xerosis – starts as superficial punctate keratopathy in lower nasal quadrant, later xerosis with development of a plaque
- Corneal ulcer – punched out, usually in lower half, may be bilateral, may be associated with secondary bacterial infection and hypopyon
- Keratomalacia – colliquative necrosis of corneal stroma; may be localised or involve whole cornea, may cause scarring, descemetocoele, staphyloma, phthisis bulbi
- Corneal scars – typically symmetrical and inferior
- Fundal changes – rare; white punctate lesions in peripheral and equatorial retina, due to mottled depigmentation of retinal pigment epithelium, reversible on treatment

Pathology

- Conjunctival xerosis – keratinising squamous metaplasia, loss of goblet cells, chronic inflammatory infiltrate of substantia propria
- Bitot's spots – mass of keratin, xerotic bacilli (Corynebacterium xerosis), and fungal elements; may become self-perpetuating
- Corneal xerosis – focal areas of keratinised epithelium
- Keratomalacia – colliquative necrosis of stromal collagen

Investigations

- Serum retinol – degree of decrease correlates with severity of disease

Treatment

- Systemic vitamin A deficiency is a medical emergency with an untreated mortality of 50%
- Vitamin A 200 000 IU orally stat, repeat following day, repeat 2–4 weeks later

Prophylaxis

- Vitamin A 200 000 IU every 6 months orally

Conjunctival degenerations

Pingueculum

- Due to UV exposure
- Degeneration of collagen fibres of conjunctival stroma, thinning of

3

overlying epithelium, occasional calcification
- Degeneration of collagen when it takes on the characteristics of elastic tissue → elastoid degeneration or elastosis
- Yellow white deposit on bulbar conjunctiva adjacent to nasal or temporal limbus

Pterygium

- Due to UV exposure, dust and a dry climate
- Pathology similar to pingueculum
- Triangular sheet of fibrovascular tissue adjacent to nasal limbus, invades cornea
- Iron deposit (Stocker's line) occurs in epithelium anterior to advancing head
- Distinguish from pseudo pterygium
- Treat by surgical excision ± mitomycin C adjunct or radioactive strontium plaque application to decrease recurrence

Concretions

- Occur in palpebral conjunctiva of elderly

Retention cyst

- Thin-walled, asymptomatic

Normal aging

- Loss of transparency with age
- Vessels become more prominent, telangiectatic
- Conjunctivochalasis – redundant, loose, non-oedematous conjunctiva
- Sclera → lipid deposition → yellow colour

Conjunctivitis

Symptoms
- Discomfort (itching = allergy, scratching = corneal involvement)
- Redness, discharge, photophobia

Signs
- Discharge – watery, mucoid, purulent, mucopurulent
- Injection
- Subconjunctival haemorrhage
- Follicular reaction – lymphoid hyperplasia in stroma; typically seen in viral infection, chlamydial infection, Parinaud's syndrome, hypersensitivity to topical medication
- Papillary reaction – hyperplastic conjunctival epithelium, non-specific
- Oedema (chemosis)
- Scarring
- Lymphadenopathy

Aetiology
- Viral – herpes, adenovirus, rubeola, rubella, mumps, variola, vaccinia, varicella, molluscum contagiosum
- Chlamydial – trachoma, inclusion
- Bacterial – Staph aureus, Strep pneumoniae, Strep pyogenes, Neisseria, Klebsiella, Haemophilus, Moraxella sp, Proteus, Escherichia sp
- Fungal sp
- Allergic
  - Severe – vernal or atopic
  - Mild – seasonal allergic (pollen) or perennial allergic (house dust mite)
- Toxic – drugs, chemicals

Simple bacterial conjunctivitis

- Bacterial overgrowth + infiltration of the conjunctival epithelium + stroma

Incidence
- More common in children

Pathogenesis
- Direct inoculation or spread from organisms in nasal/sinus mucosa

Aetiology
- Staph epidermidis, Staph aureus, Strep pneumoniae (most common), haemophilus influenzae (young children), Moraxella lacunata

Treatment

- Mostly empiric
- Antibiotic drops – fusidic acid, chloramphenicol, fluoroquinolone
- Antibiotic ointments – chloramphenicol, fucidic acid
- Haemophilus – polymixin B-trimethoprim
- Supplemental oral antibiotics for ENT symptoms, children with Haemophilus sp

Adult gonococcal keratoconjunctivitis

Clinical

- Purulent conjunctivitis, massive exudation, chemosis, corneal infiltrates and melting, perforation; 15–40% incidence of keratitis

Treatment

- Without corneal involvement
  - Outpatient
  - Ceftriaxone 1 g IMI once
  - Topical erythromycin, bacitracin, gentamicin, ciprofloxacin
- With corneal involvement
  - Admit for treatment
  - Ceftriaxone 1 g 12-hourly × 3 days
  - Topical antibiotics
  - Normal saline conjunctival lavage every 30–60 mins
  - One third have concurrent chlamydial disease → doxycycline 100 mg 12-hourly × 1 week

Neonatal gonococcal keratoconjunctivitis

Incidence

- Low because of prophylactic antibiotic ointment on delivery

Clinical

- Ophthalmia neonatorum
  - Within first 5 days post-delivery → gonococcus
  - Day 3 to 2 weeks → chlamydia

Treatment

- Non-disseminated – ceftriaxone 125 mg IMI once
- Disseminated – ceftriaxone 125 mg 12-hourly × 3 days
- Chloramphenicol ointment
- Normal saline lavage

Causes of neonatal bacterial conjunctivitis

- Chlamydia trachomatis
- Streptococcus viridans
- Staphylococcus aureus
- Haemophilus influenzae
- Group D streptococcus
- Moraxella catarrhalis
- Escherichia coli
- Neissaria gonorrhoea

Viral conjunctivitis

Adenoviral keratoconjunctivitis

- One of three classic syndromes
  - Simple follicular conjunctivitis (multiple serotypes) – self-limited, care often not sought
  - Pharyngoconjunctival fever (serotypes 3 + 7) – fever, headache, pharyngitis, adenopathy
  - Epidemic keratoconjunctivitis (types 8, 19, 37) – can have significant corneal involvement; preceded by upper respiratory tract infection

3

Clinical

- Bilateral, severe follicular conjunctivitis
- Punctate epithelial keratitis, petechial conjunctival haemorrhage, large conjunctival haemorrhage + chemosis
- Preauricular adenopathy
- Membranes, pseudomembranes
- Geographic corneal erosions
- Viral shedding persists for 10 days beyond start of symptoms

Treatment

- Lubricants, antibiotics for superinfection, manual removal of membranes
- Topical nonsteroidal anti-inflammatories ineffective
- Topical steroids for reduced vision, membranes, pain/photophobia (prolongs course)

Molluscum contagiosum conjunctivitis

- Direct contact from infected individuals
- Follicular conjunctivitis
- In association with molluscum skin lesions

Herpes simplex conjunctivitis

- Herpetic skin vesicles
- Follicular conjunctivitis

Other viruses

- Enterovirus + coxsackievirus
- Epstein-Barr virus
- Measles, mumps, rubella, influenza

Chlamydial conjunctivitis

Chlamydia trachomatis serotypes

- Trachoma → A to C
- Adult + neonatal inclusion conjunctivitis → D-K
- Lymphogranuloma venereum → L 1 to 3

Adult chlamydial keratoconjunctivitis

- A sexually transmitted disease found in conjunction with urethritis or cervicitis
- Follicular conjunctival response, lower tarsal conjunctiva
- Preauricular adenopathy
- Epithelial infiltrates, micropannus
- Treat with oral doxycycline or erythromycin × 3 weeks
- Poor response to topical antibiotics

Neonatal chlamydial keratoconjunctivitis

- No follicular response, more mucopurulent discharge, membranes
- Treat with erythromycin 12.5 mg/kg orally or IVI 6-hourly × 14 days; topical antibiotics

Trachoma

- Infectious disease – poor hygiene
- 150 million people affected
- Vector → house fly

Clinical

- Foreign body sensation, redness, tearing, discharge
- Follicular reaction, especially superior tarsal conjunctiva, limbus
- Follicles get necrotic, heal by scarring or produce pits → Herbert's pits
- Stellate, linear scarring of tarsal conjunctiva → Arlt's line
- Cornea – epithelial keratitis, stromal infiltrates, pannus
- Keratoconjunctivitis sicca from scarring
- Trichiasis
- Corneal opacification

Treatment

- Topical + oral erythromycin or tetracycline (3 weeks)
- Surgical management of complications

Parinaud's oculoglandular conjunctivitis

Definition

- Unilateral granulomatous conjunctivitis and enlarged regional lymph node

Aetiology

- Cat scratch disease (Bartonella henselae) → most common cause
- TB, syphilis, tularaemia
- Sporotrichosis, other fungi
- Mumps, infectious mononucleosis

Cat scratch disease

- Bartonella henselae lives on cats and their fleas
- Regional lymphadenopathy, may progress to suppuration
- Associated fever, malaise, erythema multiforme
- Optic neuritis + neuroretinitis reported
- Recovers after 2–3 months
- Treat with doxycycline, erythromycin, azithromycin, rifampicin (no ideal regimen yet)

Allergic conjunctivitis

Allergic rhinoconjunctivitis

- Type 1 hypersensitivity to airborne antigens
- Seasonal (pollen) or perennial (house dust mite, animal dander)
- Treat with sodium chromoglycate drops, antihistamine drops, steroids

Vernal keratoconjunctivitis

- Severe allergic conjunctivitis involving cornea and conjunctiva
- Type I and IV hypersensitivity to airborne allergens
- Worse in spring and early summer
- Geographic, hereditary, and environmental factors may contribute
- More common in warmer climates
- Seen in children and young adults
- Male > female
- 75% have associated atopy (asthma, eczema)
- Symptoms – itching, tearing, foreign body sensation, discomfort
- Two forms – palpebral + limbal
    - Palpebral conjunctival changes – hyperaemia, papillary hypertrophy, cobblestones
    - Limbal conjunctival changes – mucoid nodules, Trantas dots (more common in Africans and Asians)
- Corneal changes – punctate epitheliopathy, macro erosion (shield ulcer), plaque, subepithelial scarring, pseudogerontoxon
- May be associated with keratoconus

Treatment

- Sodium cromoglycate drops
- Antihistamine drops
- Steroid drops
- Cyclosporin 0.2% drops in severe cases
- Supratarsal steroid injections

Atopic keratoconjunctivitis

- Seen in children and young adults with atopic disease
- Features are similar to vernal keratoconjunctivitis
- Treatment as for vernal keratoconjunctivitis
- Other ocular associations are keratoconus and presenile cataract

Contact dermatoblepharitis

- Topical ophthalmic medications, make-up
- Type IV hypersensitivity (cell mediated, delayed) 24–72 hours later
- Type I hypersensitivity (anaphylactic) occurs within minutes of application

Miscellaneous inflammations

Superior limbic keratoconjunctivitis

Aetiology

- Unknown, possibly autoimmune
- Possibly trauma from eyelid

3

Pathology

- Keratinisation of conjunctiva in superior limbal area, with polymorph infiltrates

Clinical features

- Uncommon, usually self-limiting
- Chronic + recurrent
- Affects middle aged women
- 20–50% have associated thyroid dysfunction
- Bilateral, chronic, remissions and exacerbations
- Non-specific symptoms of foreign body discomfort and photophobia
- Papillary hypertrophy and inflammation of superior tarsal conjunctiva and superior limbus
- Punctate epithelial erosions of superior cornea
- Corneal filaments
- Keratoconjunctivitis sicca
- Micropannus

Differential diagnosis

- Trachoma, marginal infiltrates, vernal keratoconjunctivitis, phlyctenulosis

Treatment

- No ideal regimen
- Vitamin A drops
- Silver nitrate local application
- Recession, resection, cautery of bulbar conjunctiva
- Pressure patching
- Soft contact lens

Ligneous conjunctivitis

- Rare, chronic, affects all ages
- Unknown aetiology
- Formation of firm, woody, yellowish fibrinous membranes on the conjunctival surface
- Linked to severe deficiency of type I plasminogen
- Recurs after excision
- No satisfactory treatment; success with topical cyclosporin reported
- Eventually resolves over several months to years

Mucous fishing syndrome

- Patients traumatise the conjunctival epithelium while removing mucous strands from their eyes, usually in keratoconjunctivitis sicca patients

Toxic conjunctivitis from medications

- Usually due to the preservative benzalkonium chloride → severe epithelial changes with loss of microvillae, plasma membrane disruption, subsequent cell death
- Usually occurs over prolonged application periods
- May take months to completely resolve

Giant papillary conjunctivitis

Pathogenesis

- Not fully understood, may be multifactorial → allergic, dry eye, infectious, immune, repeated mechanical trauma
- Abnormal immunoglobulins, mast cells, basophils, eosinophils

Clinical

- Redness, itching, mucoid discharge
- Worse with extended wear
- Papillary reaction, superior tarsal conjunctiva
- Punctate epithelial erosions
- Peripheral corneal infiltrates and vascularisation
- Giant papillary conjunctivitis is at the severe end of the spectrum
- More frequent in soft contact lens wear

Management

- Try new lenses → frequently resolves the problem; daily wear better than extended; 1 month contact lens-free holidays; reduce daily lens time; some do better with low water content lenses

- Improve lens hygiene; use preservative-free solutions
- Topical sodium chromoglycate, antihistamines, steroids

Chronic progressive conjunctival cicatrisation

Aetiology

- Physical – avulsion or laceration, heat
- Chemical – alkalis, acids
- Infection
- Trachoma
- Membranous conjunctivitis
  - Bacterial – Diphtheria, Strep, Staph, Gonococcus
  - Viral – herpes simplex, adenovirus 8
  - Fungal – Candida
- Oculocutaneous disorders
  - Cicatricial pemphigoid
  - Stevens-Johnson syndrome
  - Toxic epidermal necrolysis
  - Linear IgA bullous dermatosis
  - Epidermolysis bullosa
  - Dermatitis herpetiformis
  - Pemphigus vulgaris
- Other associated systemic disorders
  - Rosacea
  - Sjögren's syndrome
  - Inflammatory bowel disease
  - Graft vs host disease
  - Immune complex disease
  - Paraneoplastic syndromes – lymphoma, leukeumia, carcinoma of bronchus
- Drug induced
  - Systemic – practolol
  - Topical – long-term glaucoma treatment, idoxuridine
- Idiopathic

Pathophysiology

- Ulceration of epithelium – heals by subepithelial scarring
- Shrinkage of scar tissue → obliteration of fornices, symblepharon, ankyloblepharon, entropion with trichiasis, ectropion, xerophthalmia from goblet cell loss and blockage of lacrimal gland ducts
- Corneal involvement secondary

Benign mucous membrane pemphigoid/cicatricial pemphigoid

Epidemiology

- Rare, idiopathic, chronic, progressive, autoimmune
- Females > males 2 : 1, usually age > 60, rarely < 30

Pathophysiology

- Circulating antibody binds to basement membrane, complement fixation, inflammatory infiltrate, scarring
- May be a cyctotoxic type II hypersensitivity
- Pseudopemphigoid → topical drop related

Clinical features

- Bilateral, may be asymmetrical
- Insidious onset, recurrent attacks
- Conjunctiva involved in 70%
- Blisters and bullae of mucous membranes and skin
- Early non-specific chronic conjunctivitis, conjunctival thickening, subepithelial fibrosis, obliteration of fornices, symblephara (adhesions between palpebral and bulbar conjunctiva), ankyloblephara (adhesions between lids at the outer canthi), dry eye
- Sequelae
  - Eyelids – aberrant lashes, entropion, trichiasis, lagophthalmos, abnormal blinking, exposure
  - Ocular surface – decreased tear production, squamous keratinising, metaplasia, infection, secondary scarring and vascularisation of cornea
  - Stage I – subepithelial fibrosis, chronic red eye

  - Stage II – transient bullae, loss of goblet cells, shortening of fornices
  - Stage III – symblepharon
  - Stage IV – restricted ocular motility with extensive adhesions between lids and globe

Pathology
- Biopsy from actively affected conjunctiva → immunofluorescent or immunoperoxidase staining

Management
- Topical immunosuppression – intensive short-term topical steroids during acute exacerbations
- Systemic immunosuppression (steroids, dapsone, cyclophosphamide) – all effective but systemic side effects are a problem
  - Dapsone → initial drug of choice
  - Cyclophosphamide (cytoxan) → mainstay in severe disease
  - Methotrexate + azathioprine can be used → less effective
- Topical vitamin A – has been shown to reverse a degree of keratinisation
- Symptomatic treatment – lid surgery contraindicated → exacerbates the disease process
  - Mucosal grafting
  - Electroepilation of lashes
  - Artificial tears
  - Punctal occlusion
  - Treat secondary infections
- Immunoglobulin – under investigation

Stevens-Johnson syndrome

- Immune complex deposition in the dermis and conjunctival stroma

Causes
- Drugs – sulphonamides, proparacaine, penicillin, barbiturates, phenolphthalein, isoniazid
- Infections – herpes, measles, mycoplasma
- Sera – serum sickness
- Other – malignancy, physical agents, toxins

Clinical features
- Acute onset in young people
- Self-limiting, severe, mucocutaneous, vesiculo-bullous disease
- Acute vasculitis, affects skin in 100% and conjunctiva in 90%
- Fevers, malaise, arthralgia, skin eruptions (target lesions), vesiculo-bullous lesions, mucosal lesions (conjunctivitis, stomatitis)
- Conjunctivitis may be catarrhal, purulent, pseudomembranous
- Individual lesions have 2 week life cycle
- Entire disease lasts 6 weeks
- Cornea may be involved early but usually involved in late complications
- Symblepharon, metaplastic lashes, epiphora, dry eye, keratopathy
- Toxic epidermal necrolysis – the most severe form of Stevens-Johnson syndrome

Management
- Lubricants
- Steroids – systemic and topical
- Acyclovir – systemic, if herpes simplex is suspected
- Treat secondary infections
- Prevent symblepharon formation – rodding, scleral shell (long-term results disappointing)
- Surgery – divide adhesions, lid surgery, avoid intraocular surgery
- Treat dry eye syndrome
- Ocular surface reconstruction with amniotic membrane and limbal stem cells

Graft vs host disease

- Complication of allogenic bone marrow transplantation
- Grafted cells attack patients tissues → eye, skin, gastrointestinal tract, liver, etc.
- Conjunctival disease ± subepithelial fibrosis

- Severe keratoconjunctivitis sicca due to lacrimal gland infiltration
- Treat with aggressive lubrication, punctal occlusion, mucolytics (10% acetylcysteine), ± systemic cyclosporin

Tumours of the conjunctiva

Tumours of the conjunctiva	
Non-pigmented	
■ Benign	□ Papilloma – peduncutlated, sessile
	□ Choristomas/dermoids – dermolipoma, dermoid cyst, limbal choristoma
	□ Angiomas – haemangioma (capillary or cavernous), lymphangioma
	□ Neurofibroma/schwannoma/neuroma
	□ Lymphangiectasia + lymphangioma
	□ Lymphoid hyperplasia
■ Premalignant	□ Carcinoma in situ (conjunctival intraepithelial neoplasia)
■ Malignant	□ Mucoepidermoid cell carcinoma
	□ Mucoepidermoid carcinoma
	□ Lymphoma
	□ Kaposi's sarcoma
	□ Metastases
Pigmented	
■ Benign – derived from epithelial melanocytes	
	□ Epithelial melanosis
	□ Benign acquired melanosis
	□ Pigmented naevus
■ Benign – derived from subepithelial melanocytes	
	□ Ocular melanocytes
	□ Primary acquired melanosis
■ Malignant	□ Malignant melanoma

Other sources of conjunctival pigmentation

- Haemachromatosis (iron)
- Alkaptonuria (ochronosis)
- Addison's disease (melanin in melanocytes)
- Drugs – epinephrine (adrenochrome), silver nitrate (silver)

Conjunctival papilloma

- Pedunculated – due to infection with human papilloma virus types 6 and 11
- Sessile – non-infectious

Epibulbar choristoma

- Choristoma – congenital overgrowth of normal tissue in an abnormal location

Dermoid

- Seen in children but may not be apparent until later in life
- Commonly at limbus
- Associated with Goldenhar syndrome
- Treat by excision

Lipodermoid

- Seen in adults
- Commonly at lateral canthus

- Surgical excision may be complicated by scarring, ptosis, ocular motility problems

Angioma

- Haemangioma – capillary + cavernous, rare
- Naevus flammeus – port wine stain, may occur alone or part of Sturge-Weber syndrome
- Associated with secondary glaucoma

Neurofibroma

- Conjunctiva or eyelid → neurofibromatosis

Lymphangiectasia and lymphangioma

- Irregular, dilated lymphatic channels
- Developmental or due to trauma, inflammation
- Intralesional haemorrhage → chocolate cyst
- Surgical excision may lead to uncontrolled haemorrhage and exenteration

Lymphoid hyperplasia

- May represent a low-grade B-cell lymphoma
- Minimally elevated, salmon coloured
- Treat with local excision, topical steroids, irradiation

Conjunctival intraepithelial neoplasia

- Rare, unilateral
- Analogous to actinic keratosis of the eyelid
- Associations – human papilloma virus, UV light, HIV
- Starts near limbus, spreads to fornices and cornea
- Papilliform, gelatinous, leukoplakic
- Rarely becomes malignant
- Treat by surgical excision and cryotherapy
- Topical mitomycin C, 5-fluorouracil → appear to completely eradicate conjunctival intraepithelial neoplastic lesions

Squamous cell carcinoma conjunctiva

Incidence

- Commonly compared to lid squamous cell carcinoma
- More common in blacks, in males, age > 30 years, in immunocompromised people, in xeroderma pigmentosa

Aetiology

- UV light, viruses, genetic factors

Clinical features

- Usually starts at the limbus; associated feeder vessels
- Well-differentiated, locally infiltrative, late metastases

Treatment

- Early
  - Excision biopsy – 4 mm of conjunctiva beyond the clinical margins
  - Adjuvant I125 plaque or cryotherapy application, mitomycin C or 5-fluorouracil drops, absolute alcohol
  - Excision alone → 20–40% recurrence (within 2 years)
  - Excision and plaque or cryotherapy → less recurrence
- Late
  - Biopsy
  - Pre-operative external beam irradiation, exenteration, post-operative external beam irradiation

Mucoepidermoid carcinoma

- Very rare
- Limbus, fornix or caruncle
- Treat with wide surgical excision, cryotherapy, radiotherapy

Lymphoma

- Monoclonal proliferation of B-lymphocytes

- Salmon pink, mobile mass
- Increased risk in HIV
- Excision if small
- Radiation – usually curative, chemotherapy – if systemic
- Referral to oncologist for systemic evaluation

Kaposi's sarcoma

- Malignant neoplasm of vascular endothelium involving skin and mucous membranes + occasionally internal organs
- Infection with Kaposi's sarcoma – associated human herpes virus 8 is responsible
- Occurs most often in the setting of HIV
- Treatment may not be curative
- Surgical debulking, cryotherapy, radiotherapy, local or systemic chemotherapy, intralesional interferon alpha 2A

Metastases

- Uncommon
- Breast, lung, kidney, cutaneous melanoma

Conjunctival epithelial melanosis

- Common in Blacks

Benign acquired melanosis

Conjunctival naevus

- Junctional, compound, deep
- Uncommon, benign
- 30% are non-pigmented

Congenital ocular melanocytosis

- Ocular melanocytosis
- Dermal melanocytosis
- Oculodermal melanocytosis (naevus of Ota) – affects Oriental females; most common in distribution of first and second divisions of V cranial nerve; iris hyperchromia may occur; increased risk of melanoma; glaucoma in 10%; iris mamillations may occur

Primary acquired melanosis

- Uncommon, unilateral
- Without atypia – benign proliferation of melanocytes
- With atypia - premalignant, 50% chance of malignant transformation within 5 years

Conjunctival malignant melanoma

Pathology
- Melanoma arising from primary acquired melanosis with atypia
- Melanoma arising from pre-existing naevus
- Melanoma arising de novo

Clinical features
- Rare
- May be pigmented or non-pigmented
- Usually presents in sixth decade
- Common site is limbus, may occur anywhere

Differential diagnosis
- Large naevus, ciliary body melanoma, melanocytoma, pyogenic granuloma, pigmented conjunctival carcinoma

Treatment
- Surgical excision with wide clearance + cryotherapy
- Six-monthly checks
- Orbital recurrences treated by local resection + radiotherapy
- Lymph node involvement treated by surgical excision + radiotherapy
- Metastatic spread treated palliatively with chemotherapy
- Two-year mortality 25%
- Poor prognostic factors are – palpebral conjunctiva, mixed cell, multifocal, tumour thickness >4 mm

3

4

Cornea and sclera

Congenital abnormalities 42
Anterior chamber cleavage syndromes 44
Iridocorneal endothelial syndrome 46
Corneal dystrophies 46
Herpes zoster ophthalmicus 51
Keratitis 52
Ocular microbiology 59
Peripheral ulcerative keratitis 60
Phlyctenular disease 63
Keratoconus 65
Climatic droplet keratopathy 68
Metabolic keratopathies 69
Miscellaneous keratopathies 73
Involutional diseases 77
Pterygium 79
Chemical burns 80
Contact lenses 82
Keratoplasty 82
Limbal stem cell transplants 85
Amniotic membrane 86
Scleritis 86
Episcleritis 88

Congenital abnormalities

General

- Inheritance – may be sporadic or inherited (sex-linked recessive, autosomal dominant or autosomal recessive)
- Associations
  - Ocular – may have associated anterior segment anomalies and glaucoma
  - Systemic – may have associated skeletal anomalies and syndromes

Posterior keratoconus

- Local crater defect, variable overlying stromal haze
- Usually sporadic
- Visual acuity usually not affected; therefore, no treatment usually required

Keratoglobus

- Rare, bilateral, globular cornea; k readings 50–60D
- Generalised thinning
- Hydrops can occur
- Appears at birth
- Non-hereditary
- Strong association with blue sclera and Ehlers-Danlos syndrome
- May represent defective collagen synthesis
- Management
  - Penetrating keratoplasty prognosis poor; rather do lamellar keratoplasty
  - Avoid contact sports

Megalocornea

- Non-progressive corneal enlargement, X-linked; male > female
- $\geq$ 13 mm diameter; normal thickness, endothelium + clarity

- Due to failure of anterior lips of optic cup to grow towards each other
- Results from spontaneously arrested congenital glaucoma with exaggerated corneal growth in relation to the rest of the eye
- Associations
  - Iris translucency, miosis, goniodysgenesis, cataract, ectopia lentis
  - Craniosyntosis, dwarfism, Marfan's, facial haemiatrophy
- Management
  - Check for congenital glaucoma
  - Treat refractive errors

Microcornea

- ≤ 10 mm diameter cornea
- Anterior microphthalmos – entire anterior segment small
- Microphthalmos – whole eye small and deformed, disorganised
- Nanophthalmos – whole eye small but otherwise normal (axial length 15–20 mm + high hyperopia)
- Due to overgrowth of anterior lips of optic cup
- Or arrest of foetal corneal growth at 5 months
- Autosomal dominant or recessive, male = female
- Higher incidence of acute angle closure glaucoma + 20% get open angle glaucoma later
- Associations: persistent foetal vasculature, cataracts, anterior segment dysgenesis, foetal alcohol syndrome, myotonic dystrophy, Ehlers-Danlos

Sclerocornea

- Non-progressive, non-inflammatory, variable vascularisation
- Corneal periphery or entire cornea
- 90% bilateral
- Usually sporadic

Congenital corneal guttata

Epibulbar dermoid

- Choristoma, straddles limbus
- May cause astigmatism
- Seen in Goldenhar syndrome, sebaceous naevus syndrome, encephalocraniocutaneous lipomatosis

Goldenhar syndrome (oculoauriculovertebral dysplasia)

- Triad of epibulbar dermoid, pre-auricular appendages, pretragal fistulae
- Also lid colobomas, vertebral anomalies, mandible hypoplasia

Cornea plana

- Severe decrease in corneal curvature, hypermetropia, shallow anterior chamber
- K readings of 20–30D
- Can have ocular problems like anterior segment dygenesis and can be associated with systemic diseases like Ehlers-Danlos syndrome
- Watch out for glaucoma + refractive errors

Vertical oval cornea

- Associated with congenital syphilis and Turner's syndrome

Blue sclera

- Due to generalised scleral thinning
- Osteogenesis imperfecta, Ehlers-Danlos syndrome

4

Congenital cloudy cornea

Causes of congenital cloudy cornea	
■ Congenital	□ Trisomy 13 + 18 + 21
	□ Turner's syndrome
	□ Mucopolysaccharidoses types 1, 4, 6
	□ Gangliosidosis.
	□ Chediak-Higashi syndrome
	□ Cystinosis
■ Traumatic	□ Birth trauma (forceps usually)
■ Inflammatory	□ Rubella
	□ Syphilis
	□ Gonorrhoea
	□ Herpes
■ Dystrophic	□ Congenital hereditary endothelial dystrophy
Malformation	□ Sclerocornea
	□ Anterior mesodermal dysgenesis (Peter's anomaly)
■ Glaucoma	

Causes of a congenital cloudy cornea

S – Sclerocornea
T – Tears in Descemet's membrane (glaucoma, trauma)
U – Ulcers/keratitis
M – Mucopolysaccaridoses
P – Peter's anomaly
D – Dystrophy – congenital hereditary endothelial

Congenital forceps injury of cornea

- Cornea cloudy at birth, then clears
- Vertical Descemet's scrolls appear
- Acute corneal decompensation may develop after several decades
- May also have periorbital forceps depressions + occipital skull depressions

Anterior chamber cleavage syndromes

- A group of embryological disorders
- Dysgenesis of structures derived from the neural crest
- Many of these conditions are associated with glaucoma

Classification of anterior chamber cleavage syndromes		
Cornea	■ Endothelium	□ Congenital hereditary endothelial dystrophy
		□ Peter's anomaly
Trabecular meshwork	■ Stroma	□ Congenital hereditary stromal dystrophy
	■ Primary goniodysgenesis	□ Trabecular dysgenesis
		□ Axenfeld-Rieger syndrome

Posterior embryotoxon

- Prominent, thickened, centrally displaced Schwalbe's ring
- Schwalbe's ring is the junction of the trabecular meshwork and the termination of Descemet's membrane
- Seen in 8–30% of normal eyes, usually autosomal dominant
- Visible by external examination
- Rest of eye usually normal
- Associations – cornea plana, corectopia, aniridia, Alagille's syndrome (arteriohepatic dysplasia)

Axenfeld-Rieger syndrome

- A spectrum of disorders characterised by
  - Posterior embryotoxon with attached iris strands
  - Iris hypoplasia, glaucoma (50%) due to trabecular meshwork dysplasia
  - Skeletal, cranial, facial and dental abnormalities (hypodontia and microdontia, redundant paraumbilical skin, mental retardation)
- Autosomal dominant or sporadic

Peter's anomaly

- Usually sporadic, autosomal dominant and autosomal recessive also reported
- Central corneal leukoma, due to absent endothelium
- Iridocorneal adhesions at the edge of the leukoma
- Lens apposition to leukoma with shallow anterior chamber
- Anterior lenticular opacity
- 60% bilateral
- Ocular associations include
  - Congenital glaucoma in 50%
  - Microphthalmos, cataract, microcornea, aniridia, persistent foetal vasculature
- Systemic associations (60%) include
  - Developmental delay
  - Cleft palate
  - Congenital heart defects
  - Skeletal anomalies
  - Craniofacial dysplasia
  - Hearing loss
- May be associated with genetic syndromes
  - Trisomy 13, 14, 15
  - Peter's-plus syndrome
  - Kivlin's syndrome
  - Pfeiffer's syndrome

4

Posterior polymorphous dystropy

- May be a form of anterior chamber cleavage syndrome

Circumscribed posterior keratoconus

- Central or paracentral
- No anterior surface abnormality
- Varying overlying stromal haze
- Unilateral, non-progressive, sporadic
- ± Astigmatism and amblyopia

Arcus juvenilus

- Lipid deposition in peripheral stroma
- Not associated with serum lipid abnormality

Sclerocornea

- Non-progressive, inflammatory sclerisation
- Periphery or entire cornea
- Cornea plana in 80%
- 90% bilateral
- Angle structures commonly malformed
- Usually sporadic, also autosomal dominant, autosomal recessive

Congenital hereditary stromal dystrophy

- Autosomal dominant, very rare
- Bilateral central superficial clouding

Posterior amorphous stromal dystrophy

- Rare, autosomal dominant, bilateral and symmetrical
- Diffuse grey-white sheets of stromal opacity

Congenital hereditary endothelial dystrophy

- Bilateral congenital corneal oedema
- Bluish-white cornea
- Autosomal recessive, at birth, stationary, nystagmus
- Autosomal dominant, first or second year, progressive, pain + tearing
- Probable endothelial dysgenesis
- No systemic association
- Gene: 20p11,2–q11,2

Iridocorneal endothelial syndrome

- Also known as primary proliferative endotheliopathy
- A group of conditions – dystrophy or dysplasia of corneal endothelium

Pathophysiology

- Degeneration of endothelial cells with proliferation of the remaining cells which encroach on the trabecular meshwork → peripheral anterior synechiae, glaucoma, iris distortion, corneal oedema

4

Corneal dystrophies

Classification of corneal dystrophies	
Anterior	Cogan's microcystic
	Reis-Bücklers
	Thiel-Behnke
	Meesman's
	Schnyder's
Stromal	Lattice 1, 2, 3, 3A
	Granular 1, 2, 3
	Avellino
	Macular 1,2
	Gelatinous drop-like dystrophy
	Fleck dystrophy
	Central cloudy dystrophy of Francois
Posterior	Fuchs' endothelial
	Posterior polymorphous
	Congenital hereditary endothelial dystrophy
Ectatic	Anterior keratoconus
	Keratoglobus
	Posterior keratoconus
	Pellucid marginal degeneration

Definition

- Group of progressive, bilateral, genetically determined (most are autosomal dominant) corneal opacifying disorders with little or no relationship to environmental or systemic factors
- They develop in the absence of inflammation, and usually present in the first to fourth decade

Corneal dystrophies – anterior

Cogan's microcystic dystrophy (corneal epithelial basement membrane dystrophy)

- Most common dystrophy seen
- In adult females, usually sporadic (may be autosomal dominant); affects 10% of people > 50 years
- An abnormality of epithelial turnover, maturation + production of basement membrane

Symptoms

- Recurrent epithelial erosions, ± decreased vision, ± corneal erosions

Signs

- Putty deposits in epithelium, round or comma-shaped; maps, dots, fingerprints, cysts

Histology

- Thickened basement membrane with extension into epithelium; cysts containing debris from degenerate epithelial cells

Treatment

- Nil or treatment for recurrent erosions
- Hypertonic saline
- Lubrication
- Epithelial debridement
- Patching
- Bondage contact lens
- Anterior stromal puncture
- Phototherapeutic keratectomy

Reis-Bücklers dystrophy

Onset

- In early childhood; autosomal dominant – chromosome 5q31

Symptoms

- Decreased vision during third decade, recurrent erosions

Signs

- Cornea progressively more cloudy with superficial reticulated opacity and epithelial defects, irregular corneal surface, decreased corneal sensation

Histology

- Degeneration of Bowman's layer, replaced by scar tissue, curly filaments on electron microscopy

Pathogenesis

- Mutation in the BIGH3 gene responsible for keratoepithelin production

Treatment

- Lamellar and penetrating keratoplasty; opacity may recur

Variants

- Anterior, geographic membrane dystrophy and honeycomb dystrophy (Thiel-Behnke) are attenuated variants

Dystrophy of Bowman's layer

- Type 1: Geographic or Reis-Bücklers
- Type 2: Thiel-Behnke dystrophy – 10q24, curly fibres on electron microscopy

Meesman's (juvenile epithelial) dystrophy

Onset

- Early childhood; rare + autosomal dominant

Symptoms

- Vision not affected; may have discomfort from rupture of cysts

Signs

- Anterior epithelial cystic opacities

Histology

- Intraepithelial cysts containing debris from degenerate epithelial cells, basement membrane may have excrescences into nasal epithelium

Treatment

- Usually nil; bandage contact lens for frequent symptoms; phototherapeutic keractomy

Schnyder's dystrophy (crystalline corneal dystrophy)

Onset

- In second decade (may be apparent in the first year of life)

Symptoms

- Decreased photopic vision, glare

Signs

- Oval area of sub epithelial crystalline opacity in a generally hazy cornea

Histology

- Accumulation of cholesterol

Treatment

- Phototherapeutic keratectomy – does not treat pan-stromal haze
- Penetrating keratoplasty – recurrences can occur

Corneal dystrophies – posterior

Cornea guttata

Onset

- In adults

Symptoms

- Decreased vision, ± pain from bullous keratopathy

Signs

- Wart-like endothelial prominences, ± with brown pigmentation → stromal and epithelial oedema, bullous keratopathy (= Fuchs' dystrophy)
- At risk for endothelial decompensation following surgery

Histology

- Excrescences of Descemet's membrane, endothelial cell degeneration

Fuchs' endothelial dystrophy

Incidence

- Common

Onset

- After the age of 50 years, more common in females, progression from guttata

Symptoms

- Decreased vision, pain from bullous keratopathy

Signs and histology

- Metabolic incompetence of endothelial cells → wart-like excrescences, endothelial cell loss, thickening of Descemet's membrane, stromal and epithelial oedema (worse in morning and high humidity), bullous keratopathy, subepithelial fibrosis and vascularisation (pannus), stromal fibrosis
- Increased incidence of chronic glaucoma and cataract; pachymetry > 650 μm → poor prognosis for cataract surgery

Treatment

- Reduce corneal oedema + relieve pain
- 5% sodium chloride drops and ointment
- Bandage contact lens
- Penetrating keratoplasty
- Descemet's stripping endothelial keratoplasty

Congenital hereditary endothelial dystrophy

Onset

- Congenital, autosomal dominant or autosomal recessive

Signs

- Bilateral early diffuse corneal oedema/haziness

Histology

- Decreased number of endothelial cells, thin Descemet's membrane

Treatment

- Penetrating keratoplasty, results poor

Posterior polymorphous dystrophy

Onset

- Birth → childhood, may be autosomal recessive; 20q11

Symptoms

- ± Decreased vision

Signs

- Vesicular lesions on Descemet's membrane, with surrounding hazy opacities; opacities may be dendritic, boomerang, circular, comma, linear, filiform
- ± Band keratopathy, anterior segment defects (peripheral anterior synechiae, abnormal iris processes), epithelial oedema

Histology

- Thickened Descemet's membrane, fibroblastic metaplasia of endothelial cells; ? represents a form of the anterior chamber cleavage syndrome

Treatment

- Usually none – most patients are stable and asymptomatic
- Penetrating keratoplasty if required

Corneal dystrophies – stromal

Granular dystrophy

- Autosomal dominant, chromosome 5q31 (along with Avellino and Reis-Bücklers)

Onset

- Type 1 in first decade, type 2 in fourth or fifth decade, type 3 late in life

Symptoms

- Decreased vision

Signs

- Opacities in superficial stroma, increase in size and number, take on appearance of Christmas tree

Type 1, 2 and 3 granular dystrophy

- Type 1
  - Most common
  - Onset early in life
  - Crumb-like opacities, broadening in teen years, not extending to limbus
  - Slowly progressive, mild to moderate visual loss
- Type 2
  - Second decade presentation
  - Fewer lesions, clear intervening areas
  - Erosions sometimes
  - VA usually better than 6/24
- Type 3
  - Presents in infancy
  - More superficial
  - Fine granular deposits confined to Bowman's or anterior stroma
  - Resembles Reis-Bücklers clinically

Histology

- Composed of extracellular hyaline material

Treatment

- Superficial keratectomy, phototherapeutic keratectomy, penetrating keratoplasty – good prognosis; may recur in graft

Avellino

- A variant of granular dystrophy
- A granular dystrophy clinically and histologically
- Some have lattice lesions as well
- Also known as – granular-lattice dystrophy

Management
- No treatment early
- Recurrent erosions → Bandage contact lens, superficial keratectomy, phototherapeutic keratectomy, penetrating keratoplasty (recurrence finer)

Lattice dystrophy

Onset
- Early, at the end of the first decade

Inheritance
- Autosomal dominant; type 1 defective gene on long arm of chromosome 5; type 2 defective gene on long arm of chromosome 9; type 3 not elucidated
- Type 1: (Biber-Haab-Dimmer) – corneal dystrophy only
- Type 2: (Meretoja's syndrome) – associated systemic familial amyloidosis
- Type 3: Like 1, but onset in fourth decade

Symptoms
- Decreased vision, corneal erosions, photophobia

Signs
- Opacities in anterior stroma – dots, spicules, and filaments (ground glass); later involvement of epithelium, decreased corneal sensation

Histology
- Amyloid deposits (form of primary localised amyloidosis)

Treatment
- Bandage contact lens for recurrent erosions
- Penetrating keratoplasty; may recur in graft
- Superficial keratectomy or phototherapeutic keratectomy

Macular dystrophy

- Least common of the three

Onset
- Autosomal recessive, clear at birth, clouding at 3–9 months

Symptoms
- Severe decrease in vision

Signs
- Diffuse clouding in superficial stroma, decreased sensation; involves corneal periphery

Histology
- Accumulation of glycosaminoglycan deposits between lamellae, ? due to abnormality of keratin sulphate metabolism

Treatment
- Penetrating keratoplasty, may recur in graft

Gelatinous drop-like dystrophy

- Primary familial amyloidosis
- Uncommon, autosomal recessive
- Source of amyloid may be the basal epithelial layer
- Similar management to lattice – high recurrence post-penetrating keratoplasty

Fleck dystrophy

- Uncommon, non-progressive, probably autosomal dominant
- Begins early, may be congenital
- Discrete, flat, gray-white, dandruff-like opacities throughout the stroma to its periphery
- Minimal symptoms, vision not reduced
- May be associated with keratoconus, dermoids, atopy

Central cloudy dystrophy of Francois

- Non-progressive, autosomal dominant
- Requires no management
- Cloudy opacity, densest centrally

Herpes zoster ophthalmicus (HZO)

Virology

- Varicella zoster human herpes virus 3
- DNA, enveloped
- Primary → chicken pox; dormant in sensory nuclei (trigeminal); reactivation → zoster

Epidemiology

- Male = female
- Mainly in sixth decade, increased with increased age
- Strong association with immunocompromise
- Va (trigeminal) affected in 15% of cases
- Globe affected in 70% of cases when Va is involved
- Three to four per 1 000 per year
- Three clinical phases – acute, chronic, relapsing

Immunology

- Temporary depression in cellular immunity; humoral immunity is normal

Pathogenesis

- Lower immunity per se is not responsible for reactivation
- Reactivation triggered by – mechanical or neural trauma, UV light, irradiation, diseases affecting neural metabolism (colds, flu, pneumonia), lymphoma, ageing of neurones, HIV

Pathology

- Viral replication in nerves and related tissues
- Infiltration with inflammatory cells
- Cell necrosis
- Resolution or continuing chronic and relapsing inflammation

Clinical features

- Flu-like illness × 1 week
- Pain over distribution Va
- Lymphadenopathy
- ± Red eye
- Rash, onset after several days of pain
- Varies in distribution, density, and severity
- Macules → papules → vesicles → pustules → crusts
- Ocular features
  - Nasociliary nerve involvement → vesicles on tip of nose and lid margins
  - Usually heralds ocular involvement (80% of cases) (Hutchinson's sign)

4

Acute lesions

- Eyelid rash
- Conjunctivitis
- Episcleritis and scleritis, trabeculitis
- Cornea
  - Involved in 40% of cases
  - Acute epithelial keratitis
  - Dendritic keratitis
  - Nummular keratitis (most common corneal lesion)
  - Disciform keratitis
  - Diffuse corneal oedema
  - Neurotrophic keratitis
- Iritis
- Choroiditis
- Retinal vasculitis
- Acute retinal necrosis (particularly with AIDS)
- Optic neuritis
- Extraocular muscle palsies; III ophthalmoplegia occurs in 30% cases, sometimes bilateral, due to retrograde spread from V nerve, may take 2 years to recover
- Associated neurological features
  - VII palsy
  - Encephalitis
  - Hemiplegia, due to cerebral vasculitis
  - Neuralgia
  - Depression

4

Chronic lesions

- Skin – scarring, recurrent rash
- Eyelids – persistent ptosis, chronic blepharitis. sequelae of scarring (entropion, trichiasis, poliosis)
- Conjunctiva – chronic conjunctivitis
- Episclera and sclera – scleritis, nodular episleritis
- Cornea
  - Nummular keratitis
  - Disciform keratitis
  - Interstitial keratitis
  - Neurotrophic keratitis
  - Lipid keratopathy
  - Iris – chronic iritis, iris atrophy
- Cataract
- Glaucoma
- Optic atrophy
- Post-herpetic neuralgia
- Ptosis, orbital oedema, proptosis – due to occlusive arteritis
- Cranial nerve involvement – within the orbit or cavernous sinus
- Systemic dissemination can occur in up to 25% of immunocompromised patients

Investigations

- HIV

Management

- Systemic
- Skin
- Eye
- Surgery

Systemic

- Systemic non-steroidal anti-inflammatories
- Systemic steroids – in severe disease, weigh against the risks, do not use in immunocompromised patients
- Acyclovir 800 mg 5 × daily × 1 week → reduces chance of systemic dissemination (best if started within 72 hours of onset of skin lesions)
- OR Famciclovir 500 mg 3 × daily, valacyclovir 1 g 3 × daily
- Analgesics – codeine or pethidine in acute stage
- Tegretol for post-herpetic neuralgia
- Antidepressants – amitryptyline

Skin

- Idoxuridine or acyclovir ointment during vesicular phase
- Post-herpetic neuralgia – massage skin, capsaicin ointment, ultrasound, transcutaneous electrical nerve stimulation, stellate ganglion block

Eye

- Acyclovir ointment; decreases the risk of rebound on withdrawal of steroids
- Antibiotic drops/ointment
- Steroid drops/ointment
- Artificial tear drops/ointment
- Oral steroids – reserve for extreme pain or associated iritis

Surgery

- Lateral tarsorrhaphy for neurotrophic ulceration
- Correction of ectropion and trichiasis
- Cataract extraction
- Glaucoma surgery
- Corneal graft; poor results, due to hypoaesthesia, tear abnormalities, lid disease, glaucoma, uveitis, vascularisation

Keratitis

Acanthamoeba keratitis

- Problem – frequent failure to recognise the disease in an early, more treatable stage

Pathogenesis

- Free-living ubiquitous protozoa in freshwater + soil
- Amoebic keratitis – 70–90% contact lens-related; rest from minor trauma

Clinical
- Severe pain (± disproportionate), photophobia, redness, epiphora
- Usually unilateral
- Protracted, progressive course
- Early – punctate epithelial erosion or dendritic → typically misdiagnosed as herpes simplex keratitis
- Central stromal infection, ring-infiltrate in the paracentral stroma
- ± Satellite lesions, corneal neovascularisation
- Radial perineuritis → enlarged corneal nerves, limbitis, scleritis
- Severe visual loss > 15%

Diagnosis
- Microscopy culture sensitivity
- Highest diagnostic yield early
- Later, organism penetrates deeper
- Giemsa or PAS stained smears
- Non-nutrient agar with e. coli overlay; blood agar (wait 2weeks before reporting negative)

Management
- Medical
- Surgical

Medical
- No optimal regime yet
- Early – epithelial debridement, 3–4 months course of anti-amoebics
- Later – stromal, 6–12 months of anti-amoebics
- Agents used topically
  - Diamidines – propamidine, hexamidine, pentamidine
  - Biguanides – chlorhexidine, polyhexamethylene
  - Aminoglycosides – neomycin
  - Imidazoles – miconazole, clotrimazole, ketoconazole, itraconazole
- Typically effective against free-living trophozoites but reduced efficacy in killing cysts
- Recent regime – chlorhexidine 0.02% + propamidine 0.1%
- Initiate hourly + taper to response (relapses common with tapering)

Surgical
- Penetrating keratoplasty – cases that progress despite maximal medical therapy, threatened perforation; not good as therapy
- High risk of recurrence if done in first year, even if quiet
- Do optical penetrating keratoplasty only after 6 months of being disease-free

4

Suppurative bacterial keratitis

Bacteriology
- Normal conjunctival flora
  - Variable, usually gram positive
  - Staph epidermidis, + some potential pathogens and fungi
- Normal defence mechanisms
  - Tears and integrity of epithelium
  - Normal healthy cornea is resistant to all organisms except Neisseria, Corynebacterium, Listeria and haemophilus
- Compromising conditions
  - Local – trauma, scarring, Staph blepharitis, climatic droplet keratopathy, dry eye, corneal exposure, allergy, trichiasis, steroids, antibiotics, contact lens wear, contaminated ocular medications
  - General – immunosuppression, malnutrition
- Causal organisms
  - Gram positive, Streptococcus pneumoniae, → haemolytic Streptococcus, Staph aureus, Staph epidermidis
  - Gram negative, Pseudomonas aeruginosa, Moraxella sp, Klebsiella pneumoniae, Proteus sp, Enterobacteriaecae (Escherichia coli)

Contact lenses
- 19–42% of bacterial keratitis caused by contact lenses in high income countries

- Extended wear soft lenses → 0.21% incidence per year
- Daily wear soft lenses → 0.04% incidence per year
- Risk increases 15 × with overnight wear

Pathology
- Acute inflammatory response in stroma with ± abscess formation
- Bacteria may produce collagenases → colliquative necrosis of stroma
- Hypopyon, if present, is usually sterile

Clinical features
- Pseudomonas
    - Diffuse, rapidly spreading, stromal necrosis with adherent mucopurulent exudate
    - Hypopyon, endothelial inflammatory plaque
- Staph aureus – round or oval
- Pneumococcus – undermined edges
- Anaerobes – slow growing
- Infectious crystalline keratopathy
    - Densely packed, white, branching aggregates of organisms in the virtual absence of a host inflammatory response
    - Seen especially in α-haemolytic Streptococcus

Differential diagnosis
- Viral
- Trophic
- Bacterial
- Toxic
- Fungal
- Nutritional
- Marginal hypersensitivity
- Traumatic

Corneal scrape

Technique
- Local anaesthetics benoxinate and proparacaine have minimal static effect
- Fungal scrape must be taken with a blade
- Culture of contact lens, eyelids

Microscopy
- Gram stain for bacteria → 60% identification rate
- Peripheral anterior synechiae stain for fungi

Culture and sensitivity
- Cooked meat medium – for anaerobes
- Thyglycollate broth – for anaerobes
- Boiled blood agar – for most aerobes and some fungi
- Chocolate agar – for Neisseria, Moraxella and Haemophilus
- Sabouraud's medium – containing chloramphenicol, for fungi

Management
- No single agent is effective against all organisms
- Antibiotics
- Mydriatic
- Collagen shield, contact lens, tissue glue
- Steroids

Antibiotics
- Hourly for 48 hours (even half-hourly at first, or every 5 mins for 30 mins loading)
- Gram positive organisms
    - Fortified cefuroxime (5%) topically
    - Subconjunctival not usually required; only for scleral spread
- Gram negative organisms
    - Gentamycin subconjunctivally
    - Fortified gentamycin (1.5%) topically
    - Ciprofloxacin topically; gives broad spectrum cover, very good as primary therapy less epithelial toxicity but less effective against Strep spp; resistance by Pseudomonas and Staph spp emerging
    - Monotherapy in children not advised
    - Systemic ciprofloxacin if there is severe keratitis with threatened spread to the sclera

Fortified topical antibiotic doses for bacterial keratitis		
Gram positive cocci	Cefazoline Vancomycin Moxifloxacin Gatifloxacin	50 mg/ml (5%) 50 mg /ml (5%) 5 mg/ml (0.5%) 3 mg/ml (0.3%)
Gram negative rods	Tobramycin Ceftazidime Ciprofloxacin	9–14 mg/ml (1%) 50 mg/ml (5%) 3 mg/ml (0.3%)

Mydriatic

- Cycloplegic

Surgical

- Collagen shield, contact lens, tissue glue
- Conjunctival flap (Gunderson)
- Penetrating keratoplasty
  - Therapeutic or optical – if there is no response, descemetocoele, perforation
  - Do a peripheral iridectomy and use interrupted sutures

Steroids

- If used, delay for 24 hours after antibiotics started, only with a known sensitivity organism and a strong response to antibiotics shown
- Contraindicated with fungal infections, use with care in pneumococcal and pseudomonas infections
- Relapse of pneumococcus shown

Failure to heal

- Combined infection – stop treatment for 24 hours, rescrape or biopsy
- Drug toxicity – use preservative-free drops

Fungal keratitis

Incidence

- Accounts for 5–60% of suppurative keratitis (5% in temperate climates → 60% in tropical climates)
- Incidence rising, due to indiscriminate use of antibiotics and steroids

Aetiology

- Thirty-five genera of fungi associated with corneal infections
  - Yeasts in compromised corneas, yeasts in temperate climates
  - Filaments in agricultural injuries, filaments in tropical climates
- Most common
  - Yeasts – Candida, Cryptococcus
  - Filamentous – Fusarium, Cephalosporium, Aspergillus
- Predisposing factors
  - Vegetable matter injury is important
  - Trauma related to contact lens wear
  - Topical steroid use
  - Systemic steroid use
  - Corneal surgery
  - Chronic keratitis – HZO, herpes simplex, vernal

Pathology

- Hyphae invade stroma parallel to collagen lamellae, may penetrate Descemet's membrane into anterior chamber
- Coagulative necrosis of corneal stroma occurs
- Satellite lesions occur

Clinical features

- Gray dirty white with feathery margins, satellite lesions, immune Wesley ring, hypopyon
- Often shows initial improvement on antibiotic treatment, then worsening

Corneal scrape

- PAS stain
- Sabouraud's or brain heart infusion culture → 50% yield
- Direct microscopy → better positive yield than culture

Management

- Antifungal medication
- Antibiotic
- Debridement

Antifungal medication

- Topical natamycin (5%) – for filaments (especially Fusarium)
- Topical flucytosine, amphotericin B (0.15–0.3%) – for yeasts + Aspergillus filaments
- Flucytosine + amphotericin are additive in combination
- Topical econazole (1%) + miconazole (1%) → broad spectrum
- Ketoconazole (200–600 mg/day) – for severe filamentous infections
- Itraconazole (200 mg/day) – good against Candida and Aspergillus, variable against Fusarium
- Oral flucytosine for intraocular Candida

Antibiotic

- Try to avoid high dose
- Mydriatic-cycloplegic

Debridement

- Enhances penetration
- Keratectomy (superficial or deep) + conjunctival flap
- Penetrating keratoplasty – therapeutic
  - Progression despite maximal therapy
  - To prevent scleral or intraocular spread
- Penetrating keratoplasty – optical

Prognosis

- Poor if the anterior chamber is invaded
- Poor in immunocompromised patients

Herpes simplex keratitis

Incidence

- Almost everyone has positive serology by middle age
- 100% of over 60s → herpes simplex in trigeminal ganglia
- One-third of people have recurrent infection

Virology

- DNA, enveloped
- Type 1 above the belt, type 2 below the belt
- 90% of the population are seropositive, most infections are subclinical

Primary ocular infection

- Typically manifests as a unilateral blepharoconjunctivitis, pre-auricular lymph nodes
- Self-limiting
- Neonatal Type 2 – from maternal genital herpes, severe
- Type 1 – at 6 months to 5 years
- From salivary contamination from an adult with labial herpes
- Acute follicular conjunctivitis, usually
- May be pseudomembranous conjunctivitis, ulcerative blepharitis, dendritic keratitis
- Treatment: topical and oral antivirals

Recurrent ocular infection

- Can affect almost any ocular tissue
- Virus reservoirs are in the trigeminal ganglion, superior cervical ganglion → iritis, lacrimal gland
- HLA B5 associated with multiple recurrences, decreased cell mediated immunity may be associated
- May be due to diminished ability of keratocytes to produce β interferon
- There are no proven trigger mechanisims (febrile illness, psychological stress, trauma, sunlight, malnutrition)

- Steroids are important in triggering a recurrence
- No difference in severity of herpes simplex keratitis found with HIV, but is associated with an increased rate of recurrence
- Localised, superficial, self-limited
- Male > female
- Decreased corneal sensation is an important sign

Classification

- Vesicular eruption of lids/blepharitis
- Follicular conjunctivitis
- Keratitis
- Uveitis
- Scleritis
- Trabeculitis
- Neurotrophic keratopathy

Causes of dendritiform ulcers

- Zoster
- Adenovirus
- Epstein-Barr virus
- Neurotrophic ulcer
- Epithelial regeneration
- Thimerosal – soft contact lens
- Topical drops
- Acanthamoeba
- Thygeson's
- Epithelial deposits – iron lines, Fabry's disease, systemic drugs

Epithelial keratitis

- Dendritic, geographic, marginal, punctate
- Treatment: Acyclovir ointment 3%, oral as effective (less local side effects but more expensive)

Epithelial trophic ulceration (metaherpetic post-infectious)

- Following epithelial keratitis, due to failure of hemidesmosome formation between epithelium and Bowman's membrane
- Epithelium is heaped up along the edges
- Distinguish from geographic ulcers by non-staining of edges with rose bengal
- Due to lack of epithelial membrane
- ? Due to mitotic arrest and inhibition of sliding
- ? Due to collagenases and proteases secreted by diseased epithelium

Stromal keratitis

Disciform (also known as endothelilitis)

- Due to vital antigen taken up by stromal cells → cell mediated response
- There must have been a previous episode of epithelial keratitis
- This may have been subclinical
- Lymphocytes adhere to endothelium → stromal oedema

Necrotising

- Due to active viral invasion of stroma → abscess
- May be indistinguishable from bacterial/fungal
- Look for stromal vascularisation
- Treatment: Very sensitive to topical steroids; topical + oral acyclovir

Interstitial

- Associated with vessel ingrowth
- Differential: zoster, acanthamoeba, Epstein-Barr virus, mumps, Lyme, sarcoid, Cogan's
- Treatment: Topical steroids + topical or oral antiviral

Stromal scarring secondary to endothelial dysfunction

Endothelitis

- Linear
- Line of keratic precipitates on endothelium
- Progresses centrally, accompanied by peripheral stromal and epthelial oedema
- Also seen in syphilis

Uveitis

- Anterior + posterior
- Mild (from immune origin) + severe (from direct viral invasion)
- Elevated IOP from trabeculitis
- Iris defects
- Treatment: oral antivirals penetrate the anterior chamber – may be beneficial

4

Scleritis

Trabeculitis

Neurotrophic keratopathy

- Neurotrophic ulcers do not stain with rose bengal, herpetic do

Special investigations

- Scrape → multinucleated giant cells, fluorescent antibody test virus culture in brain-heart infusion
- Serum antibodies – increased in primary infection, no change in secondary infection

Management

- Antiviral medication – see pharmacology
  - Topical acyclovir 6 × daily × 1 week
  - ± Oral acyclovir 400 mg 5 × daily × 1 week
  - Antibiotic if indicated
  - Mydriatic – cycloplegic if indicated
  - Steroids – in disciform stromal keratitis
- Epithelial debridement, in epithelial keratitis
- Soft contact lens and lubricants, in metaherpetic ulceration
- Keratoplasty
  - Therapeutic, for recurrent incapacitating infection
  - Optical, for corneal scarring
  - Cover with acyclovir, 15% recurrence in first year, 25% in first 5 years
  - Acyclovir causes renal failure in 0.5% over 5 years – reasonably safe
  - Do not use cyclosporin → causes renal toxicity in combination with acyclovir
  - Can use mycophenoloate – actually potentiates acyclovir

Measles keratitis

- Conjunctivitis with Koplik's spots, epithelial keratitis, ± uveitis
- Keratitis in malnourished + vitamin A deficient children may be severe → corneal scarring → blindness
- Rarely – optic neuritis, retinal vascular occlusion, pigmentary retinopathy
- ? Due to decreased cell mediated immunity

Other viral diseases of the cornea

Mumps

- Dacryoadenitis, follicular conjunctivitis, epithelial and stromal keratitis, iritis, trabeculitis, scleritis

Rubella

- Microphthalmos, corneal haze, cataracts, iris hypoplasia, iridocyclitis, glaucoma, salt + pepper pigmentary retinopathy

Epstein-Barr virus

- Ocular disease uncommon
- Most common cause of acute dacryoadenitis
- Acute follicular conjunctivitis, Parinaud's oculoglandular syndrome, epithelial corneal dendrites
- May cause a stromal keratitis
- Treatment: topical steroids in sight-threatening cases

Varicella, variola, vaccinia, adenovirus, molluscum contagiosum

Ocular microbiology

Classification of ocular microbiology			
Viruses	DNA	Herpes, adenovirus, poxviruses Papovaviruses	HSV 1 + 2, varicella-zoster, Epstein-Barr virus Epidemic keratoconjunctivitis, smallpox, molluscum contagiosum human papilloma virus
	RNA	Picornaviruses	Enteroviruses (polio, coxsackie, echo, enterovirus), rhinovirus rubella, encephalomyelitis, yellow fever
		Togaviruses orthomyxoviruses + paramyxoviruses	Influenza, mumps, measles, parainfluenza
		Retroviruses	HIV
Bacteria	Gram positive	Cocci	Staph spp Strep spp – β haemolytic → s. pyogenes Enterococcus –endophthalmitis
		Rods	Corynebacteria – acute membranous conjunctivitis Propionobacterium – chronic post-op endophthalmitis Bacillus – post-traumatic endophthalmitis
		Filaments	Mycobacteria Nocardia – keratitis Actinomyces – canaliculitis
	Gram negative	Cocci	Neisseria
		Rods	Pseudomonas – water contaminants Enterobacteriacae (e. coli, Klebsiella, Enterobacter, Salmonella, Shigella, Proteus, Serratia) Haemophilus – preseptal cellulitis → fulminant meningitis in children Bartonella henselae – cat scratch disease (scratch or fleas) Serotypes A→C cause trachoma; obligate intracellular parasites of mucosal epithelium
		Chlamydia	Treponema pallidum
		Spirochaetes	Borrelia burgdorferi – transmitted by tick bites → Lyme disease

4

Fungi	Yeasts Moulds	Candida Filamentous Non-filamentous	 Fusarium → fulminant keratitis Aspergillus Mucor, Rhizopu, Pneumocycstis carinii
Parasites	Protozoa	Acanthamoeba microsporidia Toxoplasma gondii leishmania	Cornea + brain Epithelial keratitis in immunocompromise Cats → chorioretinitis → adult or transplacental Transmitted by female sand fly → cutaneous leishmaniasis → eyelids
Helminths	Oncho-cerca volvulus Toxocara canis	Transmitted by black fly Dogs and cats	River blindness (microfilarial invasion of cornea + uvea) Visceral larval migrans, ocular larval migrans
Arthropods	Phthorus pubis Demodex spp Fly larvae	Pubic lice → lashes Colonises lashes + meibomian glands → blepharitis ophthalmomyiasis	Maggot infestation of the eye
Prions		Creutzfeldt-Jakob scrapie bovine spongiform encephalitis, Kuru	

Peripheral ulcerative keratitis

Differential diagnosis of peripheral ulcerative keratitis

Ocular

- With ulceration
  - Terrien's marginal degeneration
  - Pellucid degeneration
  - Dellen
- Without ulceration
  - Microbial – bacterial, acanthamoeba, fungal, herpetic

- Mooren's ulcer
- Exposure keratopathy
- Marginal keratitis
- Phlyctenulosis
- Ocular cicatricial pemphigoid

Systemic

- Microbial – TB, syphilis, gonococcus, Borreliosis, bacillary dysentery, zoster, AIDS, hepatitis C, helminths
- Rheumatoid arthritis
- SLE
- Wegener's
- Polyarteritis nodosa
- Relapsing polychondritis
- Scleroderma
- Sjögren's syndrome
- Behçet's
- Sarcoidosis
- Inflammatory bowel disease
- Alpha antitrypsin deficiency
- Malignancy

Terrien's marginal degeneration

- Marginal thinning of cornea – localised or extensive
- Male = female
- Usually in second or third decade of life
- Unilateral or asymmetrically bilateral
- Starts in upper cornea, rarely involves inferior cornea
- Starts with opacification and vascularisation (pannus), epithelium remains intact
- Astigmatism develops – high against the rule or oblique astigmatism; perforation is a threat
- Aetiology unknown, histology shows phagocytosis of collagen precursors by histiocytes
- Association with vernal
- Treat with steroids and cycloplegics, conjunctival flap, graft

Mooren's ulcer

Definition

- Painful deep marginal ulcer with overhanging edges, spreads circumferentially

Aetiology

- Unknown; physical or chemical trauma may precede, ? alters epithelial antigens → auto antibody formation → Ag-Ab-C complexes deposited in the limbal arcades
- Evidence for autoimmunity, ? following hepatitis C infection

Pathophysiology

- Deficiency of suppressor T-cells
- Increased IgA
- Increased plasma cells, lymphocytes, Igs + complement in adjacent conjunctiva
- Precipitating factors – trauma, surgery, parasitic infection (incidence of Mooren's is high in parasite endemic areas)
- This inflammation may change the expression of corneal or conjunctival antigens

Pathology

- Destruction of basement membrane and superficial stroma, chronic inflammatory cell infiltrate
- Healing occurs by scarring

Features

- Two types
  - Benign, unilateral, occurring in older people
  - Severe, bilateral, occurring in younger people
- Ulcer has central margin undermined and peripheral margin flat
- Spreads circumferentially and radially, may involve sclera
- Progressive, perforation rare

Treatment

- Topical steroid drops, cyclosporin drops
- Systemic steroids, cyclosporin, other immunosuppressives
- Surgery – local conjunctival excision; also resection of diseased cornea, radiation, cryo, penetrating keratoplasty, lamellar keratoplasty, conjunctival flap
- Hepatitis C – associated cases respond to interferon therapy

Pellucid degeneration

- Cornea thinned inferiorly, results in irregular astigmatism, may be related to keratoglobus and keratoconus
- Fairly common, non-hereditary, bilateral
- Aetiology unknown
- Protrusion of the cornea above the band of thinning
- Treatment
  - Contact lens early on
  - Penetrating keratoplasty – difficult + prone to rejection because close to limbus

Furrow degeneration

- Occurs in old age, asymptomatic, furrow occurs in lucid interval of arcus

Post-irradiation thinning

- After β plaque

Keratitis in rheumatoid arthritis

- Most common cause of immune peripheral ulcerative keratitis

Clinical features

- Correlates with systemic disease exacerbation ± poor disease control
- Usually unilateral and sectoral
- Initial lesion within 2 mm of limbus
- Varying degrees of vascular occlusion of adjacent vascular networks
  - Sclerosing keratitis – adjacent to scleritis
  - Peripheral corneal thinning – non-inflammatory resorption of peripheral corneal tissue
  - Acute stromal keratitis – inflammatory stromal keratitis of peripheral cornea → opacification and vascularisation
  - Acute corneal melting (keratolysis) of peripheral cornea

Treatment

- Improve wetting – often associated with sicca; decreases cytokines in tear film
- Promote re-epthelialisation – lubricants, patching, bondage contact lens, doxycycline, sodium citrate 10%
- Suppress inflammation
  - Topical – steroids (but delays re-epthelialisation, predisposes to superadded infection, exacerbates melting by inhibiting collagen production)
  - Systemic – steroids, cytotoxics, immunomodulatory, IV cyclophosphamide
- Bandage contact lens, cyanoacrylate, penetrating keratoplasty for perforations; avoid conjunctival flaps → brings vasculature closer

Keratitis in SLE

- Punctate epithelial keratopathy
- Marginal thinning
- Marginal infiltration
- Marginal ulceration with infiltration and vascularisation

Keratitis in polyarteritis nodosa and Wegener's granulomatosis

- Bilateral marginal stromal infiltrates → ulceration → circumferential spread

Ring infiltrates and ulcers

- Inflammatory
- Occur in acute leukemia, scleroderma, systemic lupus erythematosus, polyarteritis nodosa, Wegener's granulomatosis, rheumatoid arthrirtis, relapsing polychondritis, gonococcal arthritis, tuberculosis

Marginal infiltrates and ulcers

- Associated with chronic staphylococcal blepharoconjunctivitis
- Sub epithelial infiltrate → overlying staining ulcer → bridging blood vessels → resolution

Fuchs' superficial marginal keratitis

- Idiopathic, occurs in children and young adults
- Superficial marginal keratitis that spreads over cornea
- Advancing ulcer demarcated from central cornea by a sinuous grey line
- Does not reach centre of cornea
- Pseudopterygium develops in areas of recurrent keratitis, chronic course, relapses and remissions
- May resemble Terrien's

Rosacea keratitis

Rosacea

- A chronic acneiform disorder of unknown aetiology affecting skin and eyes; typically underdiagnosed

Incidence

- Common
- Female > male
- Onset at 30–60 years

Clinical

- Stage 1 – Erythema + progressive telangiectasis
- Stage 2 – Inflammatory papules and pustules
- Stage 3 – Inflammatory nodules, sebaceous gland hyperplasia, rhinophyma

Keratitis

- Occurs in 5% of cases
- Punctate epitheliopathy; of inferior two-thirds of cornea
- Peripheral vascularisation and sub epithelial infiltrates of inferotemporal and inferonasal cornea
- Thinning of cornea
- Perforation, rarely

Other ocular features

- Conjunctivitis, blepharitis, recurrent styes and chalazia
- Treatment of ocular rosacea
  - Topical steroid drops, fusidic ointment
  - Systemic tetracycline

Face

- Rhinophyma, malar rash, flushing, telangiectasias, papules + pustules

Management

- Doxycycline – alters the nature of sebum, inhibits matrix metalloproteinases, alters the interaction between meibomian glands and resident bacteria (probably best to continue a low dose indefinitely)
- Topical metronidazole 0.75% gel
- Advanced cases – treat conservatively; poor prognosis for penetrating keratoplasty

Phlyctenular disease

Phlyctenular keratoconjunctivitis

Definition

- Delayed hypersensitivity response (type 4-cell mediated) within the conjunctiva

4

and/or cornea to some antigen in a sensitised individual
- Either tuberculoprotein or staphylococcal antigen (either exotoxin or wall antigen in lysing bacteria) or other bacterial antigen
- The response is characterised by the formation of a nodule of lymphocytes

4

Pathogenesis
- May be just one of several local reactions, but notable because of the severity of the symptoms and the obvious site
- Ocular surface and specifically the limbus may be susceptible to delayed hypersensitivity phenomena
- No keratin in conjunctiva, therefore, readily penetrated by particles or macromolecules
- Conjunctival epithelium may actually phagocytose antigenic particles
- Limbal epithelium is thin and more porous
- Presensitised T and B lymphocytes, sensitised at a remote site, lie within substantia propria of the conjunctiva
- Two possible routes of stimulation of the lymphocytes – systemic and local
  - Systemic challenge is from leakage of antigen from the conjunctival vessels
  - Local challenge is from topical antigen
- Challenge of the T-cells results in blast transformation and secretion of lymphokines
- Lymphokines diffuse outwards, are absorbed by blood on conjunctival side but not absorbed over a triangular area of cornea and therefore recruit other immune cells into the area
- Release of lysozymes then leads to unceration and vascularisation
- Isolated corneal phlyctens are probably due to a humoral immune mechanism i.e. antigen in contact with a specific antibody within the cornea
- This would activate the complement cascade and inflammatory cells could be recruited from the tear film

Aetiology
- Tuberculosis
- Staphylococcus
- Other – coccidiodes, candidiasis, lymphogranuloma, pneumococcus

Pathology
- Focal subepithelial collection of lymphocytes
- Progression abscess formation → ulceration → evacuation → healing

Historical perspective
- Earliest descriptions – malnourished children with clinical TB, in which the phlycten represented an allergic response to endogenous tuberculoprotein
- Later descriptions – well nourished children with no evidence of clinical TB
- Most recent descriptions – emphasise the increasing importance of staphylococcus and other bacteria as being the causative agent, with the decrease in the incidence of TB in the communities in which it is described

Clinical features of TB phlycten
- Occurs in the first and second decades, female : male = 3 : 2
- Corneal involvement → photophobia, blepharospasm, tearing
- Phlyctens may be focal or wandering, vascularised or non-vascularised
- Corneal lesions usually bilateral and occur inferiorly

Evidence for TB association with phlyctens

Criteria for diagnosis of TB phlycten – one of the following

- Family history of TB/history of TB exposure
- Clinical evidence of TB

- Positive Mantoux
- Positive chest x-ray

Epidemiological evidence for TB association

- High incidence of positive tuberculin reactions
- High incidence of positive chest x-ray
- High incidence of history of past or present TB
- High incidence of family history of TB
- High incidence of subsequent clinical TB
- Clinical similarity to complications of ophthalmoreaction of Calmette in TB patients
- Significant incidence of previous phlyctenulosis in adults with TB
- Worldwide parallelism between incidence of TB and incidence of phlyctenulosis
- Rapid disappearance on steroid treatment
- Experimentally produced by instillation of tuberculium into conjunctival sac of tuberculin sensitised humans
- Experimentally, produced by injection of tuberculoprotein into blood stream of non-TB rabbits previously sensitised

Clinical features of non-TB phlycten

- Occurs in older people
- Less blepharospasm and photophobia
- Usually evidence of staph blepharitis or other regional infection (hordeolum, dermatitis)
- Less dramatic response to steroid treatment

Differential diagnosis

- Acne rosacea keratitis
- Trachoma
- Recurrent staphylococcal marginal ulcers
- Limbal vernal conjunctivitis
- Nodular episcleritis
- Bacterial ulcers
- Herpes simplex keratitis
- Pingueculum and pterygium

Treatment

- Topical steroids
- Rapid response if due to TB
- Less effective if due to staph; add local and/or systemic antibiotics

Mantoux interpretation

- Give 5IU purified protein derivative intradermally, read at 72 hours
- Non-reactive/no response
  - ? Error in administration
  - Or 'at risk', therefore, requires BCG
- Diameter < 10 mm – have cell mediated immunity against TB
- Diameter 10–15mm
  - 'Grey area', ? have sensitivity due to BCG
  - ? Significant and require chemoprophylaxis
- Diameter > 15 mm or ulcerating – significant; have active TB, either subclinical or clinical
- If no clinical or x-ray evidence of TB → subclinical → chemoprophylaxis to prevent adult TB; chemoprophylaxis with isoniazid × 6 months or isoniazid + pyrizanimide × 6 months
- If clinical or x-ray evidence of TB → clinical → treatment with isoniazid, rifampicin, pyrizanimide, ? ethambutol
- In patients with phlyctenular keratoconjunctivitis
  - Expect the Mantoux to be > 15 mm or ulcerating
  - Therefore, do not do Mantoux, exclude clinical TB and put on to chemoprophylaxis or treatment

Keratoconus

Incidence

- Variable, female > male
- Usually bilateral, often asymmetrical
- Usually manifests at puberty, may be earlier or later
- Common – 50 per 100 000

Aetiology and pathophysiology

- ? Due to local glucose-6-phosphate dehydrogenase deficiency, ? due to local abnormality of collagen; perhaps it is the final common pathway for a number of disorders
- Earliest change is in basal epithelial cells; these degenerate, release proteolytic enzyme, → fragmentation of basement membrane
- ? Role of heredity; familial in 6–8% – ? autosomal dominant with incomplete penetrance
- ? Locus on chromosome 21

Histology

- Every layer of cornea may be involved
- Early degeneration of basal epithelial cells
- Later disruption of basement membrane, downgrowth of epithelium into Bowman's membrane
- Fleischer ring composed of ferritin in and between epithelial cells
- Decreased number of collagen lamellae in stroma (normally 40 in centre and 60 in periphery)
- Breaks in Descemet's membrane → acute hydrops
- Abnormal endothelial cells
- Corneal scarring in Bowman's layer or in stroma

Associations

- Systemic
  - Atopic disease (eye rubbing)
  - Down's syndrome
  - Connective tissue disease (Ehlers Danlos syndrome, osteogenesis imperfecta, Marfan's syndrome, pseudoxanthoma elasticum)
  - Lawrence-Moon-Biedl syndrome
  - Neurofibromatosis
  - Noonan's syndrome
  - Icthyosis
- Ocular
  - Retinitis pigmentosa
  - Vernal conjunctivitis (7% have keratoconus)
  - Colobomata
  - Congenital cataract
  - Duane's syndrome
  - Ectopia lentis
  - Glaucoma
  - ? Hard contact lens wear

Classification

- By keratometry
  - Mild (< 48D)
  - Moderate (48–54D)
  - Severe (> 54D)
- Morphologically
  - Nipple cone (< 5 mm)
  - Oval cone (5–6 mm)
  - Globus cone (> 6 mm)

Symptoms

- Starts with regular corneal astigmatism → irregular astigmatism; progressive for 10–20 years
- Progression during adolescence, stabilisation at full growth
- But progression can occur at any time
- Photophobia, glare, decreased vision

Signs

- Myopic astigmatism
- Corneal protrusion, stromal thinning at cone apex, Fleischer ring, prominent nerves, scarring of Bowman's membrane, striae anterior to Descemet's membrane, Munson's sign
- Apex displaced inferonasally
- Ruptures in Descemet's membrane → acute hydrops; resolves with scarring after 8–10 weeks
- Some patients regain good vision following resolution of the hydrops depending largely on the extent and localisation of the scar
- Scissoring of the red reflex on retinoscopy
- Rizzutti's sign → a conical reflection on the nasal cornea when a penlight is shone from the temporal side
- Vogt lines → fine parallel striations or stress lines in the stroma

Differential diagnosis
- Keratoglobus
- Megalocornea
- Keratectasia
- Congenital anterior staphyloma

Investigatons
- Computerised videokeratography
- Placedo ring-based topography
- Orbscan

Treatment
- Spectacle correction
- Hard contact lens correction
- Keratoplasty

Spectacle correction
- For regular astigmatism

Hard contact lens correction
- For irregular astigmatism
- May be corneal contact lens or scleral contact lens
- Contact lens fitting procedure in keratoconus
  - Decide if the keratoconus is sagging or nipple
  - Sagging – base curve 1/4 between 2 k readings
  - Nipple – base curve 1/2 between 2 k readings
  - Soper lens, mini hard lens, piggyback lens may also be used

Keratoplasty
- Indicated if
  - Poor vision even with hard contact lens (< 6/12 with contact lens, < 6/18 with spectacles)
  - Inability to wear hard contact lens
  - Scarring after acute hydrops
  - Increasing cone size
  - Following perforation
  - 5–10% require keratoplasty
- Technique
  - Flatten apex with cautery
  - Place graft centrally
  - Use same size donor button to decrease post-op myopia and astigmatism
- Complications – 10% rejection rate
- Results – 98% achieve 6/12 or better; 40% achieve this unaided
- Deep lamellar keratectomy → very difficult
- Treat hydrops conservatively – cycloplegics, hypertonic saline, patching, soft contact lense

4

Non-inflammatory ectatic disorders			
	Keratoconus	Keratoglobus	Pellucid marginal degeneration
Frequency	Most common	Rare	Less common
Laterality	Usually bilateral	Bilateral	Bilateral
Age of onset	Puberty	Birth	20–40 years
Thinning	Inferior paracentral	Greatest in periphery	Inferior band, 1–2 mm wide
Protrusion	Thinning at apex	Generalised	Superior to band of thinning
Iron line	Fleischer ring	None	Sometimes
Scarring	Common	Mild	Only after hydrops
Striae	Common	Sometimes	Sometimes

Climate droplet keratopathy

- Also known as corneal elastosis, keratinoid degeneration, spheroidal degeneration, Labrador keratopathy, Bietti's nodular dystrophy, proteinaceous degeneration
- Primary age-related
- Secondary associated with ocular injury or inflammation

Definition

- Corneal degeneration due to adverse climatic conditions

Aetiology

- Exposure of cornea to excessive UV light → denaturation of plasma proteins as they diffuse through the cornea
- Damage to cornea by microparticles
- Low humidity → drying of cornea

Incidence

- Male > female
- Higher incidence and severity with age

Histology

- Droplets of altered plasma proteins occur in the superficial stroma and Bowman's layer
- Consist of an amorphous hyaline substance
- Later disruption of Bowman's layer and subepithelial fibrosis
- Later attenuation and loss of overlying epithelium, sometimes with epithelial keratinisation

Grading

- Bilateral
- Interpalpebral

Grade 1

- Small droplets close to the limbus on the medial and lateral sides with clear lacunae between
- Lie at level of anterior stroma, best seen by retroillumination
- Clear area between affected cornea and limbus

Grade 2

- Droplets occur across the whole palpebral cornea, but vision is not affected

Grade 3

- Associated impairment of vision
- Droplets are more numerous and extend further into the stroma

Grade 4

- Large yellow nodules protrude from the corneal surface
- Overlying epthelium may be thinned or absent
- Tear film abnormalities, loss of sensation, epithelial erosions, secondary bacterial ulcers all occur

Associated diseases

- Pterygium and pingueculum are rare
- Iris atrophy, pseudoexfoliation and cataract may occur in association
- Anterior lens capsule changes – frosting, plateau formation, bag formation or herniation may be associated

Differential diagnosis

- Fuchs' dystrophy
- Other causes of endothelial decompensation
- Band-shaped keratopathy
- Acute glaucoma

Management

- Prophylaxis – UV filter sunglasses
- Treatment: Removal of nodules in Grade 4 by phototherapeutic keratectomy, penetrating keratoplasty, optical iridectomy
- ? Regression may occur following lens extraction; mechanism unknown

Metabolic keratopathies

Classification of metabolic keratopathy	
■ Disorders of carbohydrate metabolism	□ Mucopolysaccaridoses □ Diabetes
■ Disorders of lipid metabolism and storage	□ Hyperlipoproteinaemias □ Hypolipoproteinaemias □ Sphingolipidoses □ Mucolipidoses □ Bietti's crystalline corneoretinal dystrophy
■ Disorders of amino acid metabolism	□ Cystinosis □ Tyrosinaemia □ Akaptonuria
■ Disorders of protein metabolism	□ Amyloidosis
■ Disorders of immunoglobulin synthesis	
■ Non-inflammatory disorders of connective tissue	□ Ehlers-Danlos □ Marfan's syndrome
■ Disorders of nucleotide metabolism	□ Gout □ Porphyria
■ Disorders of mineral metabolism	□ Wilson's disease □ Hypercalcaemia □ Haemochromatosis
■ Systemic neoplasia	□ Enlarged corneal nerves

Disorders of carbohydrate metabolism

Mucopolysaccaridoses

- Rare, inherited lysosomal storage diseases
- Eight separate syndromes with several common features – Hurler's, Hunter's, Sanfilippo's, Scheie's, Morquio's, Sly's, Vacant, Maroteax-Lamy
- Clinical – corneal clouding, pigmentary retinopathy, optic atrophy
- Cloudy cornea involves entire cornea; may be progressive from periphery to centre
- Treat with penetrating keratoplasty, but abnormal storage material may collect in the graft

Diabetes

- Non-specific corneal changes
- Punctate epithelial erosion, basement membrane changes, Descemet's folds (Waite-Beetham lines), interface changes, hypoaesthesia
- ? Due to accumulation of sorbitol
- Management before corneal surgery
  - Minimise epithelial debridement
  - Increase lubrication
  - Avoid toxic medications, bondage contact lens

Disorders of lipid metabolism and storage

Hyperlipoproteinaemias

- Common; ocular signs can help in early disease detection
- Fredrickson's 5 types – xanthelesma, corneal arcus, arcus juvenalis

Hypolipoproteinaemias

- Five disorders
  - Lecithin-cholesterol acyltransferase deficiency
  - Tangier's disease
  - Fish eye disease
  - Familial hypobetalipoproteinaemia

- Bassen-Kornzweig syndrome
- The last two do not cause corneal disease
- Rare, autosomal recessive
- Peripheral arcus, corneal clouding, neuropathy with lagophthalmos

Sphingolipidoses

- Rare, inherited disorders of complex lipids
  - Fabry's disease – x-linked recessive inheritance
  - Multiple sulphate deficiency – autosomal recessive
  - Generalised gangliosidosis – autosomal recessive
- Principally affect the retina – also periorbital oedema, cataracts, papilloedema
- Whorl-like lines in basal epithelium
- Heterozygous females may show some corneal changes
- Penetrating keratoplasty results poor

Mucolipidoses

- Inherited defects of carbohydrates + lipids combined
- Mucolipidosis 1–4, Goldberg syndrome, mannosidosis, fucosidosis
- Mucopolysaccarides accumulate in the cornea, sphingolipids in the retina and central nervous system
- Varying degrees of corneal clouding
- Penetrating keratoplasty and deep lamellar keratoplasty – poor results

Bietti's crystalline corneoretinal dystrophy

- Rare, autosomal recessive
- Peripheral corneal opacities + tapetoretinal dystrophy
- No specific treatment

Disorders of amino acid metabolism

Cystinosis

- Rare, autosomal recessive
- Accumulation of cystine within lysosomes
- Presents as an infantile, intermediate or adult form
- Crystals in the cornea and trabecular meshwork
- Treatment: cysteamine drops → decrease crystal density
- Crystals recur in penetrating keratoplasty grafts

Differential diagnosis of corneal deposits

Type	Superficial	Stromal	Deep stromal/ endothelial	Conjunctiva
Pigmented	Cornea verticillata (Fabry's disease, amiodarone) Striate melano-keratosis Pigmented (non-calcific) band keratopathy Spheroidal degeneration Adrenochrome Alkaptonuria	Phenothiazines Blood-staining Bilirubin Siderosis Corneal tattoo	Mercury Wilson's disease Chalcosis (copper) Chrysiasis (systemic gold) Argyriasis (topical silver) Krukenberg spindle	Tetracycline Adrenochrome Argyriasis

Non-pigmented	Subepithelial mucinous dystrophy Coat's white ring Calcific band keratopathy Ciprofloxacin	Granular dystrophy Macular dystrophy Fleck dystrophy Lipid deposition Mucopoly-saccaridoses	Cornea farinata PreDescemet dystrophy X-limbed Icthyosis Argyriasis (silver)	Gout (urate)
Refractile/ crystalline	Meesman's Superficial amyloid Tyrosinaemia II Gout	Lattice Schnyder's Bietti's Immuno-globulin deposits Cystinosis Infectious crystalline keratopathy	Polymorphic amyloid degeneration	Cystinosis

Tyrosinaemia

- Autosomal recessive, tyrosine accumulation
- Pseudodendrites, corneal vascularisation + scarring
- Photophobia, tearing, injection
- Restrict tyrosine + phenylalanine intake

Alkaptonuria

- Rare, autosomal recessive; defective tyrosine metabolism → alkapten accumulates
- Darkly pigmented dot opacities in corneal epithelium (ochronosis)

Amyloidosis

Accumulation of amyloid in various tissues			
Type	**Heredity**	**Ocular distribution**	**Associated conditions**
Primary localised	Non-familial Familial	Conjunctival plaque Polymorphic amyloid degeneration Lattice I + III Granular + Avellino Gelatinous drop-like	None
Primary systemic	Non-familial Familial	Skin + conjunctiva Ophthalmoplegia, ptosis, vitreous veils, dry eye, pupil abnormalities Lattice II, cranial neuropathies	Occult plasma cell dyscrasis Cardimyopathy Peripheral neuropathy Gastrointestinal disease Skin involvement Meretoja's syndrome

Secondary localised	Non-familial	Conjunctiva, skin, cornea	Trachoma, psoriasis, retinopathy of prematurity, keratoconus, leprosy, syphilis, uveitis, climate droplet keratopathy, trichiasis
	Familial	None	
Secondary systemic	Non-familial	Vitreous, conjunctiva, skin	TB, leprosy, syphilis theumatoid arthritis, SLE
	Familial	None	Multiple endocrine neoplasia IIa

Disorders of immunoglobulin synthesis

- Excess immunoglobulin synthesis by plasma cells in
  - Multiple myeloma
  - Waldenstrom's macroglobulinaemia
  - Benign monoclonál gammopathy
- Crystalline deposits in all layers of the cornea or conjunctiva
- Copper deposits – cornea
- Sludging of conjunctiva and retinal blood flow
- Scleral infilatrate, bony orbital invasion + proptosis
- No specific ocular treatment – will resolve with successful treatment of the malignancy

Non-inflammatory disorders of connective tissue

Ehlers-Danlos syndrome

- Autosomal dominant, autosomal recessive, x-linked recessive
- Brittle cornea, rupture with minor trauma, blue sclera, keratoconus, keratoglobus

Marfan's syndrome

- Megalocornea, keratoconus, cornea plana (20%)

Disorders of nucleotide metabolism

Gout

- Hyperuricaemia with deposits of urate crystals
- Acute inflammation of the sclera, episclera + conjunctiva
- Fine corneal, epithelial + stromal deposits in the absence of inflammation

Porphyria

- Porphyrin accumulation due to defective haem metabolism
- Necrotising scleritis, corneal thinning + perforation, symblepharon

Disorders of mineral metabolism

Wilson's disease (hepatolenticular degeneration)

- Autosomal recessive
- Copper deposits – liver, kidneys, brain, cornea
- Descemet's membrane deposists → Kayser-Fleischer ring (golden brown, ruby red or green pigmented ring)
- Treatment: penicillamine

Hypercalcaemia

- Band keratopathy

Prominent corneal nerves	
Enlarged corneal nerves	**More visible corneal nerves**
■ Multiple endocrine neoplasia 116 ■ Refsum's syndrome ■ Hansen's disease (leprosy, beading of nerves) ■ Riley-Day syndrome (familial dysautonomia) ■ Neurofibromatosis ■ Acanthamoeba perineuritis	■ Keratoconus ■ Ichthyosis ■ Fuchs' corneal dystrophy ■ Corneal oedema ■ Congenital glaucoma

Miscellaneous keratopathies

Interstitial keratitis

Definition

- Vascularisation and non-suppurative infiltration of corneal stroma
- Usually associated with systemic disease
- Without primary involvement of the epithelium or endothelium

Pathogenesis

- Usually a type 4 hypersensitivity response to infectious micro-organisms or antigens

Causes

- Herpes simplex most common
- Congenital or acquired syphilis – the first infection to be linked to interstitial keratitis
- TB, leprosy, sarcoid, Lyme disease
- Mumps, herpes simplex, herpes zoster, rubeola (measles), influenza
- Lymphogranuloma venereum, onchocerciasis, trypanosomiasis, leishmaniasis
- Gold toxicity, arsenic toxicity
- Cogan's syndrome, Hodgkin's disease

Syphilitic interstitial keratitis

- Congenital → bilateral (80%)
- Acquired → unilateral (but occurs very rarely)
- Manifestation in first 2 years → infectious
- Later → immune mediated
- Usually manifest at 10–20 years of age
- Progressive stage
  - Lasts 2 weeks
  - Pain, lacrimation, circumcorneal injection, vessel ingrowth
- Florid stage
  - Lasts 2–4 months, classical salmon patch
- Retrogressive stage
  - Lasts 1–2 years, clearing starts peripherally → ghost vessels remaining
  - May be complicated by glaucoma, uveitis
- Non-ocular signs of syphilis
  - Dental deformities
  - Bone + cartilage abnormalities
  - VIII deafness
  - Mental retardation

Treatment

- Steroids in active stages, penetrating keratoplasty

Cogan's syndrome

- Unknown aetiology, ? autoimmune
- Onset in young adults → middle age
- Interstitial keratitis, uveitis, vertigo, tinnitus, VIII nerve deafness
- Treat with topical and systemic (for the VIII nerve) steroids
- Cytotoxics for unresponsive cases

Disciform keratitis

- Caused by herpes simplex and zoster, mumps, varicella, variola, vaccinia
- Viral antigen is integrated into stromal fibroblast, cell mediated response occurs against those cells
- Corneal stromal and epithelial oedema in a round or oval distribution, associated with keratic precipitates
- Also known as endothelitis

Exposure keratopathy

Causes

- Lagophthalmos – VII palsy, severe proptosis, scarring of eyelids, Parkinson's, drug abuse, blepharoplasty (any disease process that limits lid closure)
- Proptosis – thyroid eye disease and others

Signs

- Inferior punctate epitheliopathy → ulceration, neovascularisation, infection
- Treatment: artificial tears, taping of lids, bandage contact lens, tarrsorrhaphy – lateral or medial, gold weights upper lid

Neurotrophic keratopathy

Causes

- V injury (surgical trauma, cerebrovascular accident, multiple sclerosis, tumours, zoster)
- Herpes simplex and zoster keratitis
- Diabetes
- Leprosy (Hansen's disease)
- Hereditary sensory neuropathy (a reduction in small myelinated nerve fibres)
- Familial dysautonomia (Riley-Day syndrome)

Pathology

- Normal corneal sensation necessary for maintaining metabolic integrity of corneal epithelium
- Also decreased tearing

Signs

- Punctate epitheliopathy → ulceration, neovascularisation, infection

Treatment

- Artificial tears, bandage contact lens, avoid benzylkonium, tarsorrhaphy, penetrating keratoplasty in inactive zoster, punctal occlusion, amniotic membrane, Gunderson flap to preserve the eye as a last resort
- Topical nerve growth factor under investigation

Thygeson's superficial punctuate keratitis

- Rare, bilateral, recurrent, ultimately self-limiting
- Unknown aetiology – many features resemble a viral infection; probably immune though
- Multiple round-oval, grey-white, granular, elevated, sub-epithelial dots
- Waxing and waning course
- Minimal conjunctival reaction in contrast to adenoviral infection
- Tearing, foreign body sensation, photophobia
- Treat with tear lubricants, steroids, bandage contact lens
- Rapid response to steroids – but steroids may prolong the entire course as long as 15 years

Recurrent erosions

Onset

- Autosomal dominant or acquired secondary to trauma

Symptoms

- Pain, photophobia, tearing; at night or on waking

Signs

- Epithelial loss, filaments
- If mild, the epithelium is often healed by the time of the examination

Pathogenesis

- Previous, sudden, sharp, abrading injury or pre-existing epithelial basement membrane dystrophy

- The initial injury heals quickly, days to years later there is a recurrence without any precipitating event
- Poor epithelial adhesion due to abnormal basement membrane + filament network

Histology

- Lack of hemidesmasomes between basal epithelium and basement membrane → epithelial loss, microcysts, bullae, filaments

Treatment

- Ointment and pad, cycloplegia, soft contact lens, hypertonic saline 5%
- Ointment at night for 6–12 months – creates an osmotic gradient, dehydrating epithelium + promoting adherence)
- Anterior stromal punctures; 40–50 punctures with bent 23-gauge needle through loose epithelium; caution in visual axis
- Epithelial debridement (painful for a few days afterwards; therefore, debride at the time a painful, recurrent episode)
- Excimer laser phototherapeutic keratectomy; very shallow to minimise refractive effects

Causes of epithelial filaments

- Filaments → strands (filaments) or clumps (mucous plaque) of mucous and degenerating epithelial cells attached to an altered ocular surface
- Keratoconjunctivitis sicca
- Superior limbic keratoconjunctivitis
- Recurrent erosions
- Prolonged occlusion, ptosis

Causes of pannus

- Superior pannus
  - Trachoma
- Sector pannus
  - Rosacea
  - Phlyctenulosis
  - Leprosy
- Micropannus
  - Childhood trachoma
  - Inclusion conjunctivitis
  - Molluscum contagiosum
  - Long-standing staphylococcal keratoconjunctivitis
  - Vernal keratoconjunctivitis
  - Superior limbic keratoconjunctivitis
  - Contact lens wear

Causes of corneal crystal deposits

- Lipid
  - Central crystalline dystrophy (stroma)
  - Tangier's disease (stroma)
  - Secondary lipid keratopathy (stroma)
- Protein
  - Cystinosis (cystine, anterior stroma)
  - Gout (urate, anterior stroma and epithelium)
  - Tyrosinosis (tyrosine, epithelium)
  - Alkaptonuria (homogentisic acid, perilimbal)
  - Multiple myeloma (? protein, stroma)
- Calcium
  - Band keratopathy (basal epithelium)

■ Copper	□	Wilson's hepatolenticular degeneration (Kayser-Fleischer ring, posterior Descemet's membrane)
	□	Adenocarcinoma lung
	□	Multiple myeloma
■ Iron	□	Stocker's line (pterygium)
	□	Hudson-Stahle line (cornea drying)
	□	Fleischer ring (keratoconus)
	□	Ferry's line (trabeculectomy bleb)
■ Drugs	□	Chlorpromazine (deep stroma)
	□	Chloroquine (subepithelial stroma)
	□	Gold (deep stroma)
	□	Indomethacim (stroma)
	□	Amiodarone (deep epithelium)
	□	Phenytoin
	□	Suranim

Causes of epithelial keratopathy

■ Viral	□	Herpes simplex + zoster
	□	Molluscum contagiosum
	□	Measles
	□	Mumps
	□	Infectious mononucleosis
	□	Adenovirus
■ Chlamydial	□	Trachoma
	□	Inclusion conjunctivitis
■ Bacterial	□	Staphylococcal
■ Traumatic	□	Post-traumatic erosion
	□	UV irradiation
	□	Exposure
	□	Trichiasis
	□	Keratoconjunctivitis sicca
■ Allergic	□	Vernal conjunctivitis
■ Nutritional	□	Vitamin A deficiency
■ Toxic	□	Drug-induced
■ Neurologic	□	Neurotrophic keratitis
■ Unknown	□	Superior limbic keratoconjunctivitis
	□	Thygeson's superficial punctate keratopathy

Causes of corneal oedema	
■ Primary endothelial dystrophies	□ Congenital hereditary endothelial dystrophy □ Fuchs' dystrophy □ ICE syndrome
■ Secondary endothelial dystrophies	□ Acute hydrops in keratoconus
■ Glaucoma (IOP → 40 mmHg, depending on endothelial status)	
■ Trauma	□ Blunt, penetrating, chemical burns
■ Intraocular surgery	□ Mechanical damage, epinephrine, air, vitreous touch, uveitis, secondary glaucoma, turbulence endotheliopathy, flat anterior chamber
■ Contact lens wear	
■ Endothelial dysfunction secondary to inflammation (uveitis, keratitis)	

Involutional diseases

Ageing

- Flatter, thinner, slightly less transparent
- Peripheral guttata – Hassall-Henle bodies
- Endothelial cell density decreases by 0.6% per year

Coat's white ring

- Small circle of discrete grey-white dots
- Superficial stroma
- Iron-containing fibrotic remnants of a metallic foreign body

Limbal girdle of Vogt

- At nasal and temporal limbus in interpalpebral zone
- Type 1
  - Early calcific band keratopathy
  - Separate from limbus
  - Composed of calcium in epithelial base
- Type 2
  - True girdle
  - Due to UV light
  - Occurs with adjacent pingueculum
  - Composed of elastotic degeneration of subepithelial collagen

Corneal arcus

- Composed of stromal cholesterol, phospholipids and triglycerides
- Senilis usually, may be juvenalis (? hypercholesterolemia)
- Labelled lipid keratopathy if it extends axially

Corneal farinata

- Age-related, flecks in deep stroma
- ? Composed of lipofuscin, asymptomatic

Descemet's striae

- Vertical striae, ? more common in diabetics

Hassall-Henle bodies (peripheral corneal guttata)

- Peripheral collagen thickenings of Descemet's membrane
- Not associated with endothelial decompensation
- Normal aging change

Corneal keloids

- White, sometimes protuberant glistening corneal mass
- Can involve entire corneal surface
- Resemble dermoids

Dellen

- Local thin spots of cornea occurring in areas of tear film instability

Crocodile shagreen (mosaic degeneration)

- May be involutional, traumatic or juvenile; may be associated loss of vision
- Anterior opacities, composed of plaques of fibrous tissue forming in areas of interruption of Bowman's layer

Pingueculum

- Nodule of degenerate conjunctiva
- UV light-induced, with subepithelial collagen elastotic degeneration
- Histologic distinction from pterygium – pingueculum has actinic changes in stroma, pterygium also in epithelium

Calcific band-shaped keratopathy

Causes

- Hypercalcaemia, long-standing eye disease, mercury preserved eye drops, gout, hereditary, silicone oil in aphakia

Features

- Calcium carbonate deposition in basement membrane, Bowman's membrane, and superficial stroma; holes where nerves penetrate

Treatment

- EDTA chelation; not phototherapeutic keratectomy because the calcium ablates at a different rate to the stroma

Systemic causes of band keratopathy

- Hypercalcaemia
- Hyperparathyroidism
- Hypervitaminosis
- Hypophosphataemia
- Renal failure
- Mercury exposure
- Milk-alkali syndrome
- Discoid lupus
- Paget's disease
- Sarcoidosis
- Tuberous sclerosis
- Icthyosis
- Progressive facial haemiatrophy

Salzman's hyaline degeneration

- Elevated bluish-white nodules, composed of hyaline plaques between epithelium and Bowman's layer
- Associated with long-standing corneal disease

Climatic droplet degeneration (spheroidal degeneration)

- Hyaline degeneration

Amyloid degeneration

- May be primary (systemic or local amyloid) or secondary (chronic ocular disease)
- Salmon-pink-white fleshy waxy nodular masses

Lipid degeneration

- May be primary (hyperlipidemia) or secondary (chronic ocular disease)
- Dense yellow-white opacity in superficial stroma, often with prominent blood vessel

Hut eye

- Recurrent exposure to smoke irritant → conjunctival hyperemia + inflammatory oedema → elastotic degeneration of subepithelial conjunctiva

Terrien's marginal degeneration

- Cause unknown; associated with vernal
- A quiet, essentially non-inflammatory, unilateral or asymmetrically bilateral, slowly progressive thinning of the peripheral cornea

- Male = female, second or third decade
- Begins superiorly and spreads circumferentially; rarely involves the inferior limbus

Treatment

- Anular lamellar keratoplasty grafts in severe cases

Pterygium

Aetiology

- UV light; belt 37 N–37 S (visible light + UVA + UVB)
- UVB is mutagenic for P53 tumour suppressor gene in limbal basal stem cells
- Also corneal drying and trauma by microparticles, wind, dust and other particles
- Without apoptosis, transforming growth factor-β is overproduced → collagen upregulation, cellular migration, angiogenesis
- Elastoid degeneration of collagen; appearance of subepithelial fibrovascular tissue + inflammatory changes
- ? Role of heredity; autosomal dominant with low penetrance

Pathogenesis and pathology

- Drying of tear film + superimposed UV light → superficial punctate keratopathy + colander degeneration of Bowman's membrane
- Elastotic degeneration of collagen
- Fibroblast and blood vessel invasion
- Stocker's iron pigment line lies ahead of apex at Bowman's membrane
- ? Mediated by the production of a pterygium angiogenesis factor

Differential diagnosis

- Pseudopterygium, pingueculum, epithelial hyperplasia, carcinoma

Treatment

- Conservative – sunglasses and drops (steroids, lubricants, astringents)
- Surgical – indicated for cosmesis, atypism, astigmatism, occlusion of visual axis, restricted movements, significant (3–4 mm) growth onto cornea
- 30–40 % recurrence – more likely in young patients, vascular pterygium, large pterygium
- Decrease recurrence by using
    - Post-op strontium 90 β-irradiation plaque 2 000 rad; inhibits vascular budding; complications scleral and corneal ulcer, dry eye, iris atrophy, cataract
    - Post-op mitomycin C 0.02% 1 drop 12-hourly for 5 days; complications include superficial punctate keratopathy, anterior chamber reaction, delayed healing, corneal necrosis, scleral necrosis, cataract, infectious sclerokeratitis, aseptic scleral necrosis (these complications can occur months or years after the use of mitomycin C)
    - Recurrence rate decreased to 10%
    - Intra-operative mitomycin C at the time of surgery; probably safer because topical → abuse

Options for wound closure

- Bare sclera
    - Just close over the medial rectus
    - Very high recurrence – 40–50%
- Simple closure – free edges sutured together only possible in small defects
- Sliding flap – L-shaped incision adjacent to the wound
- Rotational flap – U-shaped incision adjacent
- Conjunctival graft
    - Reduces risk of recurrence to 2–5%
    - Ameliorates risk of restriction
    - Must have no tenons in graft
    - Use 8-0 resorbable sutures or tissue glue
    - May take limbal stem cells

Complications

- Dellen

4

Chemical burns

Alkalis

Agents

- Important alkalis
  - Ammonium hydroxide (most damaging)
  - Sodium hydroxide
  - Potassium hydroxide
  - Magnesium hydroxide
  - Calcium hydroxide (least damaging)
- Ammonium hydroxide is biphasic; therefore penetrates rapidly rise in aqueous pH occurs within seconds

Biochemical changes

- Saponification of fat components of cell membranes → cell death in all layers (epithelium – lens)
- Degradation of collagen and proteoglycans by hydroxide, which is fixed in the stroma; ulceration therefore continues indefinitely

Burn severity

- Depends on degree of chemical penetration (nature of chemical and time of exposure) + area of chemical exposure
- Grade 1 – clear cornea + no limbal ischaemia
- Grade 2 – hazy cornea but visible iris details, < one-third limbal ischaemia
- Grade 3 – no iris details + one-third to half limbal ischaemia
- Grade 4 – Opaque cornea, > half limbal ischaemia

Clinical stages of alkaline burns	
■ Acute (0–1 week)	□ Disruption of cell membranes → loss of cells (epithelium, ciliary body and lens) □ Thrombosis → ischaemia □ Trabecular damage → rise in IOP
■ Early reparative (1–3 weeks)	□ Corneal ulceration starts □ Epithelial regeneration □ Corneal vascular and fibroblast invasion
■ Late reparative (> 3 weeks)	□ Continued corneal ulceration □ Progressive corneal vascularisation and scarring

Complications

- Symblepharon
- Tear film deficiency due to obstruction of lacrimal secretory ducts, destruction of glands of Krause and Wolfring, destruction of goblet cells, destruction of meibomian and tarsal glands
- Neurotrophic keratitis; due to loss of corneal innervation
- Persistent corneal oedema from endothelial destruction
- Trabecular injury → glaucoma
- Ciliary body injury → phthisis bulbi
- Cataract

Treatment

- First aid
- Medical
- Surgical

First aid

- Irrigation with any non-toxic liquid for 30 mins minimum
- ± Wash out anterior chamber

- ± Inject sodium hyaluronate into anterior chamber + subconjunctivally

Medical treatment

- Topical steroids
  - Decreased inflammation + decreased neutrophil infiltration
  - Decreased collagen synthesis + keratocyte migration; decreased healing
  - Use for 7–10 days, then stop
- Ascorbic acid
  - Normally secreted by ciliary epithelium, necessary for collagen production
  - Administer topically (10% drops 2-hourly) + orally (2 g 4 times daily)
- Citric acid
  - Inhibits neutrophil activity
  - Administer topically (10% drops 2-hourly)
- Tetracycline
  - Inhibits collagen and neutrophil activity
  - Administer topically (ointment) + orally (doxycycline 100 mg 12-hourly)

Surgical treatment

- Early
  - Advancement of Tenon's capsule
  - Limbal stem cell transplantation
  - Amniotic membrane grafting
- Late
  - Division of symblephara and conjunctival bands
  - Conjunctival or mucous membrane grafts
  - Correction of eyelid deformities
  - Keratoplasty; delay for at least 6 months
  - Keratoprosthesis

Acids

Agents

- Sulphuric acid (most damaging)
- Chromic acid
- Hydrochloric acid
- Nitric acid
- Acetic acid

Biochemical changes

- Effect of heating effect + explosive effect → coagulation and precipitation of proteins (collagen and proteoglycans)

Burn severity

- Less than alkalis, due to coagulation of epithelium → barrier to penetration + buffering action of corneal stroma

Clinical stages of acid burns	
■ Acute (0–1 week)	□ Coagulation and opacification of surface epithelium □ Stromal penetration → stromal, iris, lens injury □ Elevated IOP may occur due to collagen shrinkage
■ Early reparative (1–3 weeks)	□ Vessel and fibroblast invasion □ Stromal ulceration in more severe burns
■ Late reparative (> 3 weeks)	□ Usually recovered by 3 weeks □ ± Progressive vascularisation and scarring □ Complications as for alkali burns

Treatment

- As for alkali burns

4

Contact lens

Contact lens complications	
■ Lids	□ Ptosis □ Migration
■ Conjunctiva	□ Contact allergy (? thiomersal) □ Giant papillary conjunctivitis
■ Epithelium	□ Defects → mechanical, chemical □ Hypoxia → cysts, new vessels, decreased sensation □ Immune reaction
■ Stroma	□ Keratitis → bacterial, amoebic, sterile □ Tight lens syndrome → superficial punctuate keratitis □ Corneal warpage □ Lens-induced keratoconus
■ Endothelium	□ Increased size (polymegathism) □ Change in shape (polymorphism) □ Decreased pump action → all caused by toxic effects of low stromal pH due to lactic acid + CO^2 accumulation because of hypoxia

Keratoplasty

Penetrating keratoplasty

Indications

- Optical – any opaque or diseased cornea
- Tectonic – for reparative or structural purposes
- Therapeutic – bacterial, viral, or fungal keratitis
- Cosmetic

Common indications in developed and developing countries	
■ Developed countries	□ Keratoconus □ Corneal dystrophies (Fuchs') □ Pseudophakic bullous keratopathy □ Herpes keratitis
■ Developing countries	□ Trachoma □ Measles keratitis □ Xerophthalmia □ Climatic droplet keratopathy

Operative technique

- Fleiringa's ring in aphakia
- Superior rectus + inferior rectus fixation sutures
- Measure and mark recipient cornea with trephine
- Cut donor cornea – graft on teflon block with viscoelastic coating endothelium
- Trephining from the endothelial side decreases the overall size by 0.2 mm
- Cut the recipient – trephine two-thirds to three quarter thickness, enter the anterior chamber with a blade, excise the button with scissors
- The preferred recipient bed size is 8 mm
- Use the same size donor in keratoconus
- Otherwise cut the donor larger than the recipient – 0.25 mm in a phakic eye, 0.5 mm in an aphakic eye
- Decrease the size of the graft by 1 mm for each subsequent graft, down to 4 mm
- Place the graft with on viscoelastic, 4 × 10-0 nylon cardinal sutures
- Suture the graft with 10-0 nylon; continuous or interrupted (16 sutures)
- Reform the anterior chamber with balanced salt solution
- Combined procedures – with cataract extraction ± IOL, glaucoma surgery, vitrectomy, retinal procedures

Post-operative management

- Topical steroid, antibiotic and mydriatic
- Measure IOP daily with airpuff tonometer or Tono-Pen
- Taper steroids over 1–2 months; continue with 1 drop daily indefinitely in pseudophakia
- Remove sutures when the wound has healed; at 1 year in an adult with a continuous suture, at 8 weeks in a young child
- Correct refractive error when the vision has stabilised, after the sutures have been removed; with spectacles or a contact lens

Complications

- Intra-operative
    - Irregular trephination
    - Bulging lens ± subluxation
    - Bleeding
    - Endothelial injury
    - Iris injury
    - Lens injury
    - Anterior chamber collapse
    - Choroidal haemorrhage + effusion
    - Recipient Descemet's can be inadvertently left behind
- Early post-operative
    - Donor tissue failure
    - Infection
    - Hyphaema
    - Loss of anterior chamber
    - Faulty suturing
    - Iris prolapse
    - Pupil block
    - Corneal wound ectasia
    - Corneal oedema
    - Wound leak
    - Glaucoma
    - Epithelial downgrowth
    - Endophthalmitis
    - Primary endothelial failure
- Long term
    - Cataract
    - Glaucoma
    - Graft vascularisation
    - Suture abscess
    - Vitreous adhesions
    - Dehiscence following premature suture removal
    - Anterior chamber epithelialisation
    - Cystoid macular oedema
    - High astigmatism
    - Graft rejection
    - Transmission of donor disease to host
    - Recurrence of original disease (herpes simplex in 15%, dystrophies)
    - Late wound dehiscence

- Endophthalmitis
- Persistent epithelial defect
- Microbial keratitis
- Infectious crystalline keratopathy

Control of post-operative corneal astigmatism

- Severe astigmatism → decreased visual acuity, anisometropia, aniseikonia, image distortion, monocular diplopia, inability to wear contact lenses, asthenopia
- Relaxing incisions
  - Arcuate incisions inside the graft-host junction
  - Choose axis based on corneal topography
  - Choose length of incision based on nomogram
- Compression sutures
  - Opposite to the axis of the relaxing incisions
- Wedge resection
  - For high astimatism > 8D
  - More complicated + less predictable than relaxing incisions
  - 70–90 degrees of arc, maximum 1.5 mm resected tissue

Diagnosis and management of graft rejection

- Rarely occurs before 2 weeks, may occur as late as 20 years after surgery
- Three clinical forms – may occur alone or in combination
- Epithelial rejection
  - Immune response directed entirely at the donor epithelium
  - Elevated, linear epithelial ridge of lymphocytes → advances centripetally
  - May herald the onset of endothelial rejection
  - Seen early post-operatively (1–13 months)
- Subepithelial rejection – subepithelial infiltrates + iritis
- Endothelial rejection – most common form of graft rejection
  - Damaged cells cannot be replaced
  - Khodadoust line – inflammatory precipitates on the endothelial surface
- Treat with:
  - Topical steroids
  - Periocular steroids
  - Systemic steroids orally or IVI

Causes of poor vision following penetrating keratoplasty

- Cataract
- Amblyopia
- Aphakia
- Retinal detachment
- Cystoid macular oedema
- Astigmatism

Paediatric corneal transplants

- Under 2 years of age, associated with rapid neovascularisation + early suture erosion, therefore remove sutures early
- Scleral ring to prevent globe collapse
- Anterior bulging of lens-iris diaphragm
- Post-op glaucoma, strabismus, self-induced trauma, immune rejection → very common

Suture removal according to host age

- 6–9 months → 5 weeks
- 12–24 months → 6–8 weeks
- 2–3 years → 8–12 weeks
- 4–6 years → 4 months
- 10 years → 6 months
- Teens → 9 months

Corneal autograft procedures

- Rotational autograft – eccentric trephination
- Contralateral autograft – risk of bilateral endophthalmitis

Lamellar keratoplasty

Indications

- Opacities or loss of tissue that does not involve the full thickness of the cornea

- Superficial stromal dystrophies and degenerations
- Superficial scars
- Recurrent pterygium with stromal thinning
- Corneal thinning (Terrien's, pellucid)
- Superficial corneal tumours
- Congenital lesions e.g. dermoid
- Keratoconus

Advantages
- Minimal requirements for donor material (preservation of endothelium not mandatory)
- Non-penetrating
- Faster wound healing
- Reduced rejection
- Less risky in patients with surface disease, poor compliance

Disadvantages
- Restrictive indications – do not replace endothelium
- Technical difficulty

Deep anterior lamellar keratoplasty

Deep lamellar endothelial keratoplasty

- The posterior part of the cornea is dissected + replaced by donor tissue

Descemet's stripping endothelial keratoplasty

- Descemet's membrane + endothelium is stripped + replaced by donor tissue

Limbal stem cell transplants

Causes of limbal stem cell deficiency
- Stevens-Johnson syndrome
- Pemphigoid
- Multiple surgeries
- Burns
- Contact lens keratopathy
- Aniridia
- Limbal neoplasia
- Radiation
- Antimetabolites
- Severe microbial keratitis
- Topical meds
- Pterygium
- Peripheral ulcerative keratitis

Clinical features
- Wavy epithelial opacity
- Recurrent erosions
- Persistent epithelial defects
- Corneal epithelial irregularity

Limbal stem cell autograft

- 90–180 degrees of donor limbus
- Three clock hours above and three clock hours below
- Could expand them on amniotic membrane if available (cultured limbal epithelium)
- Take 1 mm of cornea + 2–3 mm of conjunctiva
- Abnormal corneal epithelium and pannus are stripped off the host cornea first

Limbal stem cell allograft

- Will need years of immune suppression afterwards
- Cadaver 360 degrees of donor limbus
- Remove host conjunctiva
- Need to cover the host limbus 360 degrees in order to block off host vessels and then use immunosuppressants
- Need two eyes from the donor to get enough tissue
- Thin the tissue out by 50%
- Suture with 10-0 nylon and cover with a bandage contact lens
- Combined penetrating keratoplasty and stem cells less successful
- Do the stem cells first, graft later
- Keratoepithelioplasty – uses peripheral cornea or corneolimbal rims from eyebank eyes

Poor prognosis for limbal stem cell transplant

- Dry eye
- Surface keratinisation
- Stevens-Johnson syndrome
- Adnexal abnormalities (sort out all lid problems first)

Immunosuppression

- Administer for at least 1 year
- Oral prednisolone for 1 month, then taper
- Oral cyclosporin or tacrolimus
- Azathioprine or mycophenolate
- Topical steroids + cyclosporin (topical cyclosporin needs to be used for 3–4 months before there is any effect)
- ± Topical autologous serum

Alternatives to stem cell transplant

- Keratoprosthesis
- Amniotic membrane transplant

Limbal stem cell failure

- Limbal stem cell exhaustion – cells start dying after several years
- Immune rejection

Amniotic membrane

- Innermost layer of foetal membranes
- Single layer of epithelium, thick basement membrane, avascular stroma
- Immunologically inert

Properties

- Anti-inflammatory
- Antiscarring + neurotropic
- Anti-angiogenic
- Physical bandage
- Antimicrobial

Clinical use

- Graft – epithelium facing up; becomes covered by host conjunctiva or corneal epithelium and is incorporated into the tissue
- Patch – epithelium facing down; reduces inflammation; eventually falls off

Corneal reconstruction

- Limbal stem cell deficiency
  - Pemphigoid, burns + stem cell transplant
  - Substrate for ex-vivo expansion of cells
- Ulcers + perforations
  - One or multiple layers
  - Small perforations
  - Neurotrophic ulcers
  - Recurrent erosions, persistent epithelial defects
- Bullous keratopathy
  - Epithelial debridement + amniotic membrane transplant

Conjunctival reconstruction

- Pterygium – controversial: some studies show increase in recurrence
- Symblepharon – fornix reconstruction

Miscellaneous

- Burns – chemical + thermal – anti-inflammatory patch
- Band keratopathy
- Large conjunctival defects
- Shield ulcers
- Glaucoma

Complications

- Blood under membrane
- Granulomatous reaction
- Failure to achieve the intended effect
- Loss of the amniotic membrane
- Potential for transmission of infection

Scleritis

Clinical differentiation from episcleritis

- Scleritis is a severe destructive disease, may cause loss of vision and perforation
- Episcleritis is a benign, self-limiting disease

History

- Episcleritis sudden in onset, scleritis gradual in onset
- Scleritis more painful

Examination

- Depth of inflammation (slit lamp) – three layers of vessels → conjunctival, superficial episcleral, and deep episcleral
- 10% phenylephrine drops → blanching of conjunctiva and episclera
- Bluish discoloration in scleritis
- Intraocular inflammation may accompany scleritis, not episcleritis

Scleritis

Incidence

- Third to fifth decade
- Very rare in children
- Female > male

Aetiology

- One-third of non-necrotising scleritis → known cause
- Two-thirds of necrotising → unknown cause
- Infective
- Non-infective

Infective

- Granulomatous – syphilis, tuberculosis, leprosy, sarcoid
- Viral – herpes, mumps
- Pyogenic – staph aureus

Non-infective

- Invasion from uveitis in sympathetic uveitis, VKH syndrome
- Seropositive – rheumatoid arthritis, SLE
- Seronegative – ankylosing spondylitis, psoriatic arthritis, Reiter's, ulcerative colitis, Crohn's, Behçet's
- Vasculitis – polyarteritis nodosa, Wegener's, giant cell, syphilis
- Other connective tissue diseases – erythema nodosa, amyloidosis, relapsing polychondritis
- Metabolic – gout, porphyria, alkaptonuria, cystinosis, hypercalcaemia
- Ophthalmia nodosum

Clinical classification

- Anterior
  - Diffuse (40%)
  - Nodular (44%)
  - Necrotising – with inflammation (10%); without inflammation (scleromalacia perforans) (4%)
- Posterior (2%)

Pathology

- Immune mediated vasculitis
- ? T-cell mediated
- ? Type III allergic reaction i.e. antigen-antibody-compliment complexes
- Fibrinoid necrosis with abnormal precipitation of glycosaminoglycan; surrounding lymphocytes, plasma cells, giant cells
- Vessels show medial necrosis and perivascular cuffing

Clinical features

- Onset over several days
- Pain is dominant; radiates, caused by distension of sensory nerves; scleromalacia perforans is painless
- Bluish discoloured inflammation, associated episcleritis
- Nodular anterior
  - Immobile, tender, elevated
- Diffuse anterior
  - Widespread
  - Sectoral in 60%, entire anterior segment in 40%
- Necrotising with inflammation
  - Localised → spreads
  - Sclera becomes transparent, uveitis and cataract may complicate
  - Staphyloma only occurs if IOP > 40 mmHg
- Necrotising without inflammation
  - No symptoms
  - Occurs over several months
  - Almost exclusively seen in rheumatoid arthritis or porphyria
  - There is actually inflammation, just not seen

4

- Posterior
  - Associated exudative retinal detachment, retinal haemorrhage, macular oedema, disc swelling, angle closure glaucoma, proptosis, ophthalmoplegia
  - Can occur in isolation or with anterior scleritis
  - B–scan → T sign
  - Often no related systemic disease is found with posterior scleritis
  - ? In same spectrum of disease as idiopathic orbital inflammation

Treatment

- Medical
  - Topical steroid or indomethacin
  - Systemic nonsteroidal anti-inflammatories (indomethacin) or steroid
- Non-necrotising
  - Indomethacin 75–100 mg daily, to start
  - Add prednisone 40–100 mg daily if necessary
- Necrotising
  - Prednisone 60–80 mg daily
  - ± Cyclosporin
  - ± Cyclophosphamide 50 mg 12 hourly × 3 months – in severe cases
- Surgical – scleral graft

Complications

- Cataract (7%)
- Keratitis (37%)
- Scleral thinning and transparency (33%)
- Uveitis in one-third of patients
- Glaucoma (18%)
- Cataract secondary to steroid or uveitis
- Exudative retinal detachment in posterior scleritis
- Optic nerve swelling

Corneal changes

- Occurs in 40% of scleritis and 15% of episcleritis
- Same aetiology, same treatment
- Sclerosing keratitis (most common)
- Acute stromal keratitis
- Limbal guttering (rare)
- Keratolysis → Descemetocoele

Special investigations

- Physicians consult
- Full blood count, ESR
- Serum uric acid
- Syphilis serology
- Plasma proteins and electrophoresis
- Collagen screen
- Chest x-ray
- X-ray sacroiliac joints

Course and prognosis

- If untreated, some scleral defect will result (increased transparency, thinning or ectasia)
- 25% of patients have decreased vision after 1 year
- In necrotising scleritis – 40% lose vision; some die of vasculitic complications

Episcleritis

- Self-limiting, benign inflammation of the episcleral tissue
- Obscure pathophysiology

Aetiology

- Idiopathic 90%
- Known 10%
  - Herpes zoster/simplex
  - Collagen diseases, including rheumatoid arthritis
  - Gout
  - Syphilis, tuberculosis
  - Allergy
  - Rosacea

Clinical classification

- Simple (diffuse) – sectoral (70%); entire episclera (30%)
- Nodular (localised mobile nodule)

Pathology

- Antigen-antibody-compliment complexes
- Lymphocyte infiltration

Clinical features

- Benign recurrent condition
- Sudden onset
- Less painful, pain localised
- Confined to episclera
- Bright red or salmon-pink compared to violaceous in scleritis

Special investigations

- Only work up if there are multiple recurrences
- ESR
- Rheumatoid factor, antinuclear factor
- Syphilis serology
- Uric acid

Treatment

- Simple – no treatment or lubricants
- Nodular
  - Steroid drops
  - Nonsteroidal anti-inflammatory drops
  - Systemic indomethacin or steroids

Course

- Resolves in 1–3 weeks; may recur, but benign

5

Glaucoma

Classification 90
Intraocular pressure 93
Disc changes in glaucoma 95
Gonioscopy 97
Primary chronic open angle glaucoma 97
Normal pressure glaucoma 100
Ocular hypertension 101
Primary angle closure glaucoma 102
Congenital glaucoma 104
Secondary glaucomas 106
Neovascular glaucoma 108
Pigment dispersion 111
Pseudocapsular exfoliation 112
Inflammatory glaucoma 113
Lens-related glaucoma 114
Post-cataract surgery glaucoma 115
Ciliary block glaucoma 116
Iridocorneal dysgenesis 117
Iridocorneal endothelial (ICE) syndrome 117
Tumours 117
Vitreoretinal surgery and corneal grafts 118
Glaucoma post-VR surgery 118
Genetics 118
Perimetery 119
Glaucoma drugs 122
Antifibrotic agents 124
Neuroprotection 124
Glaucoma imaging 124
Glaucoma in pregnancy 125
Studies in glaucoma 126

Classification

Adult glaucoma classification

Angle closure		
Primary		
■ With pupil block	□ Intermittent □ Acute □ Chronic	
■ Without pupil block	□ Plateau iris	
Secondary		
■ Anterior (pulling mechanism)	□ Contracture of membranes	– Neovascular glaucoma – ICE syndrome – Posterior polymorphous dystrophy – Trauma

	Contracture of inflammatory precipitates	
Posterior (pushing mechanism)	Aniridia	
	With pupil block	– Intumescent lens – Subluxed lens – traumatic; spontaneous – Following lens extraction – iris vitreous block – pseudophakia – Intraocular inflammation – Ciliary block glaucoma
	Without pupil block	– Following lens extraction – forward vitreous shift – Following scleral buckling – Following panretinal photocoagulation – CRVO – Intraocular tumours – malignant melanoma; retinoblastoma – Iris and ciliary body cysts – Retrolenticular tissue contracture – retinopathy of prematurity; persistent foetal vasculature

Open angle

With decreased outflow

Primary open angle glaucoma	Chronic simple glaucoma Open angle glaucoma with low tension		
Secondary open angle glaucoma	Pre-trabecular (membrane growth)	– Fibrovascular membrane (neovasuclar glaucoma) – ICE syndrome – Epithelial downgrowth – Fibrous ingrowth – Inflammatory membrane	
	Trabecular	– Clogging of meshwork	Red cells – haemorr-hagic; ghost cell Macrophages – haemolytic; phacolytic;

5

			melanomalytic Neoplastic – malignant melanoma; neurofibromatosis; juvenile xanthogranulomatosis Pigment particles – pigmentary glaucoma; uveitis; malignant melanoma Protein – pseudocapsular exfoliation; uveitis; lens induced (phacolyic); alfa chymotrypsin induced Vitreous in anterior chamber
		– Alterations of trabecular meshwork	Oedema – uveitis; scleritis; alkali burn Trauma (angle recession) Intra-ocular foreign body (siderosis, chalcosis) Steroid induced
	□ Post-trabecular (increased episcleral venous pressure)	– Carotid cavernous fistula – Cavernous sinus thrombosis – Retrobulbar tumour – Dysthyroid eye disease	
	□ Superior vena-caval obstruction		
	□ Mediastinal tumour		
	□ Sturge-Weber syndrome		
	□ Familial episcleral venous pressure elevation		
With normal outflow facility			
■ Hypersecretion glaucoma			

Congenital glaucoma classification

Primary congenital glaucoma	
Associated with congenital abnormalities	
■ Mesodermal neural crest dysgenesis	
	□ Axenfeld's anomaly □ Rieger's anomaly □ Peter's anomaly □ Marfan's syndrome □ Weill-Marchesani syndrome □ Aniridia
■ Phacomatoses/hamartomas	□ Neurofibromatosis (von Recklinghausen's) □ Encephalotrigeminal angiomatosis (Sturge-Weber syndrome) □ Angiomatosis retinae (von Hippel-Lindau) □ Oculodermal melanocytosis (naevus of Ota)
■ Metabolic disease	□ Oculocerebrorenal syndrome (Lowe's syndrome) □ Homocystinuria
■ Other	□ Trisomy 13–15 (Patan's syndrome) □ Broad thumb syndrome (Rubenstein-Taybi syndrome)

Secondary congenital glaucoma	
■ Trauma	
■ Inflammatory	□ Congenital rubella □ Uveitis
■ Neoplastic	□ Juvenile xanthogranuloma □ Retinoblastoma
■ Other	□ Persistent foetal vasculature □ Retinopathy of prematurity

Intraocular pressure

Normal IOP

- Statistical concept
- Gaussian curve, skewed to right
- Mean 15.5 mmHg ± 2.57 mmHg
- Two standard deviations (97.5% of eyes) → upper limit 20.9 mmHg
- In men > 40 years + 2SDs → 21 monthly
- In women > 40 years + 2SDs → 24 monthly

Factors determining IOP

- Rate of aqueous secretion
- Resistance encountered in outflow channels
- Level of episcleral venous pressure

Specific factors associated with IOP

- Age
  - IOP increases with increased age

  - If obesity and hypertension are excluded, then IOP decreases with age
- Gender
  - IOP in females higher than in males
- Blood pressure
  - Increased systolic BP → increased ultrafiltration → increased IOP
- Obesity
  - Obesity → increased intraorbital pressure → increased IOP
- Diurnal variation
  - IOP highest between 4.00 am and 8.00 am, lowest in the evening; increases immediately on waking; returns to normal within 2–5 mins
  - 0.9% of population show a variation of 9 mmHg
  - 30% of population show a variation of 4 mmHg
- Season
  - IOP low in summer, high in winter
- Posture
  - Standing on head → increase in episcleral venous pressure → increase in IOP
- Exercise
  - Exercise → decrease in IOP
- Race
  - Blacks have a higher mean IOP
  - Blacks have an optic nerve that is more susceptible to increase in IOP

Measurement of IOP

Schiötz tonometry

- Measures depth of indentation by a given weight
- Normal ocular rigidity 0.0215
- Ocular rigidity decreased in myopia, dysthyroid eye disease increased with age
- Low ocular rigidity → falsely low reading, and vice versa

Applanation tonometry

- Measures force to flatten a standard area of cornea
- The surface tension of tear film and the elasticity of the cornea cancel each other with a tonometer head of 3.06 mm diameter
- The force applied by the tonometer is then a measure of the IOP (Imbert-Fick principle)

Types of applanation tonometer

- Goldmann tonometer
- Perkins tonometer
- Air puff tonometer – air pulse flattens the cornea, the light reflected from the cornea is monitored, a maximal signal occurs when the cornea is flattened, the time interval for the air pulse to produce applanation is proportional to the IOP
- Tono-Pen

Errors in applanation tonometry

- Poor technique, failure to calibrate, squeezing by the patient, corneal irregularities, inadequate fluorescein

IOP and risk of glaucoma

- 33% of patients with glaucoma present with IOP < 21
- 1 reading > 21 → glaucoma risk 0.5–1% per year
- 1 reading > 25 → glaucoma risk 2–3% per year
- 1 reading > 30 → glaucoma risk 40% per year

IOP following LASIK

- Currently no accurate way of measuring IOP in eyes that have undergone LASIK
- We need more knowledge about the interplay between central corneal thickness, corneal + scleral rigidity, and IOP
- 2.5–3.5 mmHg for every 50 μ can be used
- LASIK patients have shown a wide variability in IOP change after the procedure

Dresden correction table								
Central corneal thickness	462–486	487–512	513–537	538–562	563–587	588–612	613–637	638–662
Correction (mmHg)	+3	+2	+1	0	−1	−2	−3	−4
+ 0.5 mmHg per 10 μm difference from 550 μ								

Disc changes in glaucoma

Retinal nerve fibres

- Within retina
  - Papillomacular bundle, radial nasal fibres, arcuate temporal fibres, with respect for horizontal raphe
- Arcuate fibres reaching superotemporal and inferotemporal disc are the most vulnerable – (this explains the predominance of arcuate field defects in glaucoma), papillomacular fibres are the least vulnerable
- Within optic nerve head
  - Fibres from peripheral retina are deepest in the retina and most peripheral in the optic nerve
  - Fibres from central retina are more superficial in the retina and more central in the optic nerve head

Optic nerve head

- Three layers – superficial layer, prelaminar layer and laminar layer
- Scleral canal
  - Hole in the sclera through which 1.2 million axons exit
  - Vertically oval, vertical diameter 1.75 mm
- Lamina cribrosa
  - Series of plates of collagen, perforated by 200–400 pores
  - Largest pores arranged in a vertical hourglass distribution at superior and inferior poles
- Optic cup
  - Depression in centre of optic nerve head
  - Pale due to exposure of lamina cribrosa and loss of glial tissue
  - Size is related to size of disc
- Neuroretinal rim – tissue between edge of cup and margin of disc

Pathogenesis

- There are two mechanisms proposed, with clinical and experimental evidence for each, probably both are operative
- Vascular insufficiency
- Mechanical – block of axoplasmic flow at lamina cribrosa

Vascular insufficiency

- The posterior ciliary arteries supply the disc via
  - Superficial nerve fibre layer – branches from retinal vessels
  - Prelaminar – branches from choroidal vessels (most susceptible)
  - Laminar – branches from circle of Zinn-Haller and short posterior ciliary arteries direct
  - Retrolaminar – pial branches from short posterior ciliary arteries + central retinal artery + circle of Zinn-Haller
- It is a low pressure system, susceptible to increase in IOP → decrease in prelaminar flow → neuronal degeneration
- Diastolic pulse is seen at IOP 65 mmHg, systolic arrest seen at 70 mmHg (normal ophthalmodynamometry)
- Decrease in BP → disc more susceptible (normal tension glaucoma)

5

5

Mechanical – block of axoplasmic flow at lamina cribrosa

- Lamina at 6 o'clock and 12 o'clock is weakest, with greatest displacement with rise in IOP
- Results in compression of laminae + misalignment of pores → compression of axons → obstruction to axoplasmic flow → degeneration of neurones
- Initially reversible, maximal in temporal quadrants, maximal in peripheral axons within particular bundles
- Larger retinal ganglion cells are selectively damaged

Features

- Correlate with field changes in 85% of cases
- Early disc changes missed in 35% of cases on direct fundoscopy
- Cupping and other features

Cupping

- Vertical cup:disc > 0.7 (0.3 in infants); usually < 0.4; only 2% > 0.7
- Vertical cup:disc asymmetry > 0.2
- Increase in cupping
- Cup extending to disc margin
- Sharp or undermined cup edge (excavation)
- Deep cup
- Associated pallor
- Vertical disparity of cup i.e. vertical elongation

Other features

- Exposure of lamina cribrosa
- Nasal displacement of vessels
- Baring of vessels
- Pulsation of arteries
- Dilated veins
- Splinter haemorrhages; these precede notches (especially in normal pressure glaucoma)
- Notching; at superior and inferior poles
- Bayoneting of vessels; due to double angulation as they dive into the cup
- Parapapillary atrophy
- Decreased neural rim area
- Atrophy of superficial nerve fibre layer at upper and lower poles; early slit/wedge defects → large areas of atrophy with baring of retinal blood vessels
- Nerve fibre layer defects – seen with red-free light

Evaluation of disc changes in glaucoma

- Stereo photos
- Retinal nerve fibre layer changes
- Quantitative analysis of optic disc topography – normal values and other measures
- Normal values
  - Disc area 1.84 2 mm^2
  - Cup:disk ratio 0.428
  - Rim area 1.33 mm^2
  - Cup volume 0.256 mm^3
- Other measures
  - Cup area
  - Height variation contour
  - Rim volume
  - Mean cup depth
  - Maximum cup depth
  - Cup shape

Evaluation of retinal nerve fibre layer changes in glaucoma

- Red-free fundoscopy
- Red-free photographs
- Scanning laser ophthalmoscopy

Clinically important disc signs

- Weak
  - Alpha and beta zone
  - Peripapillary zone
  - Cup > pallor
  - Narrowing of retinal arteries
- Moderate
  - ISNT rule not obeyed
- Strong
  - Notch
  - Nasal cupping
  - Large cup for small disc
  - Localised retinal nerve fibre loss

- Diffuse retinal nerve fibre loss
- Generalised retinal nerve fibre loss
- Acquired optic disc pit
- Optic disc haemorrhage
- Cup:disc ratio asymmetry > 0.2

Gonioscopy

Anatomy

- Iris/ciliary body
- Scleral spur
- Trabecular meshwork
  - Uveal
  - Corneoscleral
- Schwalbe's line
- Schlemm's canal is at junction of mid and posterior one-third of trabecular meshwork

Angle width (Shaffer Grading System)

- 0 – closed; indentation differentiates appositional closure and synechial closure
- Slit – no iridocorneal contact, no angle structures visible
- 1 (10 degrees) – narrow, closure probable (Schwalbe's line visible)
- 2 (20 degrees) – narrow, closure possible (trabecular meshwork visible)
- 3 (25–30 degrees) – open, closure impossible (scleral spur visible)
- 4 (35–40 degrees) – wide open (ciliary body visible)

Trabecular pigment

- Grade 0–4
- May be increased due to
  - Ageing
  - Disease – acute angle closure glaucoma, trauma, uveitis, diabetes, pigmentary glaucoma, pseudocapsular exfoliation
- Sampaolesi's line occurs on the corneal side of Schwalbe's line

Other features to note

- Iris processes; present in one-third of eyes
- Peripheral anterior synaechiae
- Evidence of angle injury/recession
- New vessels
- Blood in Schlemm's canal; from compression of episcleral vein by gonio lens or from pathological raised episcleral venous pressure
- Note how many degrees/clock hours are affected

5

Primary chronic open angle glaucoma

Definition

- Chronic progressive optic neuropathy
- With characteristic changes in the nerve head and visual field
- Raised intraocular pressure is the most important risk factor

Prevalence

- Whites – 1% of people over 40
- Blacks – 3–4 times higher

Pathogenesis

- Ischaemic theory – poor optic nerve head perfusion
- Mechanical theory – raised IOP and/or weakness of lamina cribrosa → collapse of laminal plates → malalignment of axonal channels → direct compression of axons

Pathology

- Impaired outflow facility at trabecular meshwork, ? due to glycosaminoglycan accumulation, ? due to parasympathetic neuropathy → decreased ciliary muscle tone → slackening of scleral spur → collapse of Schlemm's canal
- Progressive loss of axons in optic nerve head

Risk factors

- Elevated IOP
- Age

- Family history
- Race
- Other

Elevated IOP

- This is the most important risk factor for glaucomatous optic neuropathy
- Progression of disc damage and field loss correlates with IOP level and IOP control
- Threshold IOP – IOP above which ganglion cell death and field loss occurs; this loss increases exponentially above this level
- Hypertension deviation value – time during which IOP is above the threshold IOP on the diurnal curve; this correlates with the progression of field loss
- Intolerance index – difference between the threshold/target IOP and the actual IOP; if it is 4 mmHg or less, no progression of field loss occurs; if it is 5 mmHg or more, progression of field loss occurs
- The aim of treatment should be to achieve consistent IOP control to less than the threshold IOP

Age

- There is increased incidence with increased age
- Most cases present after 65 years, rare under 40 years

Family history

- Increased incidence with positive family history
- There is an increased risk with a first degree relative affected (2 × with a parent affected, 4 × with a sibling affected)
- Multifactorial inheritance
- Mendelian autosomal recessive steroid responsiveness
  - 60% – non-steroid responders
  - 35% – heterozygous moderate steroid responders (IOP 22–30 mmHg following a 6- week course of topical betamethasone)
  - 5% – homozygous high steroid responders (chronic open angle glaucoma) (IOP > 30 mmHg following a 6- week course of topical betamethasone)
  - Gene on chromosome 1q → juvenile glaucoma; transmitted as autosomal dominant

Race

- 3–4 × more common in Blacks

Other

- Diabetes, cardiovascular disease, migraine, Raynaud's, myopia

Clinical features

- Male : female ratio 1 : 1
- More common in older patients (> 40 years)
- Chronic, insidious, slowly progressive, bilateral, painless
- Features
  - Elevated IOP
  - Cupping and atrophy of disc
  - Field loss
  - Open angles
- Elevated IOP – 8% of people > 40 years have IOP > 21 mmHg
- Only 1% of people > 40 years have glaucoma
- 50% of people with glaucoma have IOP < or = 21 mmHg on one reading
- Diurnal variation in people with glaucoma may be up to 5 mmHg in 90% of cases, and phasing may be necessary to pick up an elevated IOP

Case detection

Technique

- Tonometry, disc fundoscopy, perimetry
- 50% of patients with glaucoma have an IOP less than 21 mmHg at the first examination; tonometry alone is therefore insufficient

Features for early detection

- Nerve fibre layer atrophy; seen with red-free light; this precedes field loss by 5–6 years of age
- Colour vision deficit (blue–yellow)
- Fluorescein filling defects of disc, at the upper and lower poles
- Decreased contrast sensitivity
- Decreased pattern visually evoked potentials
- Automated field examination

Current treatment options

- Lower the IOP
- For the individual patient, decide what the target IOP should be
- Target IOP = threshold IOP
- Determine the target IOP by – severity of existing damage, level of IOP, age, general health
- Progressive damage is unlikely if IOP < 16 mmHg

Options

- Medical
  - Beta-blockers
  - Carbonic anhydrase inhibitors (dorzolamide)
  - Alpha agonists (brimonidine)
  - Prostaglandins (latanoprost)
  - Prostamides (bimatoprost)
  - Cholinergics (pilocarpine)
- Laser
  - Argon laser trabeculoplasty
  - Selective laser trabeculoplasty
  - Diode laser trabeculoplasty
  - Diode laser cycloablation
- Surgical
  - Trabeculectomy
  - Viscocanalostomy
  - Deep sclerostomy
  - Drainage tube
- The efficiency of IOP control and control of field progression is surgical > laser > medical
- Medical treatment frequently fails because
  - IOP is inadequately controlled (brought to the upper 'normal' range but not to below the threshold IOP)
  - A significant proportion of patients are seriously non-compliant (about 25%)
  - Wide fluctuations in IOP occur on medical treatment
- Medical treatment may prejudice the results of trabeculectomy, due to the acccumulation of inflammatory cells in the conjunctiva
- Primary trabeculectomy may therefore be preferable

Prognosis

- Untreated
  - Progression of field loss occurs in 32% of patients each year
  - In Africa, of patients with PCOAG seen for the first time, 90% are blind in one eye + 30% are blind in both eyes
- Treated
  - On treatment, the average rate of field loss is 3% per year
  - One-third of patients have pressure dependent field loss, two-thirds have pressure independent field loss
  - 75% of patients are blind 20 years from diagnosis, despite early treatment

Future treatment options

- Neuroprotection
- This may involve
  - Lowering the IOP
  - Increasing the blood flow to the optic nerve head (calcium channel blockers)
  - Protecting the ganglion cells from neurotoxins

PCOAG in black people

Clinical features

- Increased prevalence (4% compared with 1% in people over 40 years of age)
- Decreased age of onset
- Higher mean IOPs
- Larger mean cup:disc ratios
- Increased risk of blindness

- Blindness occurs earlier
- More rapid progression

Treatment
- Medical treatment
  - Pilocarpine 8% is required to achieve the same IOP lowering as is achieved with pilocarpine 1% in light blue eyes
  - Other drugs are as effective in black people as they are in whites
- Argon laser trabeculoplasty
  - Duration of benefit in blacks is less (12 months compared with 60 months)
- Surgery
  - Increased number of fibroblasts + macrophages in conjunctiva → increased scarring → increased failure
  - Therefore, routinely use cytotoxic adjunct
  - In the absence of any cytotoxic adjunct, failure after 1 year is 30% and after 5 years is 75%
  - With mitomycin C, failure after 5 years is 25%
  - With 5-fluorouracil, failure after 5 years is 50%

Normal pressure glaucoma

Definition
- Progressive optic nerve and/or visual field changes with no documented IOP reading above 21 mmHg and no other cause for these changes
- Disc and field changes of primary chronic open angle glaucoma + normal IOP
- ? Represents one end of spectrum of typical chronic open angle glaucoma
- Or is it a different disease?

Prevalence
- Prevalence very variable between populations
- 20–30% in the West

Classification
- True
- Pseudo
- Progressive (40–60%)
- Non-progressive (40–60%)

Risk factors
- Old age
- Female gender (2 : 1)
- Asians

Aetiology
- True
- Pseudo
  - Chronic open angle glaucoma with large diurnal fluctuation, recent B-blockers, yoga, low scleral rigidity with Schiötz, thin cornea + under-reading on applanation
  - Previous hemodynamic crisis (bleed, myocardial infarct) (shock induced optic neuropathy)
  - Post secondary glaucoma – (glaucomatocyclitic crisis, steroid induced, intermittent angle closure, uveitis, pigmentary glaucoma)
  - Acute anterior ischaemic optic neuropathy
  - One-third have migraine and/or Raynaud's

Pathogenesis
- Low resistance of optic disc to pressure, due to structural weakness of lamina cribrosa
- Impaired vascular perfusion of optic nerve head, due to atherosclerosis or arteriosclerosis of carotid or ophthalmic artery (i.e. represents a slowly progressive ischaemic optic neuropathy)
- Vasopasm of optic disc vessels → impaired perfusion; 47% of patients have migraine
- Nocturnal blood pressure dip

Features
- May have a family history of chronic open angle glaucoma
- Female > male

- Often monocular, IOP often upper normal
- Discrepancy between disc appearance and field loss; disc has a thinner neuroretinal rim and more pallor
- Higher incidence of disc haemorrhages than chronic open angle glaucoma
- Scotoma are closer to central fixation, have a steeper slope and a greater depth; often occur in upper hemifield
- Other characteristics include Raynaud's, migraine and nocturnal hypotension
- Disc haemorrhages are associated with progression
- IOP < 21 mmHg
- Open angle
- Characteristic disc + field changes
- Absence of a secondary cause of glaucoma

Differential diagnosis

- Primary chronic open angle glaucoma with a large diurnal variation
- Myopic disc
- Congenital disc (pit, coloboma, tilted)
- Optic atrophy – descending optic atrophy, ischaemic optic neuropathy

Investigations

- X-ray ray skull and optic foramina, CT scan head (to exclude a retrolaminar cause)
- Cardiovascular examination

Treatment

- Exclude other causes for optic neuropathy
- Exclude risk factors
- Monitor systemic blood pressure for 24 hours; if nocturnal hypotension occurs, avoid bed time hypertensive treatment and encourage exercise
- Do multiple IOPs and diurnal phasing if possible
- Consider MRI/CT, full blood count for anaemia, syphilis serology (? relationship to tertiary syphilis), carotid doppler
- Watch for signs of field progression.
- Check red desaturation; normal in ocular hypertension; if not → ? compressive lesion
- If field progression occurs, start medical treatment
- Reduce IOP as far as possible
- If field progression continues on medical treatment, consider laser treatment or surgery
- Selective laser trabeculoplasty – less effective than in primary open angle glaucoma

5

Ocular hypertension

Definition

- Elevated IOP (> 21 mmHg) on two visits
- No disc changes
- No field changes
- Open angle
- No contributing ocular disease

Prevalence

- 8% of population > 40 years
- 25% of population > 65 years
- 10% conversion to glaucoma in 10 years

Epidemiology

- Elevated IOP associated with – increased age, female gender, black race, family history, juvenile diabetes, elevated systolic BP, myopia, pseudo-capsular exfoliation, pigment dispersion

Management if there are no risk factors

- Only 10% develop field change
- One reading > 21 mmHg → 0.5–1% risk of field changes
- One reading > 30 mmHg → 40% risk of field changes
- The treatment of elevated IOP is of unproven efficacy in preventing field loss
- Therefore:
  - IOP< 25 + risk factors – no treatment
  - IOP 25–30 + risk factors – treat
  - IOP > 30 – risk factors – treat

Risk factors
- Nerve fibre layer defects
- Disc vertical cup:disk ratio > 0.7 + presence of disc haemorrhage
- Parapapillary changes
- Vascular disease
- One eye (not a risk, but consider treating early)
- Family history
- Age > 65 (3% increase in IOP → CRVO; therefore > 65 treat → IOP < 25 mmHg)
- Poor follow-up/unreliable patient
- Black race
- Myopia (structural changes in cribriform plate)
- IOP > 30
- IOP > 26 + central corneal thickness > 555
- Vertical cup:disk ratio > 0.4 + central corneal thickness < 588

5

Primary angle closure glaucoma

Definition
- Raised IOP as a result of obstruction of aqueous outflow from closure of angle by peripheral iris
- Two mechanisms are – pupil block + plateau iris

Incidence
- Leading cause of glaucoma worldwide
- 0.64% of people have grade 1 angles
- 6% of people have grade 1 + 2 angles
- Increased risk with increased age, average age at presentation 60 years
- Male : female 1 : 3 in whites, 1 : 1 in Blacks
- Less common in blacks
- Most common in Inuits (up to 10% of people over 40 years)
- Common in Asia (up to 2%)
- Whites present with acute, blacks + Asians tend to present chronic + asymptomatic

Incidence in South Africans
- 0% in blacks
- 0.1% in whites
- 2.3% in mixed race
- 83% present with chronic glaucoma + 17% with acute glaucoma

Risk factors
- Age – rare under 40, increases with each decade over 40 (increased lens thickness + forward movement with age)
- Female gender – female : male 4 : 1
- Race – common in Inuit, Chinese, south east Asians; rare in blacks
- Family history
- Ocular biometrics – crowded anterior chamber < 2.5 mm
- Hyperopia

Pathogenesis
- Relative pupil block (90%), lens block (anterior lens movement), plateau iris
- Anatomical predisposing factors – anatomical variant; small hyperopic eyes with small anterior segments → relative pupil block; anterial chamber depth less than 2.5 mm → risk of angle closure
- Refraction is usually more than +2.5 D, corneal diameter is less than or equal to 11 mm
- Increased lens size with age → increased relative pupil block (i.e. abnormal aqueous humour dynamics)
- Miosis → increased pupil block (at mid constriction)
- Physiological precipitating factors
  - Dilator muscle theory – contraction of dilator muscle → posterior vector
  - Sphincter muscle theory – miosis to 4 mm → pupil block

Classification
- Latent
- Intermittent (subacute)
- Acute (congestive)
- Chronic
- Absolute

Latent

- Features – shallow anterior chamber (eclipse sign), convex lens – iris diaphragm, close proximity of iris to cornea, grade 1 angle
- Treatment – laser iridotomy

Intermittent

- Features – last $\frac{1}{2}$ hour to 2 hours; discomfort, corneal oedema; precipitated by posture, light intensity, sympathetic stimulation
- Resolve spontaneously, classically during sleep-induced miosis
- Treatment – laser iridotomy

Acute

Features

- Venous congestion
- Corneal oedema
- Haloes
- Pain
- Anterior chamber flare and cells
- Mydriasis
- Peripheral anterior synechiae
- Autonomic stimulation
- Sector atrophy of iris
- Glaucomflecken (small anterior subcapsular lens opacities due to ischaemia)

Chronic

- Gradual increased closure; two-thirds closure → increase in pressure; may be symptomatic or asymptomatic; permanent peripheral anterior synechiae are present
- 'Creeping angle closure' → the gradual formation of peripheral anterior synechiae
- Eyes are small, as for acute glaucoma; otherwise resembles primary chronic open angle glaucoma

Provocative tests

- To detect patients with narrow, occludable angles
- Only positive in 50% of eyes at risk, change in angle is more important than increase in IOP
  - Dark room × 1 hour; IOP increases by 8 mmHg or more (physiologic provocative test)
  - Prone × 2 hours; IOP increases by 8 mmHg or more (physiologic provocative test)
  - Mydriatic – cyclopentolate 0.5% 2 drops; IOP after 1 hour increases by 8 mmHg or more
  - Pilocarpine – 2% 2 drops; IOP after 1 hour should decrease
  - Water drinking – 1 litre of water; after 1 hour IOP increases in all glaucomatous eyes

Treatment of acute angle closure

- Medical
- Surgical

Medical

- Acetazolamide
- 500 mg IVI, then 250 mg orally 6 hourly
- Pilocarpine 2–4% 6 hourly.; only effective if IOP less than 45 mmHg
- Oral glycerol 1 ml 50% solution per kilogram body weight in iced orange juice
- Recheck IOP after 1 hour
- If still not coming down – IVI mannitol 20% 12 mg per kilogram body weight over 30 mins; catheterise
- ± Retrobulbar anaesthetic
- ± Morphine and anti-emetics
- There is a 50% chance of a second acute attack while on medical treatment

Surgical iridectomy

- Ideally, this should be after 1–2 days
- It may be necessary after 6 hours if the IOP is not controlled or the angle is not opened
- 50% of fellow eyes develop acute angle closure within 5 years; therefore, treat both eyes

- Complications – flat anterior chamber, persistent fistula, hyphaema, peripheral synechiae, cataract, ciliary block glaucoma, infection

Trabeculectomy

- If peripheral anterior synechiae involve more than 75% of the angle
- If the angle has been closed for more than 1 year
- If there is advanced cupping and field loss

Primary angle closure glaucoma without pupil block (plateau iris)

Pathogenesis

- Anatomic variant; iris inserts anteriorly on ciliary body, dilatation → acute attack
- Due to anteriorly placed ciliary processes that provide structural support beneath peripheral iris
- Plateau iris is implicated in the pathogenesis of creeping/chronic angle closure glaucoma seen in black patients
- A component of pupil block is often present
- Following dilatation, the peripheral pupil bunches up, obstructing the trabecular meshwork

Features

- Plateau iris configuration
- Plateau iris syndrome
- Anterior chamber is deep, iris is flat, pupil block is minimal, angle is narrow or closed and remains so after iridectomy

Treatment

- Peripheral iridectomy for the element of pupil block
- Argon laser iridoplasty
- Miotics
- Mydriatics contraindicated

Congenital glaucoma

Primary congenital glaucoma

- Developmental glaucoma – primary congenital glaucoma + glaucomas secondary to developmental abnormalities
- Primary congenital/infantile glaucoma – evident at birth or within the first few years of life
- Juvenile glaucoma – recognised later in childhood (after 3 years of age) or early adulthood

Incidence

- One in 10 000 live births
- Male : female 2 : 1
- Bilateral in 75%
  - Neonatal 40%
  - Infantile 50%
  - Juvenile 10%
- 90% sporadic, 10% familial (autosomal recessive or multifactorial, rarely autosomal dominant)
- Second sibling has a 5% chance; child of affected parent has a 5% chance

Pathogenesis

- Developmental arrest in the late embryonic period
- Two theories:
  - Cellular or membranous abnormality of the trabecular meshwork → Barkan's membrane
  - Abnormal insertion of the ciliary muscle
- Mesodermal dysgenesis of angle (trabeculodysgenesis)
- Trabeculodysgenesis seen clinically as an absence of the angle recess, with iris inserted directly into the surface of the trabeculum
- The iris insertion may be flat or concave

Clinical features

- Classical triad: epiphora, photophobia, blepharospasm, due to corneal oedema

- Corneal oedema in 25% at birth, 60% at 6 months, initially epithelial, later stromal
- Corneal enlargement if onset < 3 years
- Normal values – horizontal diameter: Neonate 9.5 mm, 2 years 11.5 mm horizontal diameter, > 12 mm diagnostic
- Tears in Descemet's membrane (Haab's striae) initially in periphery, horizontal or concentric to the limbus
- Deep anterior chamber
- Disc cupping appears early (4–6 weeks); rapidly progressive; reversible at first, due to posterior bowing of cribriform plate, atrophy of neuroglia, shift of extracellular fluid; atrophy of nerve elements is last to occur
- Late signs: buphthalamos, subluxed lens, corneal scarring, nystagmus, myopia and strabismus

Differential diagnosis

- Causes of epiphora – lacrimal duct obstruction, corneal abrasion, conjunctivitis
- Causes of breaks in Descemet's membrane – birth trauma (vertical or oblique breaks)
- Causes of large cornea – myopia, X-linked recessive megalocornea, ? forme fruste of primary infantile glaucoma
- Causes of opaque/cloudy cornea
  - **S** – sclerocornea + skin disorders that affect the cornea (congenital ichthyosis + congenital dyskeratosis)
  - **T** – trauma
  - **U** – ulcer/intrauterine inflammation
  - **M** – metabolic/ mucopolysaccharidoses
  - **P** – Peter's anomaly
  - **E** – endothelial dystrophy (congenital hereditary endothelial dystrophy, posterior polymorphous dystrophy)
  - **D** – Descemet's, congenital glaucoma

Examination under anaesthetic

- Anaesthetic choice – halothane → drop in IOP of 15–20 mmHg; ketamine → initial increase in IOP which then drops to normal after 5 mins
- IOP – Perkins or Tono-Pen applanation
- Corneal measurement – horizontal diameter
- Gonioscopy – features are of trabeculodysgenesis; if there are associated cicatricial changes, this indicates a likely poor surgical result
- Fundoscopy – cupping, myopia
- Axial length

Management

- Medical – pre-op beta-blocker drops
- Surgical
- Follow-up examination under anaesthetic
- Squint and amblyopia – early detection and treatment
- Refraction – detect and treat myopia (due to buphthalmos), astigmatism (due to Haab's striae)

Surgical management

Trabeculotomy

- Limbal based flap, scleral lamellar flap, incise at blue white line down to Schlemm's canal, insert trabeculotome and sweep into anterior chamber
- Repeat on other side, → 100–120 degree sweep, suture flaps
- Complications – failure to find Schlemm's canal (proceed to trabeculectomy), hyphaema
- Controls IOP in 80% of cases (same results as goniotomy)

Goniotomy

- Incise trabecular meshwork in 1 quadrant with Grieshaber knife, halfway between scleral spur and Schwalbe's line, under Koeppe lens visualisation
- Incises Barkan's membrane, ? interrupts pull of ciliary muscle

5

- IOP controlled in 80% of eyes at each operation, can be repeated up to 6 times
- Then proceed to trabeculectomy or seton

Trabeculectomy

- Following failure of trabeculotomy or goniotomy
- Remove clear cornea, not scleral spur

Glaucoma drainage devices

- For failed goniotomy + trabeculotomy

Prognosis

- If untreated usually go blind, spontaneous remissions rarely occur
- The results depend on
  - Age of onset (worse earlier)
  - Delay in treatment
  - Gonioscopy findings
- Visual loss is due to
  - Amblyopia
  - Corneal scarring
  - Refractive error
  - Optic nerve injury
- Best prognosis
  - Asymptomatic at birth and symptoms develop within 24 months of age
- Worst prognosis
  - Symptoms at birth or present after 24 months of age

Anomalies associated with childhood glaucomas

Chromosomal

- Trisomy 21 (Down's syndrome)
- Trisomy 13 (Patau's syndrome)
- Trisomy 18 (Edwards' syndrome)
- Turner's

Systemic congenital disorders

- Lowe's syndrome
- Stickler's syndrome
- Zellweger's syndrome
- Hallermann-Streiff syndrome
- Rubinstein-Taybi syndrome
- Meyer-Schwickerath + Weyers syndrome
- Prader-Willi syndrome
- Cockayne syndrome
- Foetal alcohol syndrome
- Marfan's syndrome
- Neurofibromatosis
- Sturge-Weber syndrome
- Weill-Marchesani syndrome

Ocular congenital disorders

- Corneal ectropion uveae
- Congenital corneal staphyloma
- Corneal plana
- Iridoschisis
- Megalocornea
- Microcornea
- Microphthalmos
- Morning glory syndrome
- Persistent foetal vasculature
- ROP
- Sclerocornea
- Lens anomalies – dislocation, microspherophakia
- Anterior segment dysgenesis – Peter's, Axenfeld-Rieger syndrome
- Aniridia
- Congenital cataract

Secondary glaucomas

Glaucoma secondary to uveitis

Mechanisms

- Trabecular occlusion by inflammatory debris
- Decreased outflow facility by plasmoid aqueous
- Trabeculitis
- Posterior synechiae (seclusio pupillae → iris bombé)
- Peripheral anterior synechiae
- Hypotony in uveitis – due to decreased aqueous production or increased uveoscleral outflow due to ciliary oedema

Glaucomatocyclitic crisis (Posner-Schlossmann syndrome)

- Recurrent bouts of markedly raised IOP + low grade anterior chamber inflammation
- Aetiology – ? mediated by prostaglandins, ? allergic in nature
- Pathology – ? trabeculitis
- Features
  - Unilateral, recurrent, lasts 2 hours to 2 weeks, normal in between
  - High IOP (40–60), eye white or minimally injected, corneal oedema, haloes, 1+ cells flare and keratic precipitates, open angle, male > female
- Treatment – antiglaucoma medication, topical steroid, oral indomethacin, no evidence to support chronic suppressive therapy

Lens induced glaucoma

- Phacomorphic glaucoma – lens intumescence → pupil block in old age or cataract
- Phacolytic glaucoma
  - Leakage of proteins through lens capsule in hypermature cataract
  - Engulfed by macrophages
  - Macrophages and lens proteins block trabecular meshwork
- Lens particle glaucoma – following cataract surgery or penetrating trauma
- Phacoanaphylactic uveitis – rare; granulomatous uveitis from exposed previously isolated lens protein, particularly seen if nucleus is lost into vitreous, or in second eye following cataract surgery
- Lens subluxation – pupil block by lens or vitreous; this may be traumatic or spontaneous
- Pseudoexfoliation syndrome

Steroid induced glaucoma

- Steroid response automal recessive
- General population steroid response: 5% high, 35% moderate, 60% no response
- Primary open angle glaucoma patients: 90% high, 10% moderate, 0% none
- Correlates with phenylthiocarbamide non-taste
- High risk for steroid response – chronic open angle glaucoma, family history of glaucoma, diabetes, myopia
- Steroids may be
  - Endogenous
  - Exogenous – topical, periocular or systemic
- Elevated IOP may occur after 1 week to 2 years
- May occur after 1 drop
- Steroids → ? glycosaminoglycan deposition in trabecular meshwork, by stabilisation of lysosomal membranes
- Steroids ? inhibition of endogenous phagocytosis by trabecular endothelium

Treatment

- Stop steroids, IOP decreases after few days to weeks
- Medrysone and fluoromethalone have less IOP effect for the same anti-inflammatory effect

Ghost cell glaucoma

- Degenerated red blood cells (tan cells) from vitreous haemorrhage block trabeculum
- Starts after 2–3 days, lasts 1–2 weeks
- IOP 60–70, ± pain, eye white, tan cells seen in vitreous, anterior chamber and angle
- Occurs in 3 settings – cataract extraction complicated by vitreous haemorrhage
- Pre-existing vitreous haemorrhage, then cataract extraction
- Vitreous haemorrhage in an aphakic eye

Red cell glaucoma

- With traumatic hyphaema
- Blockage of trabecular meshwork by red blood cells → secondary elevation of IOP
- Hyphaema < 5 mm → 4% risk of elevated IOP
- Hyphaema > 5 mm → 85% risk of elevated IOP

Treatment

- Medical
- Surgical evacuation of blood if
  - IOP > 50 for 2 days
  - IOP > 35 for 7 days
  - Corneal blood staining
  - Total hyphaema for more than 5 days

Schwartz syndrome

- Retinal detachment usually → hypotony
- Open angle glaucoma associated with retinal detachment may be due to
  - Angle recession from trauma
  - Associated iritis
  - Photoreceptor outer segments in aqueous

Glaucoma following panretinal photocoagulation

- Lasts 2–7 days
- Increased fluid in suprachoroidal space → movement of ciliary body forward → narrowing of angle

Tumour induced glaucoma

- Tumour involvement of angle
- Tumour metastasis to angle
- Forward displacement of lens

Epithelial downgrowth

- Following perforating injury or surgery
- Results in glaucoma
- Treat by photocoagulation, surgical excision, cryodestruction, intracameral 5-fluorouracil

Hypersecretion glaucoma

- Very rare
- Intermittent, occurs in hypertensive middle-aged females

High myopia and glaucoma

Associated problems

- Decreased ocular rigidity
- Little cupping
- Myopic atrophy → field loss

Glaucoma secondary to trauma

Early angle closure

- Subluxed or swollen lens (phacomorphic)
- Pupil block due to hyphaema

Late angle closure

- Posterior synechiae secondary to uveitis
- Peripheral anterior synechiae secondary to uveitis or collapse of anterior chamber
- Lens induced (phacolytic, phacoanaphylactic, lens particle)

Early open angle

- Hyphaema
- Ghost cell glaucoma secondary to vitreous haemorrhage
- Uveitis

Late open angle

- Angle recession (concussion or contusion injury)

Cyclodialysis

- Secondary to trauma (cyclodialysis cleft)
- Rarely secondary to a surgical procedure

Neovascular glaucoma

Causes of rubeosis iridis

- Retinopathies (retinal ischaemia)
- Inflammatory
- Neoplastic
- Post-op
- Idiopathic

Retinopathies (retinal ischaemia)

- Central retinal vein occlusion (100 day glaucoma); 36% of cases of rubeosis iridis; in 50% of cases of central retinal vein occlusion
- Diabetic retinopathy; 32% of cases of rubeosis iridis
- Branch retinal vein occlusion; 4% of cases of rubeosis iridis; in 4% of cases of branch retinal vein occlusion
- Central/branch retinal artery occlusion; 4% of cases of rubeosis iridis; in 2% of cases of retinal artery occlusion
- Carotid artery occlusion
- Aortic arch syndrome
- Carotid cavernous fistula
- Giant cell arteritis
- Eale's disease
- Coat's disease
- Sickle cell retinopathy
- Retinopathy of prematurity
- Persistent hyperplastic primary vitreous
- Longstanding retinal detachment

Inflammatory (0.5% of cases of rubeosis iridis)

- Chronic uveitis

Neoplastic (1% of cases of rubeosis iridis)

- Retinoblastoma
- Malignant melanoma of uvea

Post-op

- Cataract extraction
- Vitrectomy
- Retinal detachment surgery

Staging

- I new vessels around pupil
- II new vessels over iris
- III new vessels in angle with peripheral anterior synechiae formation
- Rubeosis iridis
- Secondary open angle glaucoma
- Secondary synechial angle closure

Pathogenesis

- Ischaemic retina → angiogenic factor(s)
- ? Lens extraction → removal of physical barrier
- ? Vitrectomy → removal of vitreous inhibitor

Pathology

- New vessel formation starts around the pupil margins, extends to the angle
- Contraction of fibrovascular membrane → peripheral anterior synechiae and ectropion uveae
- May take days to years to develop

Features

- Iris rubeosis, ectropion uveae
- Aqueous flare
- Features of acute glaucoma

Management

- Rubeosis iridis
  - Panretinal photocoagulation
  - Intravitreal anti-VEGF
- Secondary neovascular open angle glaucoma
  - Medical treatment of glaucoma
  - Topical steroid + atropine
  - Pan-retinal photocoagulation
- Secondary neovascular angle closure glaucoma
  - Medical treatment of glaucoma
  - Topical steroid + atropine
  - Panretinal photocoagulation
  - ± Seton
  - ± Cyclocryotherapy or transcleral laser cycloablation
  - ± Retrobulbar chlorpromazine
  - ± Enucleation

Disorders leading to rubeosis iridis

Systemic vascular disease

- Carotid occlusive disease (13%)
- Carotid cavernous fistula
- Giant cell arteritis
- Takayasu
- Blood dyscrasias

Ocular vascular disease

- Diabetic retinopathy (32%)
- CRVO (36%)
- BRVO
- CRAO
- Sickle cell disease
- Coat's disease
- Syphilis
- Eale's disease
- ROP

Other ocular diseases

- Chronic uveitis (0.5%)
- Chronic retinal detachment (1%)
- Endophthalmitis
- Stickler syndrome
- Retinoschisis

Intraocular tumours (1%)

- Uveal melanoma
- Metastatic ca
- Retinoblastoma

Ocular therapy

- Post-vitrectomy in diabetes
- Radiation therapy

Trauma

Acute neovascular glaucoma

Clinically

- Extreme pain, nausea and vomiting
- Extensive injection, corneal oedema, bullous keratopathy
- Profound decrease in visual acuity
- IOP 50–70 mmhg
- Hyphaema
- Cataract
- Gonioscopy
  - Angle rubeosis, amount of angle involved
  - Peripheral anterior synechiae
- Fundoscopy
  - Usually no view
  - CRVO, proliferative diabetic retinopathy, etc.

Emergency management

- Anaesthesia – consider in-office sub-Tenon lignocaine/macaine
- Diode laser cyclophotocoagulation
- Anterior chamber paracentesis
  - Consider in-office
  - Remove 1 ml aqueous at slit lamp
  - Short-term measure
- Inflammation
  - G. dexamethasone 2-hourly
  - G. atropine 1% bd
- Glaucoma
  - Acetazolamide 250 mg qid po
  - Topical antiglaucoma treatment – avoid miotics
- Retinal ischaemia
  - Fundus visible – panretinal photocoagulation
  - No fundal view – retinal cryoablation (peritomy, cryoablate in all 4 quadrants between extraocular muscles in a 'triangular 3, 2, 1' manner from posterior to anterior, 15 second duration with each freeze)
  - Good PRP/cryo resolves rubeosis in 10–14 days

Long-term glaucoma management

- IOP control may occur with panretinal photocoagulation and cryo alone
- Eye with glaucoma and good visual potential
  - Trabeculectomy with mitomycin C if no rubeosis left at all
  - Otherwise drainage device
- Eye with poor visual potential – cyclodestructive procedures
  - Cyclocryoablation (peritomy, cryoablate 4 mm from the limbus for 1 minute, 3 times in each quadrant; start with 180 degrees, a further 90 degrees if response inadequate)

- Laser cyclophotocoagulation
- Painful blind eye
  - Consider enucleation

Subacute/chronic neovascular glaucoma

Clinically

- Moderate, nagging pain, IOP 30–50 mmHg

Management – not as an emergency

Inflammation

- G. dexamethasone
- G. atropine

Glaucoma

- Acetazolamide 250 mg qid po
- Topical antiglaucoma treatment – avoid miotics

Retinal ischaemia

- Fundus visible – panretinal photocoagulation
- No fundal view – retinal cryoablation
- Good panretinal photocoagulation/ cryopexy resolves rubeosis in 10–14 days

Long-term glaucoma management

- As for acute neovascular glaucoma

General investigations to consider

- Blood pressure
- Full blood count
- ESR
- Glucose
- Coagulation profile
- Hb electrophoresis
- Syphilis serology
- Rheumatoid factor
- c-ANCA
- Anti-nuclear antibodies

Pigment dispersion

Pathophysiology

- Reverse pupil block in young myopic eye → posterior bowing of iris
- Loss of pigment from pigment epithelium of iris in midperiphery from rubbing on zonules → pigment dispersion
- Accumulation of melanin in trabecular meshwork → transient rise in IOP
- Melanin phagocytosed by endothelial cells → endothelial cells autolyse → trabecular beams denuded, undergo degeneration, sclerosis and collapse → development of secondary open angle glaucoma

Features

- Pigment dispersion syndrome
  - Occurs in young (20–30 years) white myopic males
  - May be autosomal dominant with variable penetrance
  - Bilateral; often exercise induced; may have episodes of acute rise in IOP with corneal oedema (haloes) and headaches
  - Midperipheral iris concave → towards zonular fibres
  - Zentmeyer's line – pigment deposits on the zonules and anterior and posterior capsule near lens equator
  - Radial transillumination defects of the iris, pigment dispersion on the lens, iris, cornea (Krukenberg spindle; vertical; caused by aqueous convection currents and subsequent phagocytosis of pigment by the corneal endothelium), trabecular meshwork (dense uniform pigmentation)
- Pigmentary glaucoma
  - Onset at 40 years, male : female 2 : 1
  - Chronic glaucoma
  - 25–50% of people with pigment dispersion syndrome develop pigmentary glaucoma

- Tends to resolve as get older
- High IOP after dilating or exercise because of pigment release

Differential diagnosis

- Other causes of glaucoma – primary chronic open angle glaucoma, pseudocapsular exfoliation
- Other causes of trabecular pigmentation – uveitis, IOL with pigment dispersion, trauma

Management

- Prophylaxis
  - YAG peripheral iridotomy, to overcome reverse pupil block → efficacy not established
- Medical
  - β-blocker
  - Pilocarpine 1% before exercising
- Laser – do well with argon laser trabeculoplasty (50% 5 year success)
- Surgical – try and avoid, as they often improve, but it is successful

Risk factors for glaucoma in pigment dispersion syndrome

- Male, black
- Severe myopia
- Krukenberg spindle

Pigmentary glaucoma in blacks

- Elderly, hypermetropic, female, no iris transillumination defects
- Also have Krukenberg's spindle and heavily pigmented trabecular meshwork, ? due to rubbing of lens on back of iris

Pseudocapsular exfoliation

- A generalised basement membrane disorder

Incidence

- Variable in different population groups, first described in Scandinavia (30% of eyes undergoing lens extraction in Finland), common in blacks
- Increased incidence in chronic open angle glaucoma population compared with normal population (50–80% pseudo capsular exfoliation eyes have glaucoma)
- Increased incidence with age
- Male : female 1 : 1
- Unilateral in 50%

Pathophysiology

- The material is fibrillin (elastin precursor); histologically resembles amyloid
- Multifocal origin – lens epithelium, ciliary body epithelium, iris pigment epithelium, trabecular endothelium
- Flecks clog trabecular meshwork → secondary open angle glaucoma
- All eyes with pseudo capsular exfoliation will eventually develop glaucoma
- Represents a disease of all tissues, involving extracellular matrix
- May be associated with development of abdominal aortic aneurysm

Features

- Flecks occur on corneal endothelium, pupil border, lens anterior capsule (central disc and peripheral girdle; flecks only observed in peripheral lens in 25%)
- Pigment floaters in anterior chamber aqueous
- Pigmented trabecular meshwork; this pigmentation is irregular and splotchy
- Scalloped line of pigment deposition anterior to Schwalbe's line → Sampaolesi's line
- Flecks may be visible in the trabecular meshwork
- There may be pigment loss around the iris sphincter with patchy transillumination defects
- Flecks also occur on the zonules, ciliary processes, and anterior vitreous face

- Increased IOP occurs in 50–80%, tends to be higher than in primary chronic open angle glaucoma
- Phacodenesis, iridodenesis
- Increased zonule fragility + decreased pupil dilatation → increased risk during cataract surgery

Differential diagnosis
- Pigment dispersion
- True lens exfoliation (glass blowers)

Management
- Follow-up – every 6 months, to watch for development of glaucoma
- Medical treatment of glaucoma
- Laser treatment of glaucoma; do well with argon laser trabeculoplasty
- Surgical treatment of glaucoma

Risks and progression in pseudo-exfoliative glaucoma
- Incidence: 7% in SA Blacks over 40
- 18% of over 70s
- 10% will have open angle glaucoma
- Incidence varies in different populations
- It is a systemic disease

Inflammatory glaucoma

- Secondary open angle glaucoma and secondary angle closure glaucoma caused by acute iridocyclitis, episcleritis, scleritis, keratitis, posterior uveitis

Pathogenesis
- Clogging of trabecular meshwork by inflammatory precipitate
- Increased viscosity of aqueous humour
- Trabeculitis
- Posterior synechiae, seclusio pupillae, iris bombé
- Inflammatory exudate in angle, organises, pulls iris forward into peripheral anterior synechiae
- Ischaemia, new vessels, neovascular glaucoma
- Uveal effusion, anterior rotation of the ciliary body, shallow anterior chamber and angle closure
- Exudative retinal detachment, forward displacement of lens-iris diaphragm, angle closure

Clinical
- Keratic precipitates, ± peripheral anterior synechiae, posterior synechiae, bombé

Treatment
- Avoid miotics – inflammation may be aggravated
- Care with steroids → steroid response

5

Glaucoma in Fuchs' cyclitis

- Iris heterochromia, cataract + low-grade iritis
- Mostly unilateral
- Dark irisis go lighter, light irises darker
- Mild iritis – no posterior synechiae or peripheral anterior synechiae
- Diffuse, fine, stellate keratic precipitates
- Fine new vessels in angle
- Glaucoma difficult to control, does not correspond with degree of inflammation

Management of uveitic glaucoma
- ± 25% will have raised IOP at some stage
- 5–27% will have glaucoma
- 20–30% will need surgery
- Control of the inflammation is the key to success
- Argon laser trabeculoplasty (ALT) does not work due to synaechiae + other complications
- High rate of complications in cyclophotocoagulation but it's used in the limited form by some
- Immunosuppressives are key
- Shown in trials to be effective
    - Birdshot → cyclosporin
    - Juvenile idiopathic arthritis → methotrexate
    - Behçets, multifocal choroiditis → cyclosporin, azathioprine

- Serpiginous + Wegener's alkylating agents, steroids
- Trabeculectomy – 50% success alone, 60–80% with mitomycin C
- Treat the uveitis and cure the glaucoma

Lens-related glaucoma

- Open or closed

Phacolytic glaucoma

- Leakage of lens proteins from hypermature cataracts, trabecular meshwork blocks with
    - Macrophages + high molecular weight lens proteins
    - Anterior chamber inflammation, + pain
    - Definitive treatment is cataract surgery

Lens particle glaucoma

- After cataract surgery with retained lens material or penetrating injury with ruptured lens capsule
- Definitive treatment is cataract surgery

Phacoanaphylaxis

- After penetrating trauma or surgery
- Patients become sensitised to their own lens proteins
- Granulomatous inflammation
- Definitive treatment is cataract surgery

Phacomorphic glaucoma

- Swollen, intumescent lens/cataract → pupil block
- Definitive treatment is cataract surgery

Lens subluxation

- Partial zonular dehiscence e.g. in Marfan's or homocystinuria
- Treatment: Laser peripheral iridotomy, cataract surgery

Microspherophakia

- Congenital disorder of globular/spherical lens
- May occur in Weill-Marchesani, Marfan's
- Pupil block and angle closure
- Treatment: Cycloplegics to flatten the lens, pull it backwards, and break the pupillary block

Aphakic and pseudophakic glaucoma

- Vitreous face causes pupil block
- Treatment: Cycloplegics, aqueous suppressants, osmotic agents
- Treatment: Peripheral iridectomy

Anterior chamber IOLs

- Pupil block or angle damage/obstruction by haptics

Post-cataract surgery glaucoma

Causes of post-cataract surgery glaucoma	
Open angle	
■ Early onset	□ Pre-existing primary open angle glaucoma
	□ Early post-op rise in IOP
	□ A-chymotrypsin induced
	□ Sodium hyaluronate
	□ Hyphaema
■ Intermediate onset	□ Vitreous filling anterior chamber
	□ Hyphaema
	□ Inflammation
	□ Lens particle
	□ Steroid induced
	□ Ghost cell
■ Late onset	□ Primary open angle glaucoma
	□ Ghost cell
	□ Epithelial ingrowth
	□ Fibrous proliferation
Closed angle	
■ Early onset	□ Pre-existing peripheral anterior synechiae
	□ Air block
	□ Pupil block
	□ Vitreociliary block
■ Intermediate and late onset	□ Pupil block
	□ Neovascular

Transient post-op rise in IOP

- Due to
  - Plasmoid aqueous
  - Trabecular oedema

Sodium hyaluronate induced

- In the first 24 hours
- Either wash it out or give prophylactic acetazolamide

Pupil block

Causes

- Wound leak
- Inflammation
- Incomplete iridectomy
- Lens remnants
- Posterior vitreous detachment

Pathogenesis

- Posterior synechiae to anterior IOL surface or hyaloid face

Differential diagnosis

- Wound leak
- Choroidal detachment
- Vitreociliary block

Prevention

- Iridectomy
- Adequate wound closure
- Steroids, mydriatics/miotics

Treatment

- Mydriatics/miotics
- Steroids
- Iridectomy
- Anterior vitrectomy

Ciliary block glaucoma

- Misdirection of aqueous into the vitreous cavity

Aetiology

- Phakic
  - Following surgery for primary angle closure glaucoma (2–4% of cases) – there is an increased chance if the angle is closed at the time of surgery; it may develop after months
  - Following surgery for chronic open angle glaucoma
  - Following laser procedures
  - Following miotic therapy
  - Arising de novo
- Aphakic
  - Following lens extraction; may develop after months

Pathogenesis

- Block to anterior movement of aqueous; ? ciliary processes in contact with/adherent to lens equator, ? vitreous face too far forward, ? decreased permeability of vitreous to aqueous flow
- Increased force applied to vitreous gel → forward flow of aqueous through gel → compaction, dehydration, decreased conductivity of gel → movement forward of gel with anterior chamber flattening → iris-lens diaphragm displaced anteriorly
- Occurs mostly in patients with pre-existing angle closure
- Hyperopic eyes at greater risk

Pathology

- Aqueous collects in, behind or beside vitreous cavity, or in the suprachoroidal space (forme fruste of expulsive haemorrhage)

Features

- Flat anterior chamber
- Raised IOP
- Absence of pupil block

Differential diagnosis

- Suprachoroidal effusion or haemorrhage
- Pupil block

Medical

- Mydriatic – cycloplegic drops → tightening of zonules → pulling of lens back against vitreous
- Atropine 6-hourly and phenylephrine 10%
- Acetazolomide 250 mg 6-hourly
- Beta-blocker 12-hourly
- Hyperosmotic agents (mannitol and glycerol)
- Continue until the anterior chamber reforms/IOP decreases, or for 5 days
- 50% respond
- If successful, taper

Laser treatment

- ND:YAG of the anterior vitreous in aphakic + pseudophakic eyes → rupture of hyaloid face
- Argon laser photocoagulation of the ciliary processes

Surgical management

- Is the iridectomy patent or not?
  - If not, do a second iridectomy
  - If the anterior chamber deepens, this confirms pupil block
- Is suprachoroidal fluid/blood present or not?
  - Make 2 radial sclerotomy incisions 3 mm long centred 3.5 mm from limbus + paracentesis into anterior chamber; drain fluid and deepen anterior chamber
  - Vitreous aspiration 1–1.5 ml vitreous aspirated via 18 gauge needle inserted 12 mm; anterior chamber reformed with balanced salt solution and large air bubble; post-op atropine and steroids
- Vitrectomy

Management of the fellow eye

- Avoid miotics
- Prophylactic iridectomy at surgery
- Full cycloplegic treatment post-op

Iridocorneal dysgenesis

- Congenital anterior segment defects due to mesodermal dysgenesis

Axenfeld-Rieger syndrome

- Spectrum of changes
- Glaucoma in 50%
- Mostly autosomal dominant, mutation in PAX6 on chromosome 4, 10, 11, 13
- Axenfeld's anomaly – thickening and anterior displacement of Schwalbe's line (posterior embryotoxon), with adherence of iris stromal processes to the line
- Axenfeld's syndrome – if glaucoma is present
- Rieger's anomaly – same abnormalities as Axenfeld's anomaly plus extensive iris abnormalities e.g. loss of iris stroma + corectopia
- Rieger's syndrome – presence of associated skeletal and dental abnormalities, redundant periumbilical skin, hypospadias, pituitary anomalies

Peter's anomaly

- Unilateral or bilateral central corneal opacification with absent Descemet's membrane centrally
- Degree of corneal opacification varies from total lack of involvement to total opacification, scarring + vascularisation at birth
- Iris processes adhere to cornea at edge of defect in Descemet's
- ± Cataract, keratolenticular adhesion, angle closure glaucoma, posterior segment abnormalities, systemic abnormalities

Iridocorneal endothelial (ICE) syndrome

- A group of disorders characterised by abnormal corneal endothelium, causing varying degrees of iris atrophy, secondary angle closure glaucoma, corneal oedema
- Aetiology – ? viral; ? Epstein-Barr virus or herpes simplex
- Three variants
  - Chandler's syndrome (50%)
  - Essential/progressive iris atrophy
  - Iris naevus/Cogan-Reese syndrome
- Unilateral
- Presents 20–50 years of age
- Female > male
- Glaucoma in 50%
- Fine, beaten metal appearance of endothelium
- Decreased vision, pain, corneal oedema, secondary angle closure, abnormal iris
- The unaffected eye may have subclinical corneal endothelial abnormalities
- High peritheral anterior synechiae extending to Schwalbe's line → angle closure
- Varying degrees of iris abnormality – heterochromia, corectopia, ectropion uveae, stromal atrophy
- Asymmetrical loss of endothelium + abnormal cell morphology

Treatment

- Hypertonic saline; aqueous suppressants
- Surgery – trab with mitomycin C, seton, ciliary ablation
- Argon laser trabeculoplasty contraindicated → increases peripheral anterior synechiae
- Penetrating keratoplasty for extensive corneal oedema

Tumours

- Open or closed mechanism
- Direct tumour invasion of anterior chamber angle

- Rotation of the ciliary body or anterior displacement of the lens-iris diaphragm
- Intraocular haemorrhage
- Angle neovascularisation
- Tumour cell deposition in the angle
- Adults – uveal melanoma, metastases, lymphoma, leukaemia
- Children – retinoblastoma, juvenile xanthogranuloma, medulloepithelioma

Vitreoretinal surgery and corneal grafts

Glaucoma post-corneal graft

- 30% early IOP rise, 28% late IOP rise

Risk factors

- Aphakia
- Pre-existing glaucoma
- Triple procedure
- Repeated penetrating keratoplasty
- Tectonic graft for perforation

Early

- Same mechanisms as any intraocular surgery
- Trabecular meshwork collapse due to decreased zonular tension + incision into Descemet's
- Angle compression – tight sutures

Late

- Gradual AC flattening, therefore, do a prophylactic peripheral iridotomy
- Rejection
- Pigment dispersion
- Steroid response
- Peripheral anterior synechiae
- Epithelial ingrowth

Prevention

- Minimise angle compression – larger donor size
    - Looser sutures or shorter bite
    - Smaller trephine
- Meticulous wound closure
- Extensive post-op steroids

Glaucoma post-VR surgery

Pars plana vitrectomy

- Incidence – 20%
- Day 1
    - Air or SF6 gas – expansion of gas
    - Oil overfill
- Week 1
    - Hyphaema, ghost cell, haemolytic
    - Phacolytic
    - Uveitis
    - Pre-existing glaucoma
    - Fibrin pupil block – treatment: YAG
- Weeks 2–4
    - Neovascular
    - Silicone oil – pupil block or emulsification
    - Treatment: inferior peripheral iridotomy

Scleral buckling

- Anterior chamber shallowing – vortex vein compression, ciliary body congestion, choroidal effusion
- Treatment: atropine/steroids
- Remove band
- Drain effusion

Panretinal photocoagulation

- ? Aetiology of open angle
- Closed angle due to choroidal effusion + angle narrowing

Genetics

- 10–50% primary open angle glaucoma family history
- Twins – 98% primary open angle glaucoma
- Nine loci for glaucoma mapped

Nomenclature

- GLC-1: primary open angle glaucoma, loci A–F
- GLC-2: CACG, locus not found yet
- GLC-3: Congenital, loci A–C

Primary open angle glaucoma (POAG)

- GLC-1, loci A–F
- High genetic heterogenicity
- GLC–1A: The MYOC/TIGR gene (myocilin/trabecular meshwork inducible glucocorticoid response)
- Chromosome 1q
- 5% of primary open angle glaucoma
- Transmitted autosomal dominant, variable penetrance
- GLC-1B: Middle-aged, moderate IOP
- GLC-1C: Young, high IOP
- GLC-1D: Middle-aged, moderate IOP
- GLC-1E: Normal tension

Myocilin

- A stress protein
- Creates resistance to aqueous outflow at the TM when acticated
- Normal role unknown
- Found in most ocular tissue
- Increased staining for myocilin in most primary open angle glaucoma eyes
- Increased basal production in the TM in most primary open angle glaucoma eyes
- Inducible by the application of steroids

Congenital glaucoma

- GLC-3, three loci – A, B, C
- Primary congenital glaucoma – autosomal recessive with variable penetration
- Familial in 10–40%
- The CYPIBI gene codes for the cytochrome P450IBI enzyme
  - Expressed in the AC of the eye
  - Gene mutations interfere with the enzyme which participates in normal AC development
- ELAM-1gene
  - Present in the TM endothelial cells

Pigment dispersion

- 7q35
- Close to the locus for taste of phenylthiocarbamide
- Therefore, there is a high incidence of PHTC non-taste in pigment dispersion glaucoma

Rieger's syndrome

- RIEG 1 gene at 4q25
- Autosomal dominant

Aniridia, Peter's anomaly, autosomal dominant keratitis

- PAX-6 gene

5

Perimetry

Humphrey perimetery

- Static perimetry
- A stationary test target of variable intensity
- Slower than kinetic
- Tests differential light sensitivity i.e. the ability to distinguish the test light from the background light
- In pathological areas, the light might have to be up to 1 000 times brighter to be seen
- The threshold is halfway between the brightest light seen and the dimmest seen in that area

Reliability indices

- Fixation losses – detected by presenting stimuli in blind spot
- Response → fixation loss
- False positives – stimulus accompanied by sound
- Response with sound alone → false positive
- High false positive = trigger happy patient
- False negatives – stimulus presented that is much brighter than threshold
- Failure to respond → false negative
- High false negative = inattentive patient

Displays

- Numerical display – gives threshold (dB) for all points checked

- Number in brackets is the value at the same point checked a second time if the threshold at 1 point is at least 5dB less sensitive than expected
- Graphic display – each step in the pattern corresponds to a 5dB change in sensitivity i.e. the boundary between the tones is analogous to isopters measuring every 5dB

Total deviation

- Upper numerical display shows difference (dB) between patient's results and age-matched normals
- Lower graphic display shows difference as grey symbols

Pattern deviation

- Similar to total deviation, but adjusted for any generalised depression due to other factors like lens opacities or miosis or age

Global indices

- Mean deviation (MD) – measure of patient's overall field from normal reference, either up or down
- Lower p has greater significance
- Pattern standard deviation (PSD)
    - Indicates degree to which patient's visual field departs from an age matched reference field
- Short-term fluctuation
    - Indicates the consistency of the patient's responses
- Corrected pattern standard deviation
    - Measures how much the overall shape of the patient's hill of vision deviates from age matched normals

Features

- Arcuate fibres reaching the superotemporal and inferotemporal aspects of the optic nerve head are the most vulnerable to glaucomatous damage
- Glaucoma field is a nerve fibre bundle defect, i.e. follows the nerve fibre pattern in the retina → central or cecocentral scotoma (not seen usually), nasal arcuate scotoma with step, temporal sector scotoma
- Isolated paracentral scotoma are the earliest defects; occur in 5–15 degree isopters, later connect to give arcuate scotoma
- Baring of the blind spot
- Arcuate/Bjerrum scotoma; scimitar shaped, extends from the blind spot in 5–15 degree isopters to 5 degrees nasal to fixation, above and/or below, with a nasal step
- Temporal sector defect
- Generalised peripheral constriction, especially nasally
- Peripheral breakthrough of nerve fibre bundle defect
- Terminal central island + temporal island, ultimately lost

Interpretation

- Correlates with cupping
- Cupping precedes field loss; 20–30% of fibres are lost before a field defect is evident
- Colour loss precedes field loss
- In myopia, cupping is decreased, ocular rigidity is decreased and the blind spot is increased
- Progressive scotomata have sloping edges

Colour vision in glaucoma

- Blue-yellow defect occurs (tritan defect)
- Occurs early, before a disc or field defect is evident
- It is therefore useful to distinguish between ocular hypertension and glaucoma

Efficient threshold strategies

- Objective of perimetry – to get valid + reliable information in a reasonable time period
- Staircase strategy used in initial static automated perimeters

- Problem is that the more reliable the test, the longer it is
- The most accurate test on the Humphrey – 4dB step size, reduced to 2 dB on the first reversal – 'full threshold' testing takes 15–20 mins
- A less rigorous strategy uses 3dB step size – FASTPAC – lasts 8 mins → less reproducible + underestimates severity

Swedish Interactive Threshold Algorithm (SITA)

- Substantially reduces exam time without compromising quality
- Developed for the Humphrey
- Two available algorithms – SITA standard (7 mins) + SITA fast (4 mins)
- Intended to replace the full threshold + FASTPAC
- Reduces the fatigue effect
- Unlike the staircase tests using discrete intervals to step towards a threshold, SITA uses a logical 'best guess' to get to threshold
- The intensity of the first stimulus is derived from normal age statistics
- Depending on the patients response to this 1st stimulus, the intensity of subsequent stimuli is modified
- This reduces stimulus presentations by 30%
- SITA fast is less conservative and accepts higher threshold measurement errors
- Fixation quality – uses 'gaze tracking' during the test – monitoring the corneal reflex relative to pupil position is monitored; presented as a line on the bottom of the printout
- Downward deflections = reflection interrupted by upper eyelid
- Thin upward deflections = eye movements
- Thick upward deflections = head misalignment
- SITA also measures timing of patient responses to pace the test
- SITA fast → for routine screening
- SITA standard for definitive diagnosis + monitoring

Tendency-oriented perimetry

- Similar to SITA
- For the Octopus machine

Short Wavelength Automated Perimetry (SWAP)

- Large, M-cells appear to be damaged first in glaucoma
- Uses blue light spots
- Detects field defects 3–5 years earlier than standard automated perimetry
- More sensitive in detecting progression
- Use for high risk individuals suspects + high risk of progression
- Not good for routine testing because of lengthy duration + learning effect
- Confirm abnormalities with a retest
- Media opacities can be a problem, absorbing blue light
- SITA-like strategy may be added in future

Frequency Doubling Technology (FDT) perimetry

- When a low spatial frequency sinusoidal grating undergoes high temporal frequency
- Counterphase flicker, the grating appears to have twice as many light bars as dark
- Said to be 'frequency doubled'
- This is an M-cell task
- Measures contrast detection thresholds
- 17 points are tested over the central 20 degrees of field
- Stimulus is a series of white + black bands flickering at 25 Hz
- Patients have to use distance correction because the grating is at optical infinity
- Short test time
- Resilient to refractive errors up to 6D
- Screening version only 90 secs
- Good for monitoring progression

Pearls

- Initial defects should always be confirmed by a retest
- Use a new 'baseline test' if you change test types or algorithms
- FDT good for screening
- Threshold perimetry only tests up to the central 30 degrees
- Testing the more peripheral field is unhelpful – difficult to test + not very reliable

Glaucoma drugs

Beta-blockers (beta-adrenergic antagonists)

Pharmacology

- Compete with catecholamines → blockage of beta 1 (heart) and beta 2 (bronchus) receptors
- Non-selective are equipotent at beta 1 and beta 2 receptors
- Cardioselective are more potent at beta 1 than at beta 2 receptors
- Mechanism of action in the eye is unknown
- Decreased aqueous production → decreased IOP
- Additive to miotics + carbonic anhydrase inhibitors, slightly additive to adrenergic agents
- Beta-blocker effects may reduce after prolonged use

IOP reduction

- 22–26%

Side effects

- Cardiovascular (bradycardia, hypotension, reduced exercise tolerance)
- Bronchospasm
- Lethargy, mood changes, impotence, allergy, increased serum lipids

Preparations

- Timolol (non-cardio selective)
- Levobunolol (non-cardio selective)
- Betaxolol (the only cardio selective → useful in bronchospastic disorders; may be less effective)

Alpha agonists (sympathomimetics)

Pharmacology

- Mechanism of action in the eye is unknown
- Decreased aqueous production + increased uveoscleral outflow → decreased IOP

IOP reduction

- 25–26%

Preparations

- Brimonidine
- Apraclonidine

Side effects

- Ocular allergy – 15%, dry mouth, lethargy, headache, blurred vision

Contraindications

- Severe cardiovascular disease, small children → systemic hypotension

Cholinergic agonists (para-sympathomimetics/miotics)

Pharmacology

- Open angle glaucoma – contraction of longitudinal muscle of ciliary body → opening of trabecular meshwork → increased aqueous outflow → decreased IOP
- Closed angle glaucoma – contraction of sphincter pupillae muscle → opening of angle → increased aqueous outflow → decreased IOP

Side effects

- Miosis → reduced visual acuity, constriction of visual field, impaired night vision
- Spasm of accommodation → myopia, headaches
- Aggravation of iritis
- Red eye

Preparations
- Pilocarpine (drops, gel, sustained release) – direct acting, cholinergic agonist
- Carbachol – indirect acting, anticholinesterase agent

Prostaglandin analogs

Pharmacology
- Mechanism of action unknown
- Increased uveoscleral outflow → decreased IOP
- IOP reduction 30–35%

Side effects
- Conjunctival hyperaemia, foreign body sensation
- Iris pigmentation – in all preprations
- Eyelash elongation – in all preparations
- Aggravation of cystoid macular oedema in uveitis

Preparations
- Latanoprost
- Travoprost
- Bimatoprost

Carbonic anhydrase inhibitors

Pharmacology
- Carbonic anhydrase inhibition → decreased aqueous production → decreased IOP
- May also increase ocular blood flow

Side effects
- Paraesthesia, metallic taste, gastritis
- Malaise symptom complex – caused by a metabolic acidosis
- Gastrointestinal symptom complex
- Other complications – Stevens-Johnson syndrome, blood dyscrasias, renal stone formation, idiosyncratic aplastic anaemia
- Problems with co-existing renal disease
- Potassium + supplements in healthy patients not necessary
- Topical – hyperaemia, stinging, beta-blocker effects

Contraindications
- Relative – renal impairment, lung impairment, liver disease
- Full blood count, renal function before initiating in high risk groups
- Sulphonamide sensitivity

Drug interactions
- Asprin – acidosis + central nervous system disturbance
- Potentiates warfarin, hypoglycaemics, oral anticoagulants
- Thiazide (potassium losing) diuretics → be careful of hypokalaemia

Preparations
- Acetazolamide (tablets, injection)
- Dorzolamide (drops)
- Dorzolamide + timolol additive fixed combination

5

Hyperosmotic agents

Pharmacology
- Increased blood osmolality → osmotic gradient → dehydration of vitreous → decreased IOP
- Mannitol takes 30–60 mins, lasting 4–8 hours
- Glycerol takes 10 mins, lasting 4–5 hours

Side effects
- Cardiovascular overload
- Urinary retention

Drug interactions
- Potentiates the ototoxic effects of aminoglycosides
- Enhances neuromuscular blockers, excretion of lithium
- Decreases action of anticoagulants

Contraindications
- Pulmonary oedema, cardiac failure, renal impairment, intracranial bleeds, diabetics (glycerol)

Preparations
- Glycerol (oral or topical)
- Isosorbide (oral)
- Mannitol (intravenous)

Antifibrotic agents

- 5-Fluorouracil – 50 mg/ml
- Mitomycin C – 0.2 mg/ml
- Risk factors for failure: neovascular glaucoma, previous failed surgery, inflammation, aphakia, uveitis, Black race, previous topical polypharmacy, age < 40, inferior bleb

MorFlo (Moorfields-Florida) protocol

Low risk

- No risk factors or black race, use of topical meds, age < 40
- Use nothing, or intra-op 5-fluorouracil 50 mg/ml or post-op 5-fluorouracil 5 mg subconjunctiva daily for 5 days

Intermediate risk

- Combined surgery, previous conjunctival scarring, use of topical polypharmacy
- Intra-op: 5-fluorouracil 50 mg/ml or mitomycin C 0.2 mg/ml or beta irradiation

High risk

- Neovascular glaucoma, uveitis, failed surgery, aphakia, chronic conjunctival inflammation
- Intra-op: mitomycin C 0.4 mg/ml

Neuroprotection

- Glaucoma is a neurodegenerative disease, a progressive optic neuropathy resulting in characteristic cupping, with raised IOP being an important risk factor
- Neuronal death – axonal injury → death of injured neuron → secondary degeneration of other previously undamaged neurons
- Neuronal protection – preservation of those healthy neurons from the toxic stimuli released by the damaged cells
- Causes of ganglion death
    - Ischaemia – increased IOP → decreased pulsatile flow to optic nerve head
    - Excitotoxicity – increased glutamate → toxic response in adjacent cells; mediated by N-methyl-D-aspartate (NMDA) + increased intracellular calcium
    - Mitochondria – apoptosis caused by the glaucoma
    - Decreased trophic support – decreased axoplasmic flow, blocked at the lamina cribrosa
    - Inflammation – nitric oxide damage
- Neuroprotective factors
    - NMDA antagonists e.g. memantine
    - Nitrous oxide inhibitors e.g. aminoguanidine
    - Increased retinal ATP – flupirtine
    - Ca channel blockers – betaxolol, nifedipine
    - Antioxidants – Vitamin E
    - Ginkgo bilboa extract – free radical + nitrous oxide + glutamate scavenger
    - Cannabinoids – NMDA antagonism
    - Melatonin – anti-oxidant
    - Brimonidine – in experimental animals

Glaucoma imaging

Laser scanners

- Scanning laser ophthalmoscopy, laser polarimetry
- Measures nerve fibre layer thickness by measuring the change in the rotation of a polarised beam of diode laser light reflected from the retinal surface

Optic nerve head

- HRT (Heidelberg Retina Tomograph) + Talia
- Measures heights at different points + gives a colour coded map
- Moorfields classification is then used to interpret
- Very sensitive but not very specific
- I.e. if there is no change, it is probably true – no progression

- But if there is a change that may or may not be progression

Nerve fibre layer exam

- GDx
- New derivation → the GDxVCC (variable corneal compensation)
- Allows for any corneal reflection bias
- Does not show up disc haemorrhages
- In 25% of people it shows abnormally thick NFL readings and these people just cannot use GDx
- Not good for screening – < 85% specificity

Optical coherence tomography (OCT)

- Measures nerve fibre layer + cup:disk ratio
- Good sensitivity + specificity
- Corresponds well with visual fields
- No statistical difference in sensitivity has been found in studies between GDx, HRT and OCT with their own normative databases

Glaucoma in pregnancy

- No clinical studies of safety + efficacy of drugs in pregnancy
- All antiglaucoma meds have been shown to carry risks for the foetus in animal studies

Surgery

- Argon laser trabeculoplasty/selective laser trabeculoplasty can be a useful temporising measure
- Trabeculectomy + setons may be necessary
- Bupivicaine used in local block may cause foetal bradycardia
- Probably best to use only lignocaine
- Try to defer surgery until after the first trimester
- Avoid antimetabolites
- Position patient with lateral tilt to get gravid uterus off aorta

Medical – during pregnancy

- Timolol can cause foetal bradycardia + bronchspasm → discontinue
- Acetazolamide → teratogenic – sacrococcygeal teratoma
- Brimonidine has potential to cause bradycardia, hypertension, hypothermia, apnea → probably avoid during pregnancy
- Apraclonidine avoid during pregnancy
- Pilocarpine appears to be acceptable
- Prostaglandins promote labour + delivery; use with caution in the first and second trimesters

Medical – during breastfeeding

- Administer drops immediately after nursing because levels highest in the blood after 30–120 mins
- β-blockers – avoid
- Brimonidine – probably avoid or use with caution; not known if it appears in breast milk
- Acetozolamide appears in breast milk → however very low and compatible with breast feeding

Studies in glaucoma

Ocular Hypertension Treatment Study

- To evaluate safety + efficacy of topical hypotensives in preventing delaying onset of field loss and/or optic nerve damage in ocular hypertension

Results

- Topical hypotensives found to be effective in delaying onset of primary open angle glaucoma
- Treatment group – 22.5% decrease in IOP → 4.4% developed primary open angle glaucoma at 5 years
- Control group – 4% decrease in IOP → 9.5% developed primary open angle glaucoma at 5 years

Insignificant factors found

- Myopia, diabetes, family history, high or low blood pressure, migraine
- Ocular hypertensives have thicker corneas than in the general population
- Blacks had thinner corneas than Whites
- Central corneal thickness may influence accuracy of applanation
- Repeat testing failed to confirm visual field abnormalities in 604 (85.9%) of 703 reliable but abnormal fields

Conclusions

- Treat high risk cases
- Fields must be repeated several times for accuracy
- Central corneal thickness must be ascertained to get an accurate reflection of true IOP
- Reducing IOP by 20% decreases the risk of developing primary open angle glaucoma by 60%

Management of ocular hypertension

High risk (start treating → 20% reduction reasonable)

- Nerve fibre layer defects
- Parapapillary changes
- IOP ≥ 30 mmHg
- IOP ≥ 26 mmHg + central corneal thickness < 555 μ
- Cup:disk ratio ≥ 0.4 + central corneal thickness < 588

Moderate risk (withhold treatment until damage found, annual check-ups)

- IOP 24–29, no nerve fibre layer defects
- Cup:disk ratio > 0.3 + central corneal thickness > 588
- Family history of primary open angle glaucoma in a first degree relative
- High myopia

Early Manifest Glaucoma Trials (EMGT)

- To compare IOP lowering vs observation in newly diagnosed primary open angle glaucoma
- Betaxolol + argon laser trabeculoplasty vs observation
- 53% of all patients had progressed at 6 years
- Progression risk halved by treatment
- Progression risk decreased by 10% with each 1 mmHg IOP reduction

Collaborative Initial Glaucoma Treatment Study (CIGTS)

- To determine whether new open angle glaucoma patients
  are better treated with medicine or surgery
- Early field loss greater in surgery group, but similar over 5 years
- Quality of life impact similar
- Mean IOP with medicine 17–18 mmHg
- Mean IOP with surgery 14–15 mmHg
- Rate of cataract surgery higher in surgery group

Advanced Glaucoma Intervention Study (AGIS)

- A long-term study looking at the clinical course + outcome in glaucoma eyes not doing well on medication alone
- To compare two treatment sequences: ALT-Trab-Trab (ATT sequence) vs Trab-ALT-Trab (TAT sequence)
- AGIS 4
  - Blacks less combined VA + field loss with ATT
  - Whites less combined VA + field loss with TAT at 7 years

- AGIS 5
  - Encapsulated blebs more common in males + previous ALT
  - By 1 year, and with topical treatment, IOP same as others
- AGIS 7: IOP a major contribution of AGIS < 18 mmHg → significantly less field loss
- AGIS 8: Trab increases risk of cataract by 78%
- AGIS 9: Trab retards progression more effectively in blacks
- AGIS 11
  - Argon laser trabeculoplasty failure associated with younger age + higher IOP
  - Trab failure associated with younger age, higher IOP, diabetes, marked post-op inflammation and/or IOP elevation

Collaborative Normal Tension Glaucoma Study (CNTGS)

- To determine if aggressive IOP lowering halts optic nerve damage and field loss in normal tension glaucoma + to determine the risks and side effects of the treatment required to achieve low IOP
- Study found
  - IOP is part of the pathology
  - IOP lowering by at least 30% slowed field loss
  - This IOP was achieved with medicines alone in 50%
  - Surgery increased cataract
  - Rate of field progression slow in normal tension glaucoma even if untreated
  - Prognostic factors for progression – disc haemorrhage, migraine, female gender
  - Number needed to treat = 17 (i.e. IOP needs to be lowered by 30% in 17 CNTGS-like patients in order to prevent field loss in 1)

6

Lens

Classification of cataracts 128
Congenital lens defects 128
Ectopia lentis 129
Senile cataracts 131
Secondary cataracts 131
Pre-operative evaluation 132
Biometry 133
Intraocular lenses 134
Viscoelastics 135
Surgical complications 136
Endophthalmitis 138
Post-operative astigmatism 139
Developmental cataracts 139
Cataract surgery in special situations 141
Cataract surgery in uveitis 142
Lens-induced uveitis and glaucoma 144

Classification of cataracts

■ Developmental	□ Congenital □ Infantile (first 3 months)
■ Juvenile	□ Aetiology and morphology as for developmental
■ Presenile	□ Aetiology and morphology as for senile
■ Senile/age-related	
■ Secondary	□ Traumatic □ Ocular diseases □ Systemic diseases □ Metabolic diseases □ Drug induced

Congenital lens defects

Congenital aphakia

- Rare
- Primary – failure to form from surface ectoderm
- Secondary – spontaneous lens absorption
- Usually associated with other ocular abnormalities

Lenticonus

- Localised cone-shaped deformity
- Posterior more common than anterior
- Posterior – usually unilateral and axial
- Anterior – often bilateral and associated with Alport syndrome
- Oil droplet appearance on retroillumination
- Defect and surrounding cortex may opacify

Lentiglobus

- Abnormal globular shaped lens
- 95% unilateral
- May involve the entire lens or just the posterior aspect

Coloboma

- Primary – peripheral lens; isolated anomaly
- Secondary – flattening or indentation of lens periphery due to lack of ciliary body + zonule development
- Usually inferior
- May be associated with uveal colobomas and localised cataract

Mittendorf's dot

- Common remnant of the tunica vasculosa lentis
- Small, dense white spot inferonasal to the posterior pole
- Marks the place where the hyaloid artery came into contact with the posterior lens surface in utero

Epicapsular star

- Common remnant of the tunica vasculosa lentis
- Star-shaped distribution of brown/golden flecks (chicken tracks) on the central anterior capsule

Peter's anomaly

- Part of the mesenchymal dysgenesis syndrome spectrum
- Cenral/paracentral corneal opacity (leukoma)
- Thinning or absent adjacent endothelium and Descemet's membrane
- May have
  - Lens-corneal adhesions
  - Cortical or polar cataract
  - Misshapen lens with anterior displacement in anterior chamber
  - Microspherophakia

Microphakia

- Small lens, normal shape

Microspherophakia

- Lens small in diameter and spherical in shape
- High myopia (lenticular)
- Isolated or in association with Weill-Marchesani syndrome, Peter's anomaly, Marfan's syndrome, Apert, Lowe's syndrome, congenital rubella
- Can have pupil block glaucoma worsened by miotics
- Treatment: Mydriatics, peripheral iridotomy

Aniridia

- A panocular syndrome
- Complete or partial iris absence
- Anterior and posterior lens opacities at birth
- Cortical, subcapsular + lamellar cataracts develop in 50–85% within the first and second decades
- ± Ectopia lentis

6

Ectopia lentis

Definitions

- Displacement of lens – congenital, developmental or acquired
- Subluxation → partially displaced
- Luxated/dislocated → lens completely displaced from pupil

Associated findings

- Decreased vision
- Astigmatism
- Monocular diplopia
- Iridodenesis
- Cataract
- Displacement of lens into the anterior chamber or vitreous
- Pupil block glaucoma

Causes

- Isolated genetic
  - Simple ectopia lentis
  - Ectopia lentis and pupillae
- Systemic associations
  - Marfan's syndrome
  - Homocystinuria
  - Weill-Marchesani syndrome
  - Hyperlysinaemia
  - Sulphite oxidase deficiency

- Ehlers-Danlos syndrome
- Mandibulofacial dysostosis
- Crouzon's disease
- Refsum's disease
- Sturge-Weber syndrome
- Ocular associations
  - Trauma (most common cause)
  - Congenital anomalies (persistent hyperplastic primary vitreous, aniridia, Rieger's syndrome, megalocornea)
  - Buphthalmos
  - High myopia
  - Inflammation/uveitis
  - Mature cataract
  - Retinitis pigmentosa

Isolated genetic

- Simple – autosomal dominant, congenital or late onset
- Ectopia lentis et pupillae
  - Autosomal recessive, pupil ectopic and slit-shaped
  - Lens and pupil displaced in opposite directions

Marfan's syndrome

- Autosomal dominant, variable penetrance
- Mutations in fibrillin gene on chromosome 15q
- 15% no family history, ?increased paternal age a factor
- Defect of collagen metabolism
- Skeletal
  - Arachnodactyly, scoliosis, pectus excavatum, high arched palate
- CVS
  - Aortic dilatation, dissecting aortic aneurysm, floppy mitral valve
- Ocular
  - Myopathic facies, enophthalmos, refractive errors, strabismus in 20% exo > eso, increased corneal diameter, angle abnormalities, increased iris transillumination, ectopic lens superotemporal in 50–80%, retinal detachment
- 50–80% have ectopia lentis
  - Usually bilateral, symmetric + superotemporal
  - Usually congenital and stable but may progress
  - Treatment: Spectacles or contact lenses usually satisfactory
  - May need mydriasis
  - Lensectomy may be necessary – associated with high rates of vitreous loss + retinal detachment

Homocystinuria

- Autosomal recessive, inborn error of methionine metabolism
- Elevated serum levels of methionine + homocysteine
- Mental retardation – in 50% cases
- Skeletal – similar to Marfan's syndrome, tall
- CVS – vessel intimal and endothelial changes → obstruction, hypertension, coronary artery occlusion, thrombotic occlusion, peripheral gangrene, retinal artery occlusion, retinal vein occlusion
- Ocular – ectopic lens inferonasally in 90%, myopia, microphthalmos, aniridia
- Ectopia occurs in 70% of cases by 8 years; bilateral + symmetric
- Zonules have high concentration of cysteine – deficiency disrupts them
- Dietary supplementation reduces incidence

Weill-Marchesani syndrome

- Autosomal recessive inheritance
- Skeletal – opposite of Marfan's syndrome
- Ocular – microspherophakia, myopia, lens ectopia inferior and forwards, anterior chamber angle abnormalities, megalocornea

Hyperlysinaemia

- Inborn error of lysine metabolism
- Mental retardation + muscular hypotony

Sulphite oxidase deficiency

- Rare, autosomal recessive disorder of sulphur metabolism
- Mental retardation + seizures

Complications

- Refractive errors (myopia, astigmatism)
- Uveitis (contact irritation, protein leakage)
- Glaucoma (variable mechanisms)
- Retinal detachment
- Cataract

Management

- Genetic conselling, refer paediatrician or physician, no contact sports
- Correct refractive error, ± aphakic correction
- Treat amblyopia
- Mydriatic, optical iridectomy
- Treat glaucoma, uveitis
- Retinal detachment repair
- Pars plana lensectomy, ± prophylactic retinal detachment surgery; indications for lensectomy – cataract, diplopia, unable to improve visual acuity, anterior chamber dislocation, lens-induced uveitis

Senile cataracts

- Pathogenesis multifactorial + poorly understood

Aetiology

- Daylight, diet, diarrhoea/dehydration, deficiency of glutathione reductase, drugs
- UV light → tryptophan oxidation → protein breakdown → decrease in enzyme activity → decrease in ATP → Na-K pump breakdown
  - Also causes climatic droplet keratopathy and pseudo capsular exfoliation; therefore, all three often occur together
  - There is limited evidence that UVB causes cortical + posterior subcapsular cataracts; there is no evidence that it causes nuclear cataracts
- Normal ageing changes – nuclear sclerosis and urochrome deposition with brunescence
- Dehydrational crisis (note: presenile) – increased capsular permeability
- Glutathione reductase deficiency – due to dietary deficiency of riboflavin
- Drugs – cadmium in tobacco smoke; vitamin C may be protective against this effect

Morphology

- Early
  - Nuclear – sclerosis and brunescence
  - Cortical/cuneiform – vacuoles → water clefts → opacities
  - Subcapsular/cupuliform – posterior subcapsular occurs more commonly than anterior subcapsular
  - Early polychromatic lustre → opacity
- Intermediate – mature
- Late
  - Morgagnian cataract (liquefied cortex)
  - Hypermature (cortex leaks out and capsule shrinks; may contain iridescent cholesterol crystals)

Prevention

- UV protection
- Vitamin E and C supplements → free radical scavengers
- Aspirin – ? acetylation of lens proteins → protection against glycation and carbamylation

Secondary cataracts

Complicated cataract

- Iridocyclitis/uveitis
- Fuchs' heterochromic iridocyclitis (70%)
- Ocular degenerations – high myopia, retinal dystrophy, retinal detachment,

6

essential iris atrophy, absolute glaucoma, intraocular neoplasia, ocular ischaemia, retinitis pigmentosa

Traumatic cataract

- Heat (infrared) – glassblowers – outer layers of the lens capsule peel off as a single layer
- Microwave
- Chemical injuries
- Electric shock – protein coagulation
- Irradiation – up to 20 years later
- Concussion injury
- Perforating injury
- Retained IOFB (Fe → siderosis bulbi and Cu → chalcosis)
- Vossius' ring – blunt trauma

Drug induced

- Corticosteroids – systemic, topical, subconjunctival, nasal sprays, eyelid steroid creams
  Study of patients followed for 1–4 years
  - 10 mg/day → 11% had cataract
  - 10–15 mg/day → 30% had cataract
  - 15 mg/day → 80% had cataract
  - 50% of patients post PK, receiving 2.4 drops/day for 10.5 months
- Pilocarpine – up to 20%; posterior cortical + nuclear
- Phenothiazines – pigment deposition in the anterior lens epithelium (dose + duration dependent)
- Amiodarone – rarely significant
- Statins – only in excessive doses

Systemic associations

Musculoskeletal
- Myotonic dystrophy
- Dwarfism
- Mandibulofacial dysostosis
- Craniofacial dysostosis
- Lawrence-Moon-Biedl syndrome
- Osteogenesis imperfecta
- Hallermann-Streiff syndrome
- Stickler syndrome

Metabolic
- Diabetes
  - True
  - Early senile (10% of patients with senile cataract have diabetes)
- Hypocalcaemia
- Hypoglycaemia
- Wilson's disease (sunflower cataract)
- Lowe's syndrome (oculocerebrorenal syndrome)
- Homocystinuria
- Hypothyroidism
- Galactosaemia (cataract may disappear on treatment) (20% of presenile cataract are heterozygous for galactosaemia)
- Aminoaciduria
- Phenylketonuria
- Hurler's syndrome
- Refsum's disease
- Fabry's disease

Skin
- Atopic dermatitis (25%) – shield-like plaques
- Rothmund's syndrome
- Werner's syndrome
- Congenital iccthyosis
- Incontinentia pigmenti

Lifestyle and nutrition
- No relationship to a healthy lifestyle
- Slight decreased incidence of cataract with > twice a week ingestion of cooked spinach

Ischaemia
- Can occur in Takayasu arteritis, Buerger's disease, anterior segment ischaemia

Pre-operative evaluation

- Evaluation of patient
  - Visual acuity related to lifestyle
  - General medical condition (suitability for anaesthesia)
- Documentation of visual function
  - Snellen acuity with best refraction

- Visual acuity for near and far; nuclear lens opacities → decreased near acuity
- Glare disability (especially PSCLO)
- Contrast sensitivity
- Myopic shift (nuclear cataracts)
- Monocular diplopia (beam splitting opacity)

- Ocular motility
  - Tropias that may decompensate
  - Unrecognised amblyopia
- Examination of lens and fundus
  - Dilate pupil; examine with slit lamp and ophthalmoscope
  - Lens opacity metre
  - Check for pseudocapsular exfoliation
  - Check lens position
- Examination of iris
  - Check colour, dilatation, PS
- Examination of cornea
  - Guttata
  - Pachymetry (> 640 μ due to stromal oedema → poor pronosis for post-op corneal clarity)
- Endothelial cell count
  - Pre-op 2 200–2 600 – no risk
  - 1 500–2 200 – risk
  - < 1 500 – high risk
  - Also look for abnormal morphology
- Assessment of macular/retinal function
  - On-off tests
    - Light perception + light projection; fix and follow light
    - Afferent pupil defect
    - Colour identification
    - Maddox rod – lost red line → large scotoma
    - Two point light discrimination
    - Purkinje's entoptic phenomena
    - Maxwell's spot
    - Haidinger brushes
    - Blue field entoptic test
    - Photostress test
  - Recorded signal tests
    - Ultrasound B scan
    - EOG + ERG
    - VER
  - Retinal acuity tests
    - Potential acuity metre; measures acuity with Snellen letters
    - Laser interferometry; measures acuity with grating charts
- Measurements
  - Refraction
  - Biometry
  - Corneal topography
  - Corneal pachymetry

6

Biometery

IOL calculation formulae

First generation

- Based mainly on IOL position in eye, therefore anterior chamber depth most important e.g. SRK I

Second generation

- Importance of axial length e.g. SRK II

Third generation

- K readings and more exact IOL position depending on lens type e.g. Holladay I, Hoffer Q, SRK/T

Fourth generation

- Corneal diameter, lens thickness, refractive error, age, IOL-specific position e.g. Holladay II

Axial length (mm) formulae	
<19 mm	Holladay II
19–22 mm (8% of eyes)	Hoffer Q
22–24.5 mm (72% of eyes)	All formulas except SRK I
24.6–26 mm (15% of eyes)	Holladay
>26 mm (5% of eyes)	SRK/T or Holladay II

- To obtain a rapid approximate IOL power – 18D + (pre-op refraction × 1.6)
- Can be used as a quick double-check
- Regression formulas based on:
  - Corneal power
  - Anterior chamber depth post-op
  - Axial length
- Anterior chamber depth is estimated from measuring eyes with IOLs similar to that planned
- SRK (Sanders-Retzlaff-Kraff)
  - P = A –2.5L –0.9K
  - The A constant has no units; it relates lens power to the axial length and Ks; it is specific for each IOL design, differing because of its intended location and orientation in the eye
  - P = power
    A = constant
    L = axial length
    K = average keratometry
- Potential calculation errors
  - L measurement errors (2.5D per mm of L error, more in short eyes)
  - K errors (1D K error → 1D refractive error)
  - Surface drying
  - High astigmatism
  - Regression formulas are linear but the power result is not linear for high myopes and hyperopes
- Immersion A scan technique – avoids pressure on the cornea → more accurate L
- Sometimes velocity of the sound waves in the eye differs from the norm, giving inaccurate L; silicone oil in the vitreous → slower → falsely long L
- IOL Master (Zeiss)
  - Optical coherence biometry
  - No touching required
  - Measures L, K and anterior chamber depth
  - Problems with dense NS and PSCLO
- Myopes never likely to be hyperopic and vice versa
- Aim for –0.50 to –1.50 because small errors either side will result in functional vision

Intraocular lenses

IOL materials

- Poly methylmethacrylate (PMMA)
- Acrylic
  - Hydrophilic
  - Hydrophobic
- Hydrogel
- Silicone
- Collamer (a co-polymer of collagen and polyHEMA)
  - Supposed to very biocompatible because it gets coated in the body's own fibronectin
- Haptics
  - PMMA
  - Polypropelene
  - Proline
  - Polyimide

Surface modifications

- Heparin, indomethacin, fibroblast growth factor, saporin

Lens designs

- Anterior chamber IOLs
  - Results may be inferior to PCIOLs
  - Considered a safe alternative to sutured-in PCIOL
  - High incidence of RD + CMO, although mostly because the surgery had been complicated, necessitating the ACIOL implant
  - Pseudophakic bullous keratopathy can occur long term
- Posterior chamber IOLs
  - Rigid or flexible
  - Biconvex
  - Laser ridges on optic facilitate YAG by separating the capsule and the lens
  - UV light absorbing chromophores → to protect the retina in theory
  - PMMA
  - Acrylic
  - Silicone
  - Collamer
  - Square-edge technology
  - Single piece and three piece

- Suture fixated IOLs
  - Eyelets moulded in the haptics for suture fixation
- Special-use IOLs
  - Opaque flanges to decrease glare in aniridia + coloboma
- Multifocal IOLs
  - Refractive
  - Diffractive
- Toric IOLs
- Blue-blocker + UV blocker IOLs
- Iris clip lenses
- Phakic IOLs
  - Sulcus fixated
  - Iris clip

Contraindications

- No absolute contraindications
- Diabetes – proliferative retinopathy → IOL no longer considered detrimental
- Uveitis – recurrent or active (except Fuchs')
- Chronic open angle glaucoma – anterior chamber IOL contraindicated
- Endothelial dystrophy – AC IOL contraindicated

Complications

- Cornea
  - Endothelial cell loss → corneal decompensation
  - ICLE → 8–12% endothelial cell loss
  - ECLE → 12–20% endothelial cell loss
  - IOL without viscoelastic → 30–70% endothelial cell loss
  - Due to mechanical trauma at the time of surgery
  - Due to intermittent endothelial touch with anterior chamber IOLs
  - Due to persistent anterior chamber inflammation
  - Pseudophakic corneal decompensation – an important indication for corneal grafting
- Anterior chamber angle
  - Erosion + damage by AC IOL footplate → secondary glaucoma
- Iris
  - Chafing + erosion → UGH syndrome (uveitis, glaucoma, hyphaema) due to disruption of blood aqueous barrier; iridodialysis, iris prolapse, peripheral anterior synechiae, pupil capture, iris tuck, pigment dispersion
- Posterior capsule
  - Opacification rate is decreased with IOL
- Retina
  - Cystoid macular oedema – no change in incidence with IOL
  - Retinal detachment – no change in incidence with IOL
- IOL position
  - Decentration, dislocation
- anterior chamber IOL following ECLE with ruptured posterior capsule
  - There is increased severity and duration of uveitis if a primary anterior chamber IOL is inserted
  - There is no change in the incidence of cystoid macular oedema or retinal detachment if an AC IOL is inserted
- Sutured IOLs
  - Choroidal detachment
  - Retinal detachment
  - Suture erosion

Viscoelastics

Uses

- To protect the endothelium from mechanical trauma
- To maintain an open intraocular space during surgery
- Integral part of surgical procedures – viscosurgery – e.g. viscocanalostomy

Viscoelastics – two types

- Cohesive – with high molecular weight, high surface tension, e.g. Healon, Provisc. Tends to be big and bulky and does not coat tissue

- Dispersive – with low molecular weight, low surface tension, e.g. Viscoat. Smooth and coats tissue
- There is a spectrum ranging from most cohesive to most dispersive

Most dispersive					**Most cohesive**
Viscoat and Ocucoat	**Provisc**	**Amvisc**	**Amvisc plus**	**Healon**	**Healon GV**

Advantages and disadvantages

- Cohesives
  - Best for maintaining anterior chamber, capsulorrhexis and creating space
  - Easy to remove because of high surface tension
  - Can lose a large amount through wound during capsulorrhexis if the wound is open
  - Tend to go away with the first vacuum; do not protect endothelium well
- Dispersives
  - Best for protecting the corneal endothelium, sealing capsular tears, holding back vitreous and keeping iris at bay
  - Do not maintain space well
  - Attract particles to endothelium and increases risk of burn
- Both cohesive and dispersive can be used together during cataract surgery
- In the soft shell technique, dispersive is first injected to coat the endothelium and cohesive injected next to fill the anterior chamber
- This improves endothelium protection in cornea with low endothelial cell count

Physical properties of viscoelastics

- Viscoelasticity
  - When transmitted at high frequency → acts as an elastic/gel compound, low frequency → acts as a viscous compound
  - It can therefore be injected via a small cannula but still maintain an intraocular space with an open incision
- Viscosity
  - Resistance to flow
  - High viscosity holds its shape better than low
  - A function of molecular weight
  - High viscosity → Healon; low → Viscoat
- Pseudoplasticity
  - Transforms from a gel to liquid when under pressure
- Surface tension
  - Coating ability
  - Low tension → better coating
- Cohesive vs dispersive

Desired properties

- Maintains space
- Spreads + protects tissues
- Coats tissues and instruments
- Non-toxic
- Non-inflammatory
- Optically clear but visible
- Neutral effect on IOP
- Protects endothelium

Surgical complications

Anaesthesia

- General anaesthetic complications
- Local anaesthesia
  - Retrobulbar haemorrhage
  - Perforation of the globe

Intraoperative

- Corneal abrasions
- Corneal wound burn
- Iris prolapse
- Iridodialysis
- Hyphaema
- Descemet's membrane detachment

- Endothelial injury
  - mechanical
  - toxic
- Zonular dialysis
- Posterior capsule tear
- Vitreous loss
- Posterior lens dislocation
- Suprachoroidal haemorrhage
- Expulsive choroidal haemorrhage

Post-operative – early

- Refractive surprise
  - myopia
  - hyperopia
- Corneal oedema
- Endophthalmitis
  - sterile
  - infectious
- Toxic anterior segment syndrome
- Wound leak/gape/dehiscence
- Iris prolapse
- Pupil distortion
- Acute anterior uveitis
- Retained crystalline lens material causing:
  - persistent uveitis
  - glaucoma
  - hypotony
- Raised intraocular pressure – secondary to:
  - retained anterior chamber viscoelastic
  - uveitis
  - pupil block
  - hyphaema
- Vitreous wick
- Ptosis
- Diplopia

Post-operative – late

- Endophthalmitis
- Endothelial decompensation
- Chronic anterior uveitis – low grade intraocular pathogens
- Cystoid macular oedema (Irivine-Gass syndrome)
- Retinal detachment – especially following vitreous loss
- Astigmatism
- Posterior capsule opacity
- IOL decentration or malposition

Cataract surgery and diabetic retinopathy

- 10% of cataract patients have diabetes
- Removal of the lens → increased risk of worsening of the retinopathy + increased risk of iris rubeosis
- Following cataract surgery, 40% show progression of retinopathy
- This is due to
  - ? Removal of chemical + mechanical angiogenic inhibitor
  - ? Posterior vitreous detachment → scaffold for new vessels
  - ? Post-operative intraocular inflammation
  - ? Decreased secretion of vasoinhibitory substances in RPE
  - ? Increased synthesis of angiogenic factors in the iris stroma
- Visual results following cataract surgery in diabetics
  - Non-diabetics + diabetics with no retinopathy – 90% achieve 6/12 or better
  - Diabetics with background retinopathy + no maculopathy – 85% achieve 6/12 or better
  - Diabetics with quiescent proliferative retinopathy + no maculopathy – 60% achieve 6/12 or better
  - Diabetics with background retinopathy + maculopathy – 40% achieve 6/12 or better
  - Diabetics with quiescent proliferative retinopathy + maculopathy – 10% achieve 6/12 or better
  - Diabetics with active proliferative retinopathy – 6% achieve 6/12 or better

Breakdown of blood aqueous barrier following cataract surgery

Causes

- Intra-operative iris injury + diabetes are the two most important factors in BAB breakdown

Prevention

- Subconjunctival steroids have no effect on preventing BAB breakdown
- Post-op steroid + indomethacin drops → decreased BAB breakdown

Prognosis

- 80% recover within 3 months

Complications

- Posterior capsule opacification, cystoid macular oedema, continued endothelial cell loss, cytological reaction on lens surface
- Cytological reaction on lens surface
  - Small cell response – fibroblasts; deposited early and then disappear; due to BAB breakdown
  - Giant cell response – epithelioid cells; deposited late (after 3 months), then disappear; due to a foreign body reaction to the IOL
- Surface modification of IOL → less cytological reaction

Possible causes of diplopia post cataract surgery

Monocular

- Macaine toxicity of extraocular muscles
- Unmasking of macular pathology
- Beam splitting opacity

Binocular

- Pre-existing squint, previously corrected by the prismatic effect of glasses
- Increase in accommodation in a previously myopic patient
- High AC/A ratio in a previously myopic patient (needed to converge previously, but not accommodate – now has to do both)
- Refractive accommodative esotropia – in hyperopes; the new refraction may cause decompensation – patient exo because does not have to accommodate any more

Endophthalmitis

Prevention

- Most organisms are from the patient's own lid flora
- No studies have demonstrated efficacy of pre-op antibiotics or antibiotics in the infusion
- 5% povidone-iodine prewash before surgery
- Drape lashes out of surgical field
- Limit intraocular instrumentation
- Meticulous wound closure
- Up to 35% of cataract surgeries result in bacterial inoculation of the anterior chamber
- Intracameral cefuroxine after surgery
- Scleral tunnel shown to have slightly lower rate of endophthalmitis than clear cornea, probably due to less wound leak

Clinical features

- May present acutely (virulent organisms) or chronically (less virulent organisms)
- Pain, loss of vision, floaters, photophobia, lid swelling, chemosis, anterior chamber reaction ± hypopyon, vitreous cells, corneal oedema, retinal haemorrhages

Diagnosis

- Acute endophthalmitis
  - Two to 5 days post-op
  - Fulminant course
- Chronic endophthalmitis
  - Weeks or months later
  - Chronic iritis or granulomatous uveitis
  - Decreased VA
  - Little or no pain

Differential diagnosis
- Non-infectious (sterile) iritis – rare
- Toxic materials in anterior chamber – Toxic anterior segment syndrome (TASS)

Endophthalmitis Vitrectomy Study
- Patients randomised to
  - Immediate vitrectomy
  - Or vitreous tap/biopsy
- Further randomised to
  - IV antibiotics (Ceftazidime + Amikacin)
  - Or no antibiotics IV
- All received
  - IVT Amikacin 0.4 mg/ml
  - Vancomycin 1 mg/ml
  - Subconjunctival vancomycin 25 mg, Ceftazidime 100 mg, Dexameth 6 mg
- Vitreous cultures positive in 69%
- Gram positive, coagulase negative staphylococci (especially staph epidermidis) – 70%
- Other gram positives – 15%
- Gram negatives – 5.9%
- Polymicrobial growth – 9.3%
- Final post-treatment VA > 6/12 in 53%, 75% > 6/36
- Final outcome same for all groups if presenting VA better than light perception
- Vitrectomy beneficial only for those presenting with LP

Treatment
- Depends on severity + duration of infection
- Severe cases with very poor vision probably warrant early vitrectomy
- Otherwise vitreous tap for culture + injection of antibiotics
- IVT antibiotics: vomcomycin 1 mg/0.1 ml Ceftazidime 2.25 mg/0.1 ml
- Aminoglycosides may cause retinal toxicity
- IVT steroids controversial
- IVT antibiotics may be repeated depending on clinical response + cultures
- ± Oral ciprofloxacin 750 mg BD – good vitreous penetration
- ± Topical steroids + atropine

Post-operative astigmatism

Aetiology
- Pre-existing
- Position of incision
  - Corneal – less late astigmatism
  - Limbal – unpredictable
  - Scleral – less early astigmatism
- Type of incision (scleral tunnel least astigmatism)
- Size of incision – smaller = less
- Suture placement and technique
- IOL → improper placement, lenticular astigmatism

Phaco
- Scleral tunnel 3.2 mm → 0.4D
- Clear cornea 3.5 mm incision → 0.75D superior, 0.5D temporal
- Minimal pre-op astigmatism → do a corneal temporal
- 0.5–1.5 with the rule astigmatism → do a superior corneal or scleral tunnel

Developmental cataracts

Incidence
- One in 4 000 to 10 000

Aetiology
- Genetic – 33%; autosomal dominant, autosomal recessive, or sex linked recessive
- Chromosomal disorders – trisomy 21 (60%), 18, 13
- Trauma, ionising radiation
- Drugs – steroids, sulphonamides, chlorpromazine
- Infections
  - Rubella, other viruses (herpes, mumps, flu, polio, CMV, measles)

6

- Syphilis, toxoplasmosis
- If due to rubella, there is viable virus in the lens; therefore treat vigorously with intra-operative and post-operative steroids to prevent uveitis

- Maternal diabetes
- Maternal malnutrition – riboflavin and tryptophan deficiency
- Metabolic
- Galactokinase deficiency → bilateral lamellar catarcts
    - Galactosaemia → oil droplet cataracts
- Other ocular associations – persistent foetal vasculature, coloboma, ectopia lentis, aniridia, microphthalmos, retinopathy of prematurity, uveitis, retinoblastoma, anterior chamber cleavage disorders
- Prematurity + low birth weight
- Systemic diseases – juvenile idiopathic arthritis, neurofibromatosis
- Idiopathic – 30–50%; most unilateral cataracts are idiopathic, and 50% of bilateral cataracts are idiopathic

Morphology

- Usually stationary, may be progressive
- Tunica vasculosa lentis remnants – anterior
    - Pupil membrane remnants
    - Epicapsular star
    - Retroiridal pigmented lines
- Tunica vasculosa lentis remnants – posterior
    - Mittendorf's dot
    - Whorls, arcuate line
- Capsular – anterior capsule, rarely posterior capsule
- Polar – anterior and posterior, of capsule and adjacent cortex, may project forward or backward
- Anterior axial embryonal – of anterior Y suture
- Anterior and posterior stellate – of Y sutures
- Pulverulent – of inner foetal nucleus (small, therefore also asymptomatic)
- Zonular/lamellar – short-term exposure to noxious influence; thickness depends on duration, location depends on age; usually outer foetal or inner adult nucleus; may have envelope and riders
- Rare types – diffuse nuclear, total, fusiform, pisciform, spirochaetiform, floriform, spear, coralliform

Work-up

- VA assessment, presence of nystagmus, pupil reflexes, fundoscopy, morphology, dysmorphism, old photographs, B-scan/CT if masquerade considered, remember abuse
- Bilateral
    - Family history
    - Paediatric evaluation
    - Torch screen
    - Urine reducing substances (galactokinase deficiency, galactosaemia → reversible early) and amino acids (Lowe's syndrome)
- Unilateral
    - Trauma history
    - Slit lamp examination of morphology (persistent hyperplastic primary vitreous, anterior polar, posterior lenticonus)
    - Torch screen (one-third of rubella cataracts are unilateral)

Bilateral cataracts

- Small, axial, visually insignificant → do not operate
- May need mydriasis only
- Fixation reflex develops by 3 months; if dense cataracts are not operated by then → nystagmus; VA seldom better than 6/60 with nystagmus
- Ideally, do both eyes before 3 months (even 6 weeks)

Unilateral cataracts

- Amblyopia is a problem
- Surgery before 6 weeks is recommended

Surgery

- Differences from adult surgery
  - Axial length changes
  - Corneal curvature changes
  - Tissues more reactive → inflammation + fibrosis
  - Sclera less rigid
  - Capsule very elastic
  - Eye smaller
  - Amblyopia potential
  - Long pseudophakic lifespan
- Superior scleral tunnel incision favoured
- ± Anterior chamber maintainer
- Suture all wounds
- High viscosity viscoelastics for capsulotomy (can use vitrector)
- Aspirate with vitrector or phaco tip or simcoe
- Posterior capsulotomy, limited anterior vitrectomy ± posterior IOL capture
- Posterior capsular opacity takes 2 years on average, therefore on do a primary capsulotomy in children who will not be YAG candidates in the next 18 months

Post-operative care

- Intensive topical steroids
- One month of cycloplegia

Complications

- Glaucoma (incidence lower in patients receiving an IOL)
- PCO
- Late retinal detachment

Prognosis

- Depends on age of onset, age at surgery, density of opacity, unilateral or bilateral, compliance with aphakic correction + amblyopia treatment
- Unilateral
  - Removed within 4 months → 6/12 or better possible
  - Removed between 4 and 12 months → 6/18 to 6/24
  - May get good vision right up to the age of 5 as long as there was some normal visual experience prior to cataract development

Correction of aphakia

- Refraction possible within 1 week of surgery because wounds small and healing fast
- Aphakic glasses: Single vision for infants (activities all near), bifocals for older
- Over-plus them
  - < 2 years – +3.00 to +4.00
  - 2 to 4 – +3.00
  - 4 – +2.50
  - 6 to 7 – +1.00
- Contact lenses
  - Soft hydrophilic daily wear
  - Weekly silicone available (increased risk of keratitis)
- IOL
  - < 1 yr – generally not recommended
  - 1–2 years – grey area
  - > 2 years – primary IOL recommended
- IOL power: Intra-op A-scan, hand held keratometer; SRK-T formula
- < 2 years – 80% of measured power
- 2 to 5 years – 90 % of measured power
- > 5 years – emmetropia
- PMMA or acrylic lens
- IOL is relatively contraindicated in microcornea, nanophthalmos, corneal endothelial dystrophy, rubella cataract, uncontrolled glaucoma, persistent foetal vasculature, uveitis

Cataract surgery in special situations

Anticoagulation/bleeding disorders

- Small additional risk of intra- and peri-operative bleeding
- Main complications – subconjunctival haemorrhage, lid ecchymosis, incisional bleeding, rarely hyphaema
- Warfarin → after stopping takes 3–5 days before normal coagulation

- Asprin → 10 days
- Topical anaesthesia, clear corneal incision + IOL in bag best

Diabetes

- Withhold oral hypoglycaemics on the morning of surgery
- Insulin should be adjusted depending on physicians
- Place first on theatre list
- Avoid silicone IOLs in case PPV with silicone oil required
- Use a large, 6 mm optic to facilitate peripheral retinal examination
- Pupil may not dilate → hooks, pupillotomy, stretching
- Focal + PRP before + after as necessary
- Protect corneal epithelium and endothelium

Obesity

- Reverse Trendelenburg
- Neck extension
- Digital massage to reduce IOP
- Phaco not ECCE

Acne rosacea and blepharitis

- Pre-op warm compresses, lid scrubs ± doxycycline

Keratoconjunctivitis sicca

- Problem of corneal melting
- Control dry eye pre-op with non-preserved tears + punctal occlusion
- Avoid prolonged post-op antibiotics + steroids
- Topical NSAIDs associated with corneal melting

Pemphigoid

- Control with steroids + immunosuppressives pre-op
- Condition may reactivate after surgical trauma

Triple procedure

- 90% clear grafts at 1 year
- 75% → 6/12 best corrected vision or better

Nanophthalmos

- Rare – eye pathologically small
- Ratio of lens volume to eye volume high
- Shallow anterior chamber, narrow angles, thickened sclera
- Risk of intra-operative or post-operative uveal effusion

Risk of expulsive haemorrhage

- Advanced age, uncontrolled glaucoma, myopia, choroidal sclerosis, hypertension, arteriosclerosis, anticoagulation therapy, bleeding diathesis, recent trauma, active inflammation, prolonged hypotony, previous expulsive haemorrhage in the fellow eye
- Do a phaco
- Use a Honan balloon
- ± Prepare conjunctiva for a posterior sclerostomy if needed

Glaucoma

- Two-thirds of glaucoma patients have a rise in IOP of 7–10 mmHg after phaco in first 24 hours
- Vitreous loss → loose zonules
- CMO → higher risk in glaucoma
- Prostaglandin analogues may be associated with increased post-op inflammation
- 30–50% of trabs fail after cataract surgery with conjunctival manipulation
- Use clear corneal, temporal approach
- Bleb survival 3 times higher in phaco-trab than ECCE-trab

Cataract surgery in uveitis

Incidence of cataract in uveitis

- Common complication of any kind of uveitis
- Chronic anterior uveitis → 80%

- Fuchs' → 50%
- Intermediate → 45%

Considerations

- The diagnosis
- Prognosis
- Appropriate surgical timing and technique
- Type of IOL
- Surgical complications
- 'Only eyes' and children common

Diagnosis

- Important to establish cause of uveitis if possible
- Clinical course, treatment, visual outcome, complications → directly related to cause
- E.g. sarcoid → very good prognosis with cataract surgery once disease inactive

Patient selection

- Visually significant cataract with inflammation controlled
- Obscured fundal view in posterior segment pathology
- Cataract that obscures posterior segment view for post segment surgery

Prognosis

- Limited by RD, optic atrophy, vitreous opacities, CMO, ERM, glaucoma, maculopathy
- Potential VA can be estimated with inferometry
- Pre-op B-scan

Pre-op inflammation control

- Abolish all active inflammation for at least 3 months prior to surgery (6 months in Behçets)
- Zero tolerance approach, except in phacoanigenic + Fuchs'
- Additional pre-op anti-inflammatory treatment – systemic steroids
- Toxo near the posterior pole → use prophylactic antiparasitics
- Recommended regimens – no universally accepted regimen

6

Peri-operative steroid options for uveitic cataracts

- Two days pre-op
  - PO prednisolone 1 mg/kg
  - G. predforte BD
  - G. acular QID
  - PO NSAID BD
- Two weeks pre-op
  - PO prednisolone 0.5 mg/kg + taper slowly
  - Over 2–3 months by 5 mg per week
- Single dose IVI methylprednisolone 30 minutes pre-op
- Oral steroids 40 mg daily x 2 weeks pre-op, taper by 5 mg weekly post-op (IVT steroids may take over)
- IV methylpred 500 mg at surgery, then 2–7 days later, then weekly PRN
- Children
  - 0.5 mg/kg x 2 weeks, 2.5–5 mg/wk taper
  - IV MP 125–250 mg – same way

Operative complications

- Uveitis exacerbation
- Macular oedema
- Corneal oedema, glaucoma, hypotony, choroidal effusion

Surgical technique

- Phaco superior – smaller wound, less inflammation, less CMO, less uveitis relapse, fewer complications
- Pupil → may need hooks
- Capsulorhexis ± tryphan blue

IOL

- Controversial in JIA
- Acrylic as safe as PMMA
- Many avoid silicone
- 'In bag' placement essential

Post-op

- Intensive topicals
- Taper treatment back to pre-op maintenance levels
- Anterior uveitis
  - 96% improved VA
  - 66% better than 6/12
  - 45% complicated
  - Severe uveitis + increased CMO post-op
  - PCO common
- Posterior uveitis
  - 81% improved vision
  - 46% better than 6/12
  - 65% complicated
  - Severe uveitis + CMO
- CMO
  - ECCE – 20%
  - Phaco – 5%
  - Treatment: Orbital floor, steroids, increased systemic steroids, additional immune suppression
- PCO
  - Very common, less with acrylic IOL
  - IOL edge design influence
  - Uveitis must be controlled before YAG to reduce risk of CMO

6

Lens-induced uveitis and glaucoma

Phacoantigenic uveitis

- Eye normally tolerant to minute amounts of lens protein
- Large amounts of antigen → inflammation
- Usually due to ruptured capsule
- May be associated with secondary glaucoma
- Late complications – cyclitic membrane, hypotony, phthisis bulbi
- Can rarely cause sympathetic
- Treatment: Lens extraction

Lens-induced glaucoma

Phacolytic

- Complication of mature, hypermature cataract
- Lens proteins leak through a permeable capsule
- Macrophages ingest → trabecular meshwork clogged
- Pain, redness, corneal oedema, white anterior chamber precipitates
- Treatment: Antiglaucoma, topical steroids, lensectomy

Lens-particle glaucoma

- Following injury, ECCE, YAG capsulotomy
- Trabecular meshwork clogged
- Treatment: anti-inflammatory + anti-glaucoma, surgical washout

Phacomorphic

- Pupil block → secondary angle closure
- Treatment: YAG PI, lensectomy

Glaukomflecken

- Grey-white epithelial and anterior cortical lens opacities following episodes of marked IOP rise e.g. in AACG (necrotic lens material)
- Due to necrosis of lens material

7

The uvea

Aniridia 145
Iridocorneal endothelial (ICE) syndrome 146
Iris degenerations and atrophies .. 146
Uveitis classification 147
Clinical features of uveitis 148
Anterior uveitis – causes 148
Arthritis and uveitis 149
Gastrointestinal diseases associated with uveitis 150
Renal diseases associated with uveitis 150
Behçet's disease 150
Sarcoidosis 152
Pars planitis 155
Vogt-Koyanagi-Harada (VKH) syndrome 155
Sympathetic uveitis 156
Fuchs' heterochromic iridocyclitis ... 157
Toxoplasmosis 158
Childhood uveitis 159
Juvenile idiopathic arthritis and uveitis 162
Bacterial endophthalmitis 164
Fungal endophthalmitis 166
Ocular tuberculosis 167
Syphilis 168
Fungal uveitis 168
Viral uveitis 169
Parasitic uveitis 170
Ocular leprosy 171
Uveitis masquerade syndromes ... 172
Uveal tumours 173
Choroidal melanoma 174
Idiopathic multifocal white dot syndromes 177
Steroids 178
Cataract surgery in uveitis 182
Ciliochoroidal detachment 184

Aniridia

Classification of Aniridia	
▪ AN-1 (isolated)	▫ Autosomal dominant → 66% of cases ▫ No systemic implications
▪ AN-2 (Miller's syndrome)	▫ Sporadic deletion of short arm of chromosome 11 → 33% of cases ▫ Associated with Wilm's tumour, genitourinary anomalies and mental retardation
▪ AN-3 (Gillespie's syndrome)	▫ Autosomal recessive, 1% of cases ▫ Associated mental retardation and cerebellar ataxia

Ocular features

- Aniridia – may vary, partial → total
- Corneal lesions – opacity, epibulbar dermoids, microcornea, sclerocornea, keratolenticular adhesions
- Lenticular changes – opacity, subluxation, congenital absence, persistent pupillary membrane
- Fundus lesions – foveal hypoplasia, disc hypoplasia, choroidal colobomas

Pathology

- Iris stump always present, ciliary body may be hypoplastic
- Abnormal iris strands extend over trabecular meshwork; increased during first and second decades

Glaucoma

7

- Occurs in 75% of cases
- Develops in childhood or adulthood
- Treatment is difficult
    - Medical – miotics
    - Surgical – goniotomy, trabeculectomy, cyclocryotherapy, seton implant
    - ? Better results with prophylactic goniotomy to separate iris and trabecular meshwork

Treatment

- Exclude Wilm's
- Cataract extraction
- Contact lens with pupil
- Corneal graft only with limbal stem cells transplant
- Treat glaucoma
- Morcher implant

Iridocorneal endothelial (ICE) syndrome

Pathogenesis

- Basic defect of corneal endothelium; synthesises abnormal collagen, degenerates → corneal oedema, growth of membrane across angle onto iris, contraction → peripheral anterior synechiae + secondary glaucoma, also → pupil distortion (corectopia), thinning of iris, hole formation in iris (pseudopolycoria)
- ? A sequel of herpes simplex virus infection

Triad

- Progressive iris atrophy – corectopia, iris atrophy and pseudopolycoria
- Chandler's syndrome – corneal oedema
- Cogan-Reese syndrome (iris naevus) – nodular lesions of iris and iris atrophy

Features

- Occurs in middle-aged white females, unilateral, no family history
- Beaten metal appearance of posterior cornea, ± corneal oedema
- Peripheral anterior synechiae + secondary glaucoma in 50% of cases
- Iris atrophy, hole formation, pupil distortion

Treatment

- Corneal oedema
    - Medical treatment – 5% NaCl drops
    - Penetrating keratoplasty if persistent
- Glaucoma
    - Medical
    - Trabeculectomy; poor results

Iris degenerations and atrophies

Classification

- Senile atrophy
- Primary atrophies
    - Iridoschisis
    - Iridocorneal endothelial syndrome
- Secondary atrophies

Senile atrophy

- Due to sclerosis of vessels
- Results in thinning of stroma, pigment dispersion, colour change
- Dilator muscle atrophy → senile miosis

Iridoschisis

Aetiology

- Idiopathic
- Senile
- Secondary to trauma, iritis, angle closure glaucoma, use of miotics

Features

- Usually bilateral and inferior
- Meridional cleavage between anterior and posterior stromal layers, anterior layer → loose shreds in anterior chamber

Complications

- Associated with primary angle closure glaucoma in 50–90% of cases
- May cause secondary glaucoma due to mechanical blockage of trabeculum

Treatment

- Medical
- Peripheral iridotomy

Secondary atrophies

- Post-traumatic
- Post-inflammatory
- Glaucomatous (acute angle closure)
- Neurogenic (neurosyphilis)
- Ischaemic (sickle cell disease, quinine toxicity)

Uveitis classification

Anatomical

- Anterior
  - Iritis (iris)
  - Iridocyclitis (iris + pars plicata)
  - Cyclitis – peripheral retinitis (pars plicata)
  - Intermediate – pars planitis (pars plana)
- Posterior
  - Retinitis
  - Retinochoroiditis
  - Chorioretinitis
  - Choroiditis
  - Diffuse – panuveitis

Clinical

- Acute (8 weeks or less)
- Subacute
- Chronic (12 weeks or more)
- Recurrent

Pathological

- Non-granulomatous (non-mutton fat keratic precipitates)
- Granulomatous (mutton fat keratic precipitates)

Aetiological

- Exogenous
  - External injury – traumatic, sympathetic
  - Invasion of micro organisms from outside
- Endogenous
  - Associated with a systemic disease – sarcoidosis, arthritis (ankylosing spondylitis, psoriatic arthritis, juvenile chronic arthritis, Reiter's, relapsing polychondritis), GIT disease (ulcerative colitis, Crohn's), diabetes
- Infections
  - Bacteria – tuberculosis, leprosy, meningococcus, streptococcus, gonococcus, brucellosis
  - Fungi – candida, histoplasmosis, coccidiomycosis, actinomycosis, blastomycosis, aspergillosis, mucormycosis
  - Viruses – herpes zoster, herpes simplex, cytomegalovirus, measles, Epstein-Barr
  - Spirochaetes – syphilis, leptospirosis
  - Protozoa – toxoplasmosis

7

    - ▫ Parasites – toxocariasis, cysticercosis, onchocerciasis, schistosomiasis, echinococcus
- Idiopathic specific uveitis entities – Fuch's, Vogt-Koyanagi-Harada, Behçet's, White Dot syndromes
- Idiopathic non-specific uveitis entities (25% of cases)

Clinical features of uveitis

Anterior uveitis

Symptoms

- Photophobia, pain, redness, decreased vision, lacrimation

Signs

- Injection – circumcorneal
- Keratic precipitates
    - Fresh (non-mutton fat + mutton fat); mutton fat = granulomatous uveitis
    - Old
- Iris nodules – seen in granulomatous uveitis
    - Koeppe nodules around pupil margin
    - Busacca nodules away from pupil margin
- Aqueous cells – light beam 3 mm × 1 mm on high magnification
    - +1 = 5–10 cells
    - +2 = 11–20 cells
    - +3 = 21–50 cells
    - +4 = > 50 cells
    - Hypopyon
- In iritis aqueous cells > anterior vitreous cells
- In pars planitis, anterior vitreous cells > aqueous cells
- Aqueous flare
    - +1 = just detectable
    - +2 = iris details clear
    - +3 = iris details hazy
    - +4 = fibrinous exudates

Intermediate uveitis

Symptoms

- Floaters, ± decreased vision

Signs

- Anterior vitreous cells > aqueous cells

Posterior uveitis

Symptoms

- Floaters, decreased vision

Signs

- Vitreous changes – cells, flare, opacities
- Choroiditis – yellow or greyish patches, ± pigmented if old
- Retinitis – may be unifocal, multifocal or geographic
- Vasculitis – phlebitis, arteritis

Anterior uveitis – causes

Acute anterior

- HLA-B27
    - Ankylosing spondylio's
    - Psoriasis
    - Reiter's syndrome
    - UC, Crohn's + Whipple's
    - Behçet's syndrome
    - Glaucomatocyclitic crisis (Posner-Schlossman syndrome)
    - Phacolytic
    - Pseudophakia
    - Kawasaki's disease
    - Herpetic disease
    - Viruses – influenza, adenovirus, EBV, congenital rubella
    - Tubulointerstitial nephritis
    - Unknown

Chronic anterior

- Juvenile idiopathic arthritis
- Chronic iridocyclitis in young girls
- Fuchs' heterochromic iridocyclitis
- Idiopathic

Arthritis and uveitis

- Ankylosing spondylitis
- Reiter's syndrome
- Psoriatic arthritis
- Enteropathic arthritis

Ankylosing spondylitis

Epidemiology and aetiology

- HLA B27 positive in 88%; ? triggered by klebsiella aerogenes strain 43
- Most common in young adult males, with 6% familial incidence

Systemic features

- Arthritis
  - Sacroiliac joint involvement; also hips, knees, ankles
  - Varies asymptomatic to severe
  - Women show little or no back disease (despite severe eye disease)
- Also – ulcerative colitis, aortitis → aortic incompetence (5%), pulmonary apical fibrosis, general ill health

Ocular features

- Uveitis – in 25–40% of patients
- Unilateral or bilateral, precedes or follows, mild or severe

Special investigations

- X-ray sacroiliac joints
- HLA typing
- ESR

Treatment

- Systemic – anti-inflammatories, physio
- Ocular – steroids and mydriatics

Prognosis

- Very good, but ongoing recurrences can become chronic

Reiter's syndrome

Definition

- Triad of
  - Non-specific urethritis
  - Polyarthritis
  - Conjunctivitis + uveitis
- Also – mucocutaneous lesions

Epidemiology and aetiology

- HLA B27 positive in 85–95%
- Most common in young adult males (but 10% female)
- May follow bacillary dysentery, may be sexually transmitted
- ? Triggered by chlamydia, salmonella, shigella, yersinia, ureaplasma or mycoplasma

Ocular features

- In 45% of cases, unilateral or bilateral, mild or severe, often recurrent
- Conjunctivitis – in 37% of cases, papillary hypertrophy and mucopurulent discharge, usually lasts 2–4 weeks
- Keratitis – subepithelial opacities and overlying superficial punctate keratopathy, resolve with no residua
- Uveitis – mild or severe, anterior, bilateral or unilateral, often recurrent
- Other – episcleritis, retinal oedema, papillitis

Systemic features

- Arthritis – usually occurs within a month of infection; polyarthritis, knee most commonly involved, sacroiliitis in 70% of patients, plantar fasciitis, achilles tendonitis, calcaneal periostitis
- Urethritis – discharge and dysuria
- Mucocutaneous lesions – keratoderma blennorhagica (thickening of plantar skin), mouth ulcers, penis ulcers

Special investigations

- HLA B27
- Cultures negative
- Chlamydial serology may be positive
- X-ray – periostitis of os calcis, sacroiliac joint arthritis

Treatment

- Arthritis – anti-inflammatories
- Uveitis – steroids and mydriatic
- Tetracycline for presumptive chlamydia

7

Psoriatic arthritis

Epidemiology and aetiology

- Affects 7% of people with psoriasis
- Males and females equally affected
- Associated with HLA B27 in 40–60%

Clinical features

- Arthritis
- Nail changes
- Ocular features
  - Conjunctivitis, acute iritis, keratitis
  - Not seen in psoriasis without arthritis

Lyme disease

Aetiology

- Spirochaete Borrelia burgdorferi; transmitted by tick Ixodes sp

7

General features

- Stage 1
  - First month post-infection
  - Erythema migrans (an elevated annular lesion at site of tick bite), flu-like illness, follicular conjunctivitis
- Stage 2: 1–4 months post-infection
  - Multisystem dissemination – neurologic disease (Bell's palsy, meningitis), myocarditis + heart block, musculoskeletal disease;
  - Keratitis, iritis, intermediate uveitis, vitritis, panophthalmitis, optic neuritis
- Stage 3: ≥ 5 months post-infection
  - Chronic/recurrent arthritis
  - Chronic meningitis
  - Acute respiratory distress syndrome
  - Keratitis

Ocular features

- Stage 1 – follicular conjunctivitis, periorbital oedema
- Stage 2 – uveitis, retinal vasculitis, optic neuritis, keratitis
- Stage 3 – episcleritis, stromal keratitis, orbital myositis

Diagnosis

- IgM + IgG ELISA; only 50% lab positive

Treatment

- Tetracycline, erythromycin, penicillin
- IVI penicillin, ceftriaxone – for neurological disease

Gastrointestinal (GIT) diseases associated with uveitis

Syndromes

- Crohn's disease – 5–10% have ocular features; uveitis, episcleritis, scleritis, keratitis; eye involvement more likely with arthritis and large bowel involvement
- Ulcerative colitis – < 5% have ocular features
- Whipple's disease – ocular features rare

Ocular features

- Iridocyclitis
- Also – conjunctivitis, episcleritis, scleritis, keratitis, vitritis, retinal vasculitis, optic neuritis, extraocular muscle palsies

Renal diseases associated with uveitis

Tubulointerstitial uveitis

- Tubulointerstitial nephritis and uveitis (TINU)
- Drug hypersensitivity reaction

IGA glomerulonephritis

- Associated ocular manifestations – iritis, keratoconjunctivitis, scleritis

Behçet's disease

Definition

- A generalised occlusive vasculitis of unknown cause

- Triad of
  - Acute hypopyon uveitis
  - Aphtous mouth ulcers
  - Genital ulcers

Aetiology
- ? Autoimmune secondary to a viral infection

Epidemiology
- 20% of referral uveitis in Japan
- Common also in Mediterranean and Middle East
- Male : female 2 : 1
- HLA B51 phenotype common in ocular form
- Genetic spread ? occurred along the old silk route

Pathology
- Basic lesion is obliterative vasculitis, with round cell infiltrate, swelling and proliferation of endothelium, and fibrinoid degeneration

Clinical features
- May be complete (all four major criteria) or incomplete
- Most serious form of posterior uveitis

Diagnostic criteria

Major diagnostic criteria
- Recurrent aphthous ulcers of mouth
- Skin lesions – erythema nodosum, subcutaneous thrombophlebitis, inflammatory reaction to pin prick
- Eye lesions
  - Anterior uveitis
  - Posterior uveitis
- Genital ulcers

Minor diagnostic criteria
- Arthralgia/arthritis
- GIT lesions
- Epididymitis
- CNS involvement (strokes, palsies, confusion)

Ocular features
- Occurs in 70–80%
- Iridocyclitis + hypopyon, in response to ischaemia from obliterative vasculitis
- Necrotising retinal vasculitis → retinal vein occlusion, retinal detachment, secondary cataract, secondary glaucoma, phthisis bulbi, AION; untreated → loss of vision occurs after 3–4 years of the disease

Special investigations
- HLA typing
- Pin prick test (prick skin with a sterile hypodermic needle → pustule forms within a few minutes)

Treatment
- Steroids
  - Local
  - Systemic
- Chlorambucil 0.1 to 0.2 mg/kg/day; continue for at least 6 months after the last exacerbation, monitor FBC
- Cyclosporin A – 10 mg/kg/day, superior to steroids
- Colchicine
- Surgery – lensectomy, vitrectomy
- Infliximab shown to be safe and highly effective

Prognosis
- Clinical course exacerbations and remissions
- Blindness occurs in 25% of patients
- Mortality 3–4%

Causes of uveitis and hypopyon

- Behçet's
- Ankylosing spondylitis
- Reiter's
- Idiopathic

7

Sarcoidosis

- Multisystem granulomatous inflammatory disorder thought to result from an exaggerated cellular immune response to a variety of self/non-self antigens
- Most common organs involved
  - Lungs
  - Lymph nodes
  - Skin
  - Eyes (25%) – lid skin, orbit, conjunctiva, intraocular structures
  - Adrenal glands are the only organs not affected

Incidence

- 50 per 100 000 in whites; 150 per 100 000 in blacks
- Female:Male = 2 : 1
- Most common in third and fourth decades

Aetiology

- Unknown
  - ? Immunologic response to unknown antigen → macrophage release cytokines, infiltration of T-helper lymphocytes, epitheloid cells, giant cells → more cytokines → more inflammatory cells → granuloma
  - ? Abnormal immune response directed against one or more antigens in individuals with hereditary or acquired abnormality in immune system
  - Inhalation antigens
  - Genetic factors – familial incidences in certain population, specific HLA association e.g. HLA-B8, HLADR3 with Löfgren's syndrome
  - Infectious agents – mycobacterium, herpes virus 8 have been implicated

Clinical spectrum

- May be asymptomatic → severe → lethal disease

Systemic features

- Erythema nodosum, arthropathy, bilateral hilar lymphadenopathy (Löfgren's)
- Heerford's syndrome – uveo-parotid fever
- Granulomata – liver, spleen, muscle
- Cutaneous lesions such as lupus pernio – 15%
- Superficial lymphadenopathy
- Constitutional symptoms – malaise, fever, weight loss
- Arthralgia
- Heart – conduction defects or pulmonary hypertension
- Renal insufficiency – secondary to nephritis, hypercalcaemia
- Cor pulmonale
- Neurological
  - Meningitis, hydrocephalus, parenchymal involvement (hypothalamus and pituitary), encephalopathy, seizures, dural venous thrombosis, vasculitis, peripheral neuropathy

Neuro-ophthalmologic features

- Orbital pseudotumor
- Optic neuropathy (direct optic nerve infiltration, contiguous inflammation, or optic nerve head granuloma)
- Neuroritinitis (disc swelling + macular star)
- Perineuritis (disc swelling without visual loss or raised ICP)
- Chiasmal/retrochiasmal visual pathway dysfunction
- Ocular motor cranial nerve palsy
- VII palsy
- Pupil abnormalities – tonic pupil, Horner's syndrome, and Argyll-Robertson pupil
- Raised ICP and papilloedema– from pseudotumor cerebri syndrome, mass effect, CSF obstruction, venous sinus thrombosis

Ocular features (25–60%)

- Most common → uveitis 30–70% and conjunctival nodules 40%
- Lids, lacrimal and conjunctival involvement – asymptomatic, diplopia, large orbital granuloma, sarcoid induced inflammatory myositis
- Acute and chronic anterior uveitis
- Vitritis with or without peripheral vasculitis
- Neovascularisation
- Chorioretinal lesions
- RPE defects
- Optic nerve granulomata
- Scleritis

Anterior uveitis

- Acute or chronic
- Chronic granulomatous uveitis (60%)
  - Mutton fat KPs
  - Iris nodules 11% (Busacca/Koeppe)
- May be complicated by
  - Cataract
  - Band keratopathy
  - Glaucoma – trabecular meshwork damage and pupillary block
  - CMO, associated with poor VA

Intermediate uveitis

- Pars planitis with vitritis
- Snow banking may occur
- More frequently – vitritis with peripheral vasculitis and snowball infiltrates

Posterior uveitis

- Inflammation of vitreous, retina, choroid– more visually disabling
- Occurs in 6–33% of sarcoidosis
- Snowballs (clumps of cells and proteinaceous debris)
- Periphlebitis – subclinical to severe
  - Typical segmental cuffing
  - Sheathing
  - Candle wax dripping
  - Perivenous exudation
- Periarterial sheathing is rare
- Small areas of peripheral venous occlusion
- Deep yellow choroidal lesions and RPE mottling
- Peripheral multifocal chorioretinitis (intraocular inflammation and multiple punched out lesions in the peripheral retina) associated with CMO, VA loss
- Association with acute multifocal placoid pigmented epitheliopathy (AMPPE) and sarcoidosis
- Arterial macroanuerysm with peripheral multifocal chorioretinitis
- Large granulomas of the choroid – may have overlying serous detachment
- BRVO/CRVO
- Preretinal granuloma (Landers sign)
- Optic disc neovascularisation
- Subretinal neovascularization
- Pigment epithelial detachment
- Optic disc swelling
- Retrobulbar neuritis without inflammation

Complications

- CMO (79%)
- Cataract (49%)
- Glaucoma (36%)
- Retinal ischaemia (16%)
- Neovascularisation (11%)

Sarcoidosis in children

- Common cause of uveitis in children under 5 years of age
- Characterised by
  - Granulomatous anterior uveitis
  - Polyarthritis
  - Rash
  - Lymphadenopathy
- Posterior uveitis and orbital disease can occur

Differential diagnosis in children

- Juvenile idiopathic arthritis
- Blau syndrome(familial granulomatosis, arthritis, uveitis, rash, camptodactyly)

Differential diagnosis in adults

- Intermediate uveitis – idiopathic, Lyme disease, MS, non-Hodgkins large B-cell lymphoma, Whipple's disease
- Small choroidal lesions – multifocal chorioretinitis with panuveitis, birdshot chorioretinopathy, TB
- Periphlebitis – Behçet's disease, TB, MS, CMV retinitis, cat scratch fever, Crohn's disease
- Syphilis
- Toxoplasmosis
- Retinal abnormality from sickle cell disease and other haemoglobinopathy
- Serpiginous choroiditis

Diagnostic criteria

- Suspected sarcoidosis
  - Hilar adenopathy
  - Erythema nodosum
  - Raised SACE
  - Positive lacrimal gland or lung Gallium67 scan
  - Raised serum globulins, calcium
  - Lymphadenopathy
  - Decreased lung diffusing capacity (40–70%) with systemic disease
- Definite sarcoidosis → histological confirmation of non-caseating granulomas; associated findings – uveitis, arthritis, neurological signs, anaemia, decreased lung function, lymphadenopathy

Diagnosis

- Biopsy skin/conjunctival nodules, lacrimal gland
- Conjunctival biopsy positive in 12% of suspected cases
- Lacrimal gland biopsy (22% positive)
- Transbronchial biopsy → up to 60% positive
- 90% positive granuloma in stage III
- CXR findings
  - Stage 0 – normal
  - Stage 1 – BHL
  - Stage 2 – BHL + pulmonary parenchyma involvement
  - Stage 3 – pulmonary infiltration
- Stage 1 resolves spontaneously in 80%, stage II 50–60%, and stage III 30%
- SACE is elevated in 50% with sarcoidosis, 60–90% in active disease
- Normal SACE levels do not exclude disease
- Raised SACE + positive gallium67 scan → specific and sensitive
- Kveim test no longer used
- Bronchi alveolar lavage → lymphocytosis with increased CD4+/CD8+ ratio– supportive of diagnosis
- Fluorescein angiography useful
- Vitrectomy may provide a tissue specimen to exclude intraocular malignancy; for persistent vitreous haemorrhage

Management

- Indications for treatment: Active pulmonary disease and/or uveitis
- Asymptomatic hilar lymphadenopathy – no need for treatment
- Steroids are the mainstay of therapy
  - Acute inflammation topical steroids + periocular steroids
  - Chronic anterior uveitis and posterior involvement may need systemic treatment
  - Neurosarcoid is an indication for systemic treatment – high initial doses to speed up remission and slow taper; prolonged low dose treatment; if prolonged use needed, can add steroid sparing agent – methotrexate low dose, cyclosporin A
- In inflammatory macular edema – treat a modest decreased in VA
  - First control inflammation
  - Consider periocular or IVT triamcinolone
  - May need PPV
- PRP in neovascularisation
- Cryoretinopexy for snow banks
- Cataract treatment as with uveitis-cataract, IOL implant is well tolerated

- Glaucoma (36%) – as opposed to 18% in other uveitis
  - Antimetabolite trabecutectomy or seton as a primary procedure; goniotomy in children
- Factors associated with poor outcome
  - Black race
  - Late onset
  - Inflammation persisting > 6 months
  - Involvement of > 3 organs
  - Stage III pulmonary disease

Pars planitis

Aetiology
- Idiopathic most common
- ? Slow virus (benign and chronic)
- ? Autoimmune (malignant)
- May be the first sign of underlying demyelinating disease (5% develop multiple sclerosis within 5 years)
- May be the first sign of sarcoidosis, Lyme disease
- May be associated with HLA DR2

Epidemiology
- Constitutes 8% of cases of uveitis
- Affects children and young adults
- Male = female
- More common under 40 years of age

Pathology
- Granulomatous inflammation of peripheral retina and uvea, peripheral retinal vasculitis

Features
- Low grade, chronic and intermittent, bilateral but asymmetrical
- Floaters, otherwise quiet
- ± Anterior chamber cells, flare, and keratic precipitates
- Vitreous cells, 'snow bank' over inferior pars plana, peripheral retinal vasculitis, snowballs

Complications
- 80% have 6/12 or better after 10 years of the disease
- Cystoid macular oedema
- Cataract
- Tractional retinal detachment
- Cyclitic membrane formation
- Glaucoma
- Band keratopathy

Special investigations
- To exclude other diseases
- Fluorescein angiogram and/or OCT, for early detection of cystoid macular oedema
- MRI if MS likely/possible

Treatment
- Only treat if cystoid macular oedema develops
- Subtenons or IVT steroids
- Cryopexy to pars plana
- Systemic immunosuppressives
- PPV for dense vitreous veils

Vogt-Koyanagi-Harada (VKH) syndrome

Definition
- Bilateral panuveitis with exudative retinal detachment, associated with skin and neurologic features
- Multisystem disease

Aetiology
- Unknown, ? autoimmune viral induced
- T-cell mediated immunity

Epidemiology
- Common in Japanese (any people with increased skin pigmentation appear to be at risk)
- Third to fourth decade, female > male; can be seen in children

Features
- Uveitis – iridocyclitis, posterior uveitis, exudative retinal detachment, papillitis, late subretinal neovascularisation (very similar to sympathetic ophthalmia)
- Alopecia, vitiligo, poliosis (usually begin only several weeks after the ocular signs and symptoms)

- Dysacousia, tinnitus, deafness (30% – temporary)
- Neurologic features – CSF increased lymphocytes, neck stiffness, hemiparesis, cranial nerve pareses, coma, psychosis, cerebellar signs

Clinical course
- Four phases
- Prodromal
  - Mimics a viral illness for a few days
  - Fever, headache, stiff neck, etc.
- Acute uveitic
  - Bilateral in 70% with a 3 day delay before second eye involvement
  - Bilateral multifocal exudative detachments, disc oedema and hyperaemia
  - White choroidal dots, Dalen-Fuchs-like nodules
  - Granulomatous anterior uveitis
- Convalescent or chronic
  - Uveal depigmentation
  - Orange-red fundal discolouration ('sunset-glow')
  - Multiple focal areas of chorioretinal atrophy
- Chronic and recurrent
  - Anterior uveitis, but posterior very uncommon

Pathology
- As in sympathetic uveitis
- Dalen-Fuchs-like nodules in retina → composed of lymphocytes, epitheloid cells, pigment-laden macrophages, altered RPE cells

Treatment
- Prompt and aggressive
- Steroids (topical, periocular, systemic) pulsed IVI for severe cases
- ± cyclosporin or other immune modulators

Prognosis
- Long-term visual prognosis is good; 66% retain 6/9 or better
- Vision threatening complications are cataract, glaucoma, and subretinal neovascularisation

Sympathetic uveitis

Definition
- Bilateral chronic granulomatous uveitis occurring after a penetrating injury (trauma or surgery)

Incidence
- 0.001–5% of penetrating injury

Aetiology
- Penetrating wounds
  - Surgical
  - Non-surgical
- Also seen with contusions, corneal ulcers, intraocular malignancies

Pathogenesis
- Retinal S-antigen, which is a component of photoreceptor membrane rhodopsin kinase, is exposed and is the exciting antigen

Pathology
- Granulomatous panuveitis, type 4 hypersensitivity
- Dalen-Fuchs nodules in retinal periphery are granulomas between retinal pigment epithelium and Bruch's membrane; composed of collections of epithelioid cells

Immunology
- Early up-regulation (increased helper and decreased suppressor T-cells)
- Late down regulation (vice versa)

Features
- Exciting eye does not recover from injury
- Sympathising eye develops granulomatous uveitis
- Onset 9 days – 66 years after injury; usually 2–12 weeks; 90% $<$ 1 year; 80% $<$ 3 months

- Dalen-Fuchs spots occur in retinal periphery
- Exudative retinal detachment, disc oedema, late chorioretinal scarring may occur
- Vitiligo, alopecia, poliosis may occur
- Fluoresein angiogram shows the same features as VKH syndrome – multiple sites of choroidal leakage, corresponding to Dalen-Fuchs spots, with late coalescence under detached retina

Complications

- Glaucoma, cataract, retinal detachment

Differential diagnosis

- Reactivation of pre-existing uveitis
- Sympathetic irritation
- Lens induced uveitis
- VKH syndrome

Treatment

- Early excision of injured eye (before 2 weeks)
- Late excision of injured eye ? contraindicated ? may be beneficial as it decreases the antigenic load
- Steroids (topical, subconjunctival, systemic)
- Immunosuppressives (cyclophosphamide, cyclosporin, chlorambucil)
- Continue treatment for 6 months after the inflammation has settled
- Surgery for cataract or glaucoma

Prognosis

- 70% controlled with steroids

Fuchs' heterochromic iridocyclitis

Aetiology

- Unknown; ? familial predisposition, ? degenerative, ? sympathetic denervation of iris, ? autoimmune
- May be the end stage of a number of different conditions
- May be related to congenital rubella

Pathology

- Narrowing of iris vessels with low grade chronic ischaemia

Features

- 3% of all uveitis cases
- Unilateral, affects young adults
- Chronic, non-granulomatous uveitis
- Occurs in quiet eyes with minimal evidence of iritis
- Stellate keratic precipitates are characteristic
- Iris stroma atrophic, iris pigment layer undergoes patchy atrophy with transillumination defects
- Rubeosis iridis, atrophy of iris sphincter with mydriasis and heterochromia
- Cataract in 50%
- Glaucoma in 25–50%, may be precipitated by cataract surgery

Treatment

- Steroids should not be used; uveitis is resistant to steroids, use may aggravate development of cataract or glaucoma
- Glaucoma may require trabeculectomy + adjunct
- Cataract surgery may be complicated by hyphaema, otherwise good results

7

Causes of heterochromia

Congenital

- Hyper
  - Retinoblastoma
  - Sturge-Weber syndrome
  - Naevus
  - Oculodermal melanocytosis
  - Waardenburg syndrome
- Hypo
  - Marfan's syndrome
  - Horner's syndrome
  - Chediak-Higashi syndrome
  - Neurofibromatosis
  - Naevus
  - Juvenile xanthogranuloma

Adult

- Hyper
  - Rubeosis
  - Naevus
  - Melanoma
  - Siderosis
  - Hyphaema
  - Post-contusion
  - Unilateral use of a prostaglandin
- Hypo
  - Horner's syndrome
  - Naevus
  - Fuchs'
  - Chronic iritis with atrophy
  - Metastatic carcinoma
  - Iris naevus syndrome

Toxoplasmosis

Aetiology and epidemiology

- Most common cause of posterior uveitis in the world, accounting for 30–50% of cases
- It is particularly common in South America
- Toxoplasma gondii, obligate intracellular protozoan
- Cat is the natural host, human may be the intermediate host
- Spread by transplacental spread or by ingestion of raw meat
- 99% congenital, 1% acquired
- Most uveitis due to recurrence around a congenital scar, due to breakdown of cysts and release of tachyzoites
- Infected pregnant woman has 40% chance of transmitting infection to the foetus
- Acquired toxoplasmosis in immunocompetent individual is benign, with transient flu-like illness
- Acquired toxoplasmosis in immunocompromised individual may be life threatening; most common lesion is intracranial space occupying lesion
- Congenital toxoplasmosis → chorioretinitis, intracranial calcification, convulsions

Features

- Focal retinitis at posterior pole with secondary choroiditis, scleritis, inflammatory exudate in vitreous ('headlight in the fog' appearance)
- Focal necrotising chorioretinitis
- Jensen's disease → active juxtapapillary toxoplasmosis

- Retinal vessels in the vicinity of an active lesion get periphlebitis and segmental arterial sheathing
- Reactivation of congenital toxoplasmosis → vitritis, acquired toxoplasmosis → little vitritis
- Iridocyclitis may occur as a 'spill over reaction'
- Typical appearance of scar
- Usually active in one eye at a time, but scars are seen in both eyes
- Resolves after 1–4 months
- In HIV – can have minimal vitritis

Differential diagnosis

- Other forms of retinitis – candidiasis, cytomegalo inclusion virus, syphilis, tuberculosis, toxocara, presumed ocular histoplasmosis

Special investigations

- Toxoplasma agglutination test
- ELISA may be more sensitive and specific
- Immune competent – 1:200 significant
- Immune compromised – any titre significant

Treatment

- Indications for treatment
  - HIV+
  - Close to major vessel
  - Close to disc or macula
  - Vitritis with VA < 6/18
- Systemic steroids – with antibiotics; if sight threatening
- Clindamycin + sulphonamide; or pyrimethamine + sulphonamide + folinic acid
- Others – cotrimoxazole, azithromycin
- Atovaquone – a newer agent; cysticidal may eradicate even the encyted form of the parasite
- Some advocate no treatment in immunocompetent individuals

Childhood uveitis

Incidence

- Rare; 5–8% of the total

Anterior (common causes)

- Idiopathic – 50%
- Trauma
- Juvenile idiopathic arthritis
- Fuch's heterochromic iritis
- Sarcoidosis
- Herpes simplex + zoster
- Tuberculosis
- Syphilis
- Lyme disease

Intermediate uveitis (common causes)

- Idiopathic – majority
- Sarcoidosis
- TB
- Toxocariasis
- Lyme disease
- Pars planitis

Posterior (common causes)

- Idiopathic – 33%
- Toxoplasmosis – most common
- Toxocariasis
- Histoplasmosis
- Tuberculosis
- Lyme disease
- Sympathetic ophthalmia
- Syphilis

Masquerade syndromes

- Retinoblastoma
- Juvenile xanthogranuloma
- Leukaemia
- IOFB
- Retinal detachment
- Malignant melanoma

Clinical approach

- Anterior
  - Usually presents as a sore red eye, sometimes quiet
  - Investigate only if chronic, recurrent, fails to respond to treatment
- Posterior
  - Presents as a red eye, poor vision, squint, leucocoria
  - Always investigate

Posterior uveitis (clinical approach)

- Posterior uveitis is an organ specific response, cw anterior uveitis, which is a systemic disease response
- Visual loss in posterior uveitis is due to
  - Cystoid macular oedema, which responds to immunosuppression
  - Macular ischaemia, in which there is no improvement on treatment
- Check fundal blood vessels; is there arterial vasculitis or venous vasculitis?

Arterial

- Systemic lupus erythematosus
- Polyarteritis nodosa
- Wegener's granulomatosis
- Acute retinal necrosis
- Eales' disease
- Syphilis

Venous

- Sarcoidosis
- Tuberculosis
- Idiopathic autoimmune
- Multiple sclerosis
- Reticulum cell sarcoma
- Pars planitis

Both

- Toxoplasmosis
- Behçet's

Treatment of immune-related paediatric uveitis

- Uveitis is the third leading cause of blindness in the USA (10%) and 5–10% of cases are paediatric
- Worldwide, 35% of uveitis patients are eventually blinded (infective causes included)
- Many 'blind years' in the paediatric population
- 12% of pauciarticular Juvenile idiopathic arthritis's go blind

Non-infective causes of paediatric uveitis

Anterior uveitis

- Idiopathic (60%)
- Juvenile idiopathic arthritis
- Sarcoidosis
- Fuchs' hetereochromic iridocyclitis
- Ankylosing spondyltis
- Other HLA-B27-related
- Psoriasis
- Inflammatory bowel disease
- Tubulo-interstitial nephritis + uveitis
- SLE
- Multiple sclerosis

Intermediate uveitis

- Juvenile idiopathic arthritis
- Pars planitis
- MS
- Sarcoidosis

Posterior uveitis

- Vogt-Koyanagi-Harada syndrome
- Inflammatory bowel disease
- Behçet's disease
- SLE
- Sarcoidosis
- PAN
- Wegener's granulomatosis

Treatment principles

- Goals – complete control of all intraocular inflammation, off all steroids, no treatment side effects
- Uveitis leads to blindness through development of maculopathy, macular oedema, optic neuropathy, glaucoma, and epiretinal membranes
- These complications are preventable in the majority
- The key is control of inflammation → zero tolerance approach
- In the past, reluctance among ophthalmologists to use immunosuppressive therapy has been fear of treatment side effects
- The ophthalmologist should employ the help of a paediatric rheumatologist if possible

- Stepladder approach
  - Topical steroids
  - Add a systemic NSAID
  - Regional steroids
  - Systemic steroids
  - Methotrexate or cyclopsporine
  - Cyclophosphamide or chlorambucil
- Approach based on a risk/reward ratio
- There are a few conditions in which we go straight to immunosuppressives e.g. Behçet's disease

Topical treatment

- Mainstay of treatment for many cases of anterior uveitis
- Adequate for many cases of anterior uveitis
- Inadequate for intermediate + posterior uveitis
- Often used in conjunction with a mydriatic cycloplegic to reduce pain and prevent posterior synaechiae

Regional treatment

- Often requires examination under anaesthetic in children
- Subconjunctival, subtenon + orbital floor long-acting steroids
- Intravitreal triamcinolone acetonide
- Valuable tool in the ophthalmology armamentarium
- May avoid the need for long-term systemic steroid
- Retinal cryopexy in pars planitis
- PPV

Systemic treatment

- Children receiving corticosteroids or immunosuppressives need special attention
- Growth retardation, infertility, carcinogenesis are possible complications
- Children receiving high dose steroids or immunosuppressives should get prophylaxis against influenza, varicella zoster, TB
- No live virus vaccines for at least 3 months after stopping treatment

7

Classification of immunosuppressives

- Antimetabolites
  - Azathioprine
  - Methotrexate
  - Mycophenolate mofetil
- T-cell inhibitors
  - Cyclosporin
  - Tacrolimus
- Alkylating agents
  - Cyclophosphamide
  - Chlorambucil

Corticosteroids

- Remain the mainstay of treatment
- Oral: 0.5–2 mg/kg/day (1 mg/kg)
- Sometimes pulsed IV methylprednisolone for faster response, more aggressive treatment required (e.g. sympathetic ophthalmia)
- Many side effects, some universal
- Dose-related suppression of growth
- Growth will cease completely at a dose greater than 2 mg/kg/day
- Height + weight should be monitored regularly e.g. 3-monthly
- Osteoporosis → Vitamin D + calcium supplemetation
- Adrenal suppression, Cushing's syndrome, hyperactivity, insomnia, avascular bone necrosis, etc.

- Mood changes, weight gain and acne problematic in teens
- Tapering of steroids important to avoid rebound inflammation and Addisonian crisis
- When do we change from steroid to immunosuppressive therapy?
    - High dose steroid required for > 1 month
    - Disease worsens on high dose steroid
    - No response after 2–4 weeks
    - Disease not completely quiet at 4 weeks high dose
    - Unacceptable adverse effects
    - Chronic prednisone requirements > 5 mg daily
    - Two to 3 relapses/exacerbations while tapering

Methotrexate

- An antimetabolite; inhibits dihydrofolate reductase
- Most common immunosuppressive used in children
- Well researched and found to be very safe in a rheumatology setting
- Clear, significant safety record above all other immunosuppressants
- Well tolerated, easy to administer
- 7.5–25 mg once weekly
- 2.5 mg folate daily may prevent nausea
- Subcutaneous injections for intolerable GI side effects
- Side effects – bone marrow suppression, GIT, hepatotoxicity, pulmonary fibrosis, stomatitis – all are uncommon + reversible
- There does not appear to be an association with malignancy in rheumatological doses
- Teratogenic
- Alcohol prohibited (liver toxicity)
- Myelosuppression with nitrous oxide exposure
- FBC, U+E, LFT 1–2 monthly
- Shown to be effective treatment for Juvenile idiopathic arthritis
- Effect takes 6 weeks to 2 months to manifest, therefore, a change in dosage is only made for 2 months at each level
- Drug withdrawal can be considered after 6 months to 1 year of complete remission – the duration uveitis is mostly limited

Cyclosporin A

- T-cell inhibitor
- 2.5–5 mg/kg/day initially; maximum 10 mg/kg/day
- Considered quite safe in children
- Efficacy proven in several small series of intermediate uveitis and panuveitis in children
- Frequent side effects – nephropathy, hirsutism, gum hypertrophy at a 6 mg/kg/day dose
- Monitor U+E, LFT, BP

Cyclophosphamide

- Alkylating agent → lymphotoxic effects
- Bone marrow suppression, haemorrhagic cystitis, malignancies (leukaemia), sterility
- Use in childhood uveitis limited
- Pulse IV cyclophosphamide in adults – limits side effects
- 1 g/m^2 IV in 250 mg normal saline piggybacked on 1L of normal saline, over 2 hours, repeated 3–4 weekly
- Monitor the response through WCC
- WCC of 3 500 to 5 000 favourable

Other

- Tacrolimus, mycophenolate mofetil, chlorambucil, azathioprine, monoclonal antibody therapy
- Experience in paediatric uveitis with these drugs is minimal
- Rarely required

Juvenile idiopathic arthritis + uveitis

Incidence

- 64–113 per 100 000 in US
- Most common cause of uveitis in children

Classification of juvenile idiopathic arthritis
■ Systemic (Still's disease); 20%; 1–3% get uveitis ■ Polyarticular; 30% (> 4 joints); 2–5% get uveitis ■ Pauciarticular; 50% (≤ 4 joints); 20–30% get uveitis

Incidence of uveitis

- Onset 2–4 years (rare before 2 years or after 12 years of age)
- Female > male
- Seronegative for rheumatoid factor, may be seropositive for antinuclear antibodies

Differential diagnosis

- Sarcoidosis, Lyme disease, psoriatic arthritis, Reiter's syndrome, IBD, AS

Clinical features

- Chronic, non-suppurative synovial inflammation; joint effusions
- Chronic anterior uveitis
- May precede or follow joint involvement
- Chronic, asymptomatic, therefore regular checks are important
- Non-granulomatous uveitis
- Fine keratic precipitate
- Bilateral in 70%
- 75% self limiting with no complications
- 25% complicated
- Complications – calcific band keratopathy, secondary cataract, posterior synechiae, macular oedema, secondary glaucoma, optic neuropathy
- Treatment: mydriatics and topical steroids
- Systemic steroids
- Immune modulators: methotrexate, mycofendate, cyclosporin
- Cataract surgery
- Anti-tunour necrosis factor drugs
- IOL implantation controversial

Risk factors for uveitis

- Female gender, pauciarticular, presence of circulating antinuclear antibodies, HLA DW5 and DPW2, < 7 years from onset of arthritis

7

American Academy of Paediatrics recommended screening schedule

Juvenile idiopathic arthritis subtype	Age at onset < 7 years	Age at onset > 7 years
Pauciarticular ANA+ < 4 years duration 4–7 years duration > 7 years duration	 3–4 months 6 months annually	 6 months annually annually
Pauciarticular ANA- < 4 years duration 4–7 years duration > 7 years duration	 6 months 6 months annually	 6 months annually annually

Polyarticular ANA+ < 4 years duration 4–7 years duration > 7 years duration	 3–4 months 6 months annually	 6 months annually annually
Polyarticular ANA- < 4 years duration 4–7 years duration > 7 years duration	 6 months 6 months annually	 6 months annually annually
Systemic	Annually (regardless of duration)	Annually (regardless of duration)

Bacterial endophthalmitis

7

Definition

- Inflammation predominantly involving the vitreous cavity and anterior chamber, usually associated with an infective process, but rarely non-infectious, sterile endophthalmitis

Clinical features

- Deceased vision, pain, hypopyon, vitritis, conjunctival hyperaemia + chemosis, lid oedema, corneal oedema, loss of red reflex, greenish hue to vitreous

Causes of bacterial endophthalmitis

Post-operative

- Incidence 0.01–0.4% (0.01% in cataract surgery)
- 80% of post-op endophthalmitis due to bacteria recovered from eyelids, conjunctiva, lacrimal system (also drops, irrigating solution, instruments)
- Usually cataract surgery but also pterygium, squint, PPV, scleral buckles, and others
- YAG capsulotomy → endophthalmitis due to release of sequestered capsular bag bugs
- 30–45% of eyes undergoing cataract surgery have positive aqueous culture at the end of the operation
- Staph epidermidis is the most common causal organism, causes 20–50%
- Three types – acute fulminant, staph epidermidis and chronic
- Posterior capsule rupture → 14 times increased risk
- Prolene haptics → 4–5 times increased risk (bacteria binds to polypropylene)

Post-penetrating injury

- Incidence 2–7% in developed countries
- Up to 12% in developing countries
- Staph epidermidis is the most common causal organism
- Also Staph aureus, Strep sp., Bacillus sp. and fungi

Embolic/endogenous
- Meningitis, pneumonia, otitis media, osteitis, endocarditis, puerperal sepsis, IV line

Bleb-associated
- 1%; especially strep + haemophilus (haemophilus → poor prognosis – only 25% achieve 6/120 or better)

Organisms
- Bacterial
  - Gram positive (Staph epidermidis, Staph aureus, Pneumococcus) – 60%
  - Gram negative (Proteus sp., Pseudomonas, Bacillus sp.) – 30%
- Fungal – Candida sp. and others: 10%

Pre-operative prophylaxis
- 5% Povidone iodine preparation of skin and conjunctiva
- Pre-op conjunctival sac culture + antibiotic treatment in high risk e.g. lacrimal drainage blockage, blepharitis
- Plastic drape over eyelid margin + lashes
- Intra-operative intracameral cefuroxime

Management
- Aqueous and vitreous tap
- Antibiotics
- Vitrectomy
- Steroids
- Mydriatic-cycloplegic

Aqueous and vitreous tap

- Anterior chamber tap with 27 gauge needle and insulin syringe; 0.1 ml withdrawn
- Vitreous tap with 22 gauge needle and 2 cc syringe or with vitrector; 3 mm from limbus; 0.1 ml withdrawn
- Vitreous tap gives the best yield for culture and sensitivity; positive in 60% of cases
- Culture on blood agar, cooked meat medium, Sabouraud's broth

Antibiotics

Post-operative
- Vancomycin
  - 1 mg intravitreal, repeat after 2–3 days if necessary
- Ceftazidime
  - 2.25 mg intravitreal, repeat after 2–3 days if necessary
  - Fortified drops alternate hourly; 50 mg/ml

Post-penetrating injury
- Amikacin: 0.4 mg intravitreal
- Vancomycin: 1 mg intravitreal

Comments on antibiotic treatment
- Poor ocular penetration with systemic dose
- Aqueous level 15% of plasma level
- Vitreous level 1% of plasma level
- Adequate vitreous level only achieved with intravitreal injection
- Intravitreal antibiotic injection provides the only means for rapidly achieving adequate levels of antibiotic within the eye; the benefit of systemic antibiotics and steroids has not been clearly demonstrated

Vitrectomy

- Advantages
  - Vitreous for MC+S
  - Bulk of infection is removed
  - Sequestered pockets of infection are eliminated

- Vitreous cavity is rendered more permeable to allow diffusion of antibiotics
- Space is created for injection of antibiotics

- Disadvantages
  - Hazardous – therefore, should not be done in every case

Steroids

- Start 24–48 hours after antibiotics
- Controversial
- Definitely not for fungal
- ± Dexamethasone 0.4 mg intravitreal
- Prednisone drops topically hourly
- Dexamethasone 4 mg subconjunctivally PRN
- Prednisone 60 mg orally daily

Mydriatic-cycloplegic

- Atropine 1% drops 12 hourly

Preparation of intravitreal antibiotics

- Ceftazidime 2.25 mg in 0.1 ml
- Gentamycin 0.4 mg in 0.1 ml
- Cephazolin 2.5 mg in 0.1 ml
- Amikacin 0.5 mg in 0.1 ml
- Vancomycin 1 mg in 0.1 ml

Chronic bacterial endophthalmitis following cataract surgery

- Onset up to 3 months following surgery, may persist for months or years
- Due to low virulence organisms – Staph epidermidis, Propiobacterium acnes, Diphtheroids
- Bacteria may adhere to IOL by production of polysaccharide glycocalyx, may sequester in capsule bag
- Adherent bacteria may be resistant to cidal concentrations of antibiotics
- Slit lamp appearance – anterior chamber cells, white plaque of bacteria on IOL or in capsule bag, keratic precipitates, vitreous cells

Aseptic post-op endophthalmitis

- Lens induced – phacoanaphylaxis
- IOL induced – polishing agent, sterilising material, polypropylene

Metastatic bacterial endophthalmitis

- Septicaemia due to meningococcus, E. coli, Haemophilus sp

Management

- Prompt high dose IVI antibiotics; blood ocular barrier is disrupted, therefore antibiotics penetrate readily
- Topical mydriatic and steroid
- ± Subconjunctival/parabulbar antibiotic prophylaxis in the uninvolved eye
- ± Intravitreal antibiotics, if there is extensive involvement of the posterior segment

Endophthalmitis following penetrating injury

- Contamination of anterior chamber occurs in 33%
- Prophylactic IV antibiotics → decreased risk of endophthalmitis

Prognosis

- Mild – good; 80% achieve 6/12 or better
- Severe – not good; 20% 6/12 or better

Fungal endophthalmitis

Incidence

- Increasing due to greater awareness and use of broad spectrum antibiotics, steroids, cytotoxics
- Constitute 10% of the total cases of endophthalmitis

Classification of fungi

- Filamentous
- Yeasts – cryptococcus
- Yeast-like – candida albicans
- Dimorphic – histoplasma

Common organisms
- Candida albicans
- Aspergillus, coccidiodes, blastomyces, sporothrix, cryptococcus, fusarium

Pathogenesis
- Exogenous
  - Longer incubation period compared with bacteria (weeks cw days), low grade inexorable progression
  - Poor vision, injection, pain, anterior chamber flare and cells, hypopyon, vitritis, posterior corneal abscess
- Endogenous
  - Poor vision, fluffy white chorioretinal lesions, associated retinal haemorrhage, snow ball opacities in vitreous
  - Patients with candida fungaemia have 1 in 3 chance of developing endophthalmitis

Diagnosis
- Aqueous tap – often negative
- Vitreous tap – for bacterial and fungal culture and sensitivity

Management
- Medical
  - Endogenous – oral fluconazole, + subconjunctival and topical miconazole
  - Exogenous – intravenous, topical and subconjunctival miconazole
- Vitrectomy
  - Allows specimen for culture, clearing of infection load, intravitreal injection

Ocular tuberculosis

Incidence
- Ocular TB occurs in 0.1–1.5% of people with TB

Pathology
- Infection with caseating or non-caseating tubercles, seen in primary TB and patients with low immunity
- Hypersensitivity to tuberculoprotein with acute exudative inflammatory reaction
- Strong affinity for oxygenated areas → lung apices and choroid
- Many patients with TB-uveitis do not have active PTB and may have a normal CXR

Features
- Lid – primary chancre, secondary lupus vulgaris, tuberculoma, blepharitis, meibomianitis
- Lacrimal sac – infection with obstruction and fistula
- Lacrimal gland – chronic dacryoadenitis
- Conjunctiva – tuberculoma, Parinaud's oculoglandular syndrome, non-specific conjunctivitis, phlyctenule
- Cornea – ulcer, interstitial keratitis, phlyctenular keratoconjunctivitis, abscess, sclerokeratitis
- Episclera and sclera – episcleritis and scleritis
- Uvea
  - Uveitis anterior or posterior, acute or chronic, granulomatous or non-granulomatous
  - Due to infection or hypersensitivity
  - 20–25% of endogenous granulomatous uveitis is due to

TB, usually chronic low grade granulomatous uveitis
  - May be miliary tubercles of choroid, may be solitary choroidal tubercles
- Retina – retinitis secondary to choroiditis, Eale's disease
- Optic nerve – optic neuritis, solitary tubercle
- CNS – meningitis, including optico-chiasmatic arachnoiditis
- Orbit – periostitis, tuberculoma
- Pleural infection – Horner's syndrome

Diagnosis

- PPD – not appropriate in endemic areas
- Two-week therapeutic trial of INH → dramatic response diagnostic

Syphilis

- Great masquerader
- Treponema pallidum
- Early syphilis < 2 years duration
- Infection → primary syphilis → secondary syphilis → early latent
- Late syphilis > 2 years
- Late latent → tertiary syphilis

Congenital

- Acquired transplacentally
- Interstitial keratitis, conjunctivitis, chronic dacryocystitis, chorioretinitis (salt and pepper fundus, pseudo retinitis pigmentosa), optic neuritis, extraocular muscle palsies

Acquired secondary

- Six to 8 months after primary infection
- Skin rash palms and soles, fever, weight loss, arthralgia
- External features – madarosis, conjunctival chancre, scleritis, interstitial keratitis
- Uveitis – unilateral or bilateral, acute or chronic, granulomatous or non-granulomatous; dilated iris capillaries (roseolae); iris nodules; unifocal or multifocal chorioretinitis; neuroretinitis

Acquired tertiary

- As for secondary, plus neuro-ophthalmic features
- Optic atrophy, Argyll-Robertson pupil, III palsy, VI palsy

Serology

- Treponemal tests – FTA-Abs + TPHA (fluorescent treponemal antibody absorption); specific and remain positive for life, may be negative very early
- Non-treponemal tests VDRL + RPR + WR – non-specific, become negative after treatment and in late tertiary disease
- Asymptomatic neurosyphilis must be ruled out with a lumbar puncture
- But syphilitic uveitis should probably be treated with a neurosyphilis regimen
- Intravenous penicillin for 10 days

Fungal uveitis

Presumed ocular histoplasmosis syndrome

Aetiology

- Histoplasma capsulatum
- Common in tropical river valleys
- Usually occurs in patients with positive serology, may have negative serology

Pathology

- Focal choroiditis in fungaemia → peripheral and peripapillary punched out scars (histo spots)
- Histo spot at macula → subretinal neovascular membrane → disciform scar

Clinical features

- Course follows exacerbations and remissions
- Occurs in second to fifth decades, bilateral in 20% of patients, second eye less severely affected

- Triad of
  - Atrophic choroidal scars in periphery (histo spots) (punched out, pigmented borders)
  - Peripapillary choroidal atrophy
  - Macular disciform lesions, resemble exudative age-related macular degeneration
- No vitreous cells

Treatment

- Steroids – oral and periocular – early stages, before maculopathy develops
- Photocoagulation – of subretinal neovascular membrane
- Management of second eye – if scars are seen in the macular area, there is a 20% chance that macular disease will develop; therefore watch and treat early
- Photodynamic therapy
- Intravitreal anti-VEGF

Candidiasis

Aetiology

- Candida albicans
- Opportunistic infection
- Three groups of patients affected
  - Drug addicts (non-sterile needles and syringes)
  - Patients with long-term indwelling catheters
  - Immunocompromised patients

Ocular features

- Focal choroiditis → multifocal retinitis → cotton ball vitritis → endophthalmitis and severe retinal necrosis → vitreoretinal traction and tractional retinal detachment

Treatment

- Oral flucytosine + ketoconazole + amphotericin B
- Vitrectomy

Other fungi causing uveitis

- Coccidiodomycosis
- Cryptococcosis
- Aspergillosis
- Mucormycosis.

Viral uveitis

- Cytomegaloinclusion virus
- Herpes simplex and zoster
- Adenovirus
- Flu, mumps, measles

CMV retinitis

- Most common opportunistic ocular infection in AIDS (15–40%)
- Usually when CD4 cells < 50
- CMV in healthy individuals is usually asymptomatic or EBV-like

Clinical

- Full thickness retinal necrosis with hard exudates + haemorrhages
- Typically spreads along the major vascular arcades
- Minimal vitritis
- Frosted branch angiitis

Diagnosis

- Clinical diagnosis
- Serology of no value

Treatment

- Ganciclovir, foscarnet, cidofovir
- Treatment actually prolongs patient survival from 6 weeks to 10 months from time of infection
- IVI ganciclovir (5 mg/kg BD × 2 weeks, then 5 mg/kg OD ongoing)
- Has toxic effects on bone marrow
- Look at border of lesion when evaluating effect
- IVT 200 μg twice a week induction, then once weekly maintenance
- Vitrasert → 4–6 month delivery of ganciclovir

Complications

- Rhegmatogenous retinal detachment – in 30%
- Occurs in active or quiescent disease

- Difficult to repair; often have multiple posterior holes
- PPV with long-term silicone oil

Acute retinal necrosis (ARN)

Aetiology

- Herpes simplex in younger patients
- Herpes zoster in older patients

Features

- Rare but devastating necrotising retinitis
- Occurs in otherwise healthy people, either gender, any age
- Uniocular in two-thirds, binocular in one-third, second eye affected within 6 weeks
- Sudden onset, rapid loss of vision with pain and redness
- Classic triad of – arteritis and periphlebitis, retinal necrosis, vitritis
- Posterior pole tends to be spared
- Lasts 4–12 weeks, resolves with residual atrophic retina, hole formation, retinal detachment (75%), proliferative vitreoretinopathy, rubeosis, ischaemic optic neuropathy

Diagnosis

- Mostly clinical
- Vitreous fluid for PCR

Treatment

- Acyclovir IVI 1 500 mg/m^2 in 3 divided doses × 7–10 days
- Heparin, then warfarin for 2–3 weeks to prevent venoocclusive disease
- Acyclovir decreases the risk of the fellow eye being involved
- Anticoagulants, to prevent arteriolar occlusion
- Periocular and systemic steroids, when starts to resolve
- Retinal detachment prophylaxis – 360 degree photocoagulation and buckle
- Laser to wall off detachments
- Retinal detachment surgery – vitrectomy and buckle; success rate 30–50%

Progressive outer retinal necrosis (PORN)

- Caused by zoster or other herpes virus
- In absence of, same time as, or subsequent to a cutaneous infection
- It may represent a form of ARN in an immunocompromised host
- Difficult to differentiate from CMV early on
- Very rapid progression in a circumferential pattern, sparing retinal vasculature
- Treatment
  - IVI ganciclovir or foscarnet + acyclovir
  - PPV for RRD → poor results
- Poor prognosis despite treatment

Herpes zoster iritis

- Occurs in 40% of ophthalmic herpes zoster
- Non-granulomatous iritis
- May become chronic, with sector iris atrophy, glaucoma, cataract

Congenital rubella

Systemic features

- 0–8 weeks gestation – 50% infection
- 9–12 weeks gestation – 33% infection
- 13–24 weeks gestation – 10% infection
- Congenital heart defects
- Deafness
- Microcephaly and mental retardation

Ocular features

- Retinopathy – most common feature; salt and pepper pigmentary disturbance
- Cataract – in 15% of cases
- Microphthalmos – in 10–20% of cases
- Glaucoma – in 10% of cases

Parasitic uveitis

- 21 parasites may cause uveitis
- Two most important are toxocara and cysticercosis

Cysticercosis

- Taenia solium (pork tapeworm)
- Most common in second decade
- Larva migrates into eye and encysts
- Two common sites are subretinal and intravitreal
- Exclude CNS disease on CT scan
- Remove by vitrectomy
- Treat with praziquantal and steroid (because larval death causes much inflammation)
- Subretinal larvae → photocoagulation

Toxocariasis

Aetiology

- Toxocara canis (dog roundworm); most puppies infected, spread to humans by ingestion of faeces or contaminated soil
- Found in 50% of healthy dogs
- Disease in humans is due to migration of second stage larvae throughout the body
- Common in children aged 6 months to 3 years

Visceral larval migrans

- Often asymptomatic; may have fever, cough, lassitude, bronchospasm, hepatosplenomegally
- Larvae wander around → eosinophilic granulomatous response (liver, lung, brain, eye, other)
- Eosinophilia, serology positive
- Treat with antihelminthics (thiabendazole)

Features of ocular toxocara

- Usually unilateral

Clinical variations

- Chronic endophthalmitis
  - Most common form; quiet white eye with anterior chamber activity and vitreous endophthalmitis
  - Posterior synechiae, iris bombé, secondary cataract, secondary glaucoma, phthisis bulbi may occur
  - May present with leucocoria and strabismus
- Posterior retinochoroiditis
  - Unilateral, hazy ill defined lesion with overlying inflammatory cells in vitreous, later glistening white or grey with traction bands to disc or macula
- Peripheral retinochoroiditis
  - In peripheral retina and ciliary body
  - Later falciform fold extends to the disc
- Other forms
  - Optic papillitis, mobile chorioretinal nematode, diffuse unilateral subacute neuroretinitis, keratitis, conjunctivitis, lens involvement, anterior uveitis

Differential diagnosis

- Of posterior uveitis
- Of leucocoria in children

Special investigations

- Ultrasound, eosinophilia, positive serology

Treatment

- Steroids – to control the inflammation; topical, subconjunctival, oral
- Antihelminthics – not effective against the ocular infection
- Cycloplegics
- Photocoagulation – of mobile larvae
- Surgery – vitrectomy for dense vitreous reaction; retinal detachment repair for traction retinal detachment

Ocular leprosy

- Mycobacterium leprae – Hansen's disease
- Mycobacterium leprae has an affinity for skin, peripheral nerves + the anterior segment of the eye
- Systemic disease with highest incidence of ocular complications
- 30% suffer some form of disability
- 5% of people with leprosy are blind

- 21% of people with leprosy have potentially sight-threatening lesions
- 25% of people 'cured' of their leprosy and discharged from follow-up still have potentially sight-threatening lesions
- Paucibacillary/tuberculoid leprosy → lagophthalmos + corneal hypoaesthesia
- Multibacillary/lepromatous leprosy → uveitis with its sequelae
- Blindness in leprosy is due to corneal opacity, iridocyclitis, cataract
- There is increased prevalence of ocular involvement if the leprosy has been present for more than 15 years

Clinical features

- Lid involvement
- Keratitis
- Uveitis

Lid involvement

- Madarosis
- Lepromatous nodules of skin, conjunctiva, sclera
- Lagophthalmos – due to nerve damage affecting VII zygomatic and temporal branches; results in lower lid ectropion
- Dermatochalasis of upper lid; may result in entropion and trichiasis

Keratitis

- Opaque corneal nerves
- Lepromatous nodules of cornea, usually limbal
- Interstitial keratitis
- Avascular punctate keratitis; in upper outer quadrant, consists of clumps of bacilli-laden cells
- Exposure keratopathy, from lagophthalmos
- Trophic keratopathy, from corneal hypoaesthesia
- Resultant corneal ulceration and scarring

Uveitis

- Acute
  - Iris and ciliary body invaded by mycobacteria
  - All the features of acute iridocyclitis, but it is not painful
- Chronic
  - Mycobacteria lodge in iris and ciliary body, persist after the skin smears are negative
  - Results in autonomic paresis → decreased pupil reaction, decreased IOP, increased IOP postural response, decreased accommodation, end stage fixed miotic pupil
  - Sequelae of uveitis – cataract, glaucoma

Treatment

- Lower lid involvement
  - Acute stage treat with systemic steroids, clofazimine, rifampicin, dapsone; may recover
  - Chronic stage treat with tarrsorrhaphy or temporalis transfer
  - Lid closure exercises, tear replacements
- Corneal involvement – protect corneas at risk
- Iris involvement
  - Treat acute iridocyclitis with steroids and mydriatics
  - Treat chronic iridocyclitis with 5% phenylephrine + atropine + steroids

Uveitis masquerade syndromes

- Conditions which can simulate uveitis

Anterior segment

- Brushfield spots
- Ischaemia
- Juvenile xanthogranuloma
- Lymphoma
- Neurofibroma

- Phenylephrine → pigment dispersion
- Pseudocapsular exfoliation
- Tan cells
- Retinoblastoma
- Leukaemia
- IOFB
- Malignant melanoma

Posterior segment

- Amyloidosis
- Angioid streaks
- Asteroid hyalosis
- Purtscher's retinopathy
- Synchisis scintillans
- Lymphoma
- Malignant melanoma
- Retinoblastoma
- Leukaemia
- Long-standing retinal detachment
- Retinitis pigmentosa

Uveal tumours

Iris naevus

- Pigmented, usually localised, may be diffuse
- Common in neurofibromatosis
- Minimal distortion, may cause ectropion iridis or sector cataract
- Composed of benign pigmented spindle cells
- May undergo malignant transformation, therefore watch

Iris melanoma

- Indicators of malignant change – ectropion iridis, sector cataract, glaucoma
- May be pigmented or non-pigmented
- May be localised or diffuse → hyperchromic heterochromia and secondary glaucoma
- Composed of spindle A or spindle B-cells
- Treat by excisional iridectomy, iridotrabeculectomy, iridocyclectomy or excision of eye
- Good prognosis, mortality 1–4%

Choroidal naevus

- Flat or minimally elevated, slate grey, indistinct margins
- May be non-pigmented, drusen, orange pigment, subretinal fluid associated
- Hypofluorescence on fluorescein angiogram
- Composed of benign spindle or polyhedral cells
- Watch for malignant change

Choroidal haemangioma

Features

- Benign, localised or diffuse, diffuse may be in association with Sturge-Weber syndrome
- Amelanotic, red orange, subretinal fluid accumulation may resemble central serous retinopathy

Histology

- Cavernous haemangioma of choroid

Special investigations

- Fluorescein angiogram → staining
- Ultrasound → high internal reflectivity

Treatment

- Nil if uncomplicated
- Photocoagulate surface if complicated by serous retinal detachment, photocoagulation → choroidal adhesion

Choroidal osteoma

- Occurs in young females
- Unilateral, juxtapapillary
- Tufts of branching vessels on surface, arising from marrow spaces within osteoma
- Ultrasound shows acoustically dense, slightly elevated tissue behind an echoic area

Juvenile xanthogranuloma

- Component of histiocytosis X spectrum
- Composed of histiocytes, Touton giant cells, and eosinophils
- Tumours of iris

- In young children
- Result in spontaneous hyphaema
- Associated skin tumours, usually resolve

Metastatic tumours

- Most common intraocular tumours
- Eye involved in 10% of malignancies
- 25% bilateral, 25% multifocal unilateral
- Carcinoma breast and carcinoma lung are the most common
- Carcinoma breast metastases to the eye in up to 40% of cases
- Posterior choroid is the usual site

Non-pigmented tumours of the iris and ciliary body

Primary

- Epithelial
    - Hyperplasia
    - Adenoma
    - Adenocarcinoma
    - Medulloepithelioma
- Non-epithelial
    - Leiomyoma
    - Haemangioma
    - Neurilemmoma (schwannoma)
    - Neurofibroma

Secondary

- Direct extension – from conjunctiva, sclera, retina, optic nerve
- Metastases – from carcinoma breast, lung, lymphoma, leukaemia

Medulloepithelioma (diktyoma)

Pathology

- Primary tumour of non-pigmented ciliary epithelium
- May be congenital or acquired
- One-third benign and two-thirds malignant
- May be teratoid (containing cartilage, muscle, neuroglia, etc.) or non-teratoid
- Composed of cords and sheets of neuroepithelial cells, slow growing

Features

- Manifest at about 4 years of age
- Ciliary body tumour → cataract, leukocoria, mass in anterior chamber, cysts in anterior chamber, secondary glaucoma

Treatment

- Iridocyclectomy or excision of eye
- ± Exenteration

Prognosis

- Good; slow growing, almost never metastasise, locally invasive

Choroidal melanoma

Incidence

- Six per million
- 98% of uveal melanomas
- Most common primary intraocular malignancy in adults
- Peak in mid-50s
- Very uncommon in non-Caucasians
- More common in fair people

Clinical features

- Ciliary body melanomas – 15%
    - Present late, ± lens astigmatism, sector cataract, dilated episcleral vessels, vitreous haemorrhage, secondary glaucoma, unexplained lower IOP, spontaneous hyphaema, subconjunctival nodule
    - May be nodular or diffuse; diffuse = ring melanoma, more aggressive
- Choroidal melanomas – 85%
    - Present earlier, typical appearance elevated dome-shaped, variable pigmentation with crescent of pigment, lipofuscin pigment accumulation in macrophages from RPE degeneration, secondary retinal detachment
    - May cause secondary cataract or secondary glaucoma
    - Extra scleral extension → proptosis or panophthalmitis

- May be dome-shaped or diffuse (flat) – diffuse has a poorer prognosis
- Pigmented or amelanotic
- Tends to metastasise to the liver
- Symptoms – loss/distortion of vision, photopsia; often asymptomatic

Pathology

- Macroscopic
- Microscopic

Macroscopic

- Choroidal mass, yellow-white to black; extension through Bruch's membrane → mushroom/collar button configuration; rarely diffuse

Microscopic

- Callendar's classification
- MacLean's modified classification

Callendar's classification

- Spindle A; slender spindle cells, best prognosis
- Spindle B; oval spindle cells
- Fascicular; palisaded spindle cells
- Mixed; spindle and epithelioid cells
- Necrotic
- Epithelioid; worst prognosis, oval, pleomorphic, mitotic figures

MacLean's modified classification

- Spindle cell naevus
- Spindle cell melanoma
- Mixed
- Epithelioid

Size

- Small: < 3 mm thickness, < 5 mm diameter
- Medium: 3–8 mm thickness, 5–16 mm diameter
- Large: > 8 mm thickness, > 16 mm diameter

Differential diagnosis

- 10% of posterior melanomas are unsuspected; diagnosis is made on histology following enucleation
- 20% of enucleations for malignant melanomas give benign pathology on histology
- Pseudomelanomas
  - Choroidal naevus; < 2 mm thick, slow growing, lipofuscin uncommon, no P32 uptake
  - Exudative haemorrhagic chorioretinopathy
  - RPE hypertrophy and hyperplasia
  - Choroidal haemangioma
  - Choroidal detachment
  - Carcinoma metastases

Choroidal naevus

- 2–6% of the normal population
- One in 5 000 become melanoma
- Clinically: ± Drusen, RPE atrophy, orange pigment, brown-grey, thickness < 2 mm

Risk factors for pigmented lesions being melanomas

To	Thickness > 2 mm
Find	Fluid – subretinal
Small	Symptoms
Ocular	Orange pigment
Melanoma	Margin within 3 mm of disc
No risks	4% chance of evolving melanoma
One risk	36%
≥ 3 risks	> 50%

Special investigations

- Fluorescein – no typical pattern; usually mottled late hyperfluorescence helpful for differentiating a choroidal haemangioma
- Ultrasound – dome or mushroom-shaped mass lesion, acoustic hollowness (central quiet zone, due to cells being closely packed), choroidal excavation (echo-free area at base of tumour), orbital shadowing
- P32 uptake – malignant cells incorporate and use phosphorus more, therefore P32 concentrated in malignant tumours
- Transocular fine needle aspiration biopsy
- Fibreoptic localisation
- Metastases search – chest x-ray, liver scan, liver enzymes
- MRI – mostly to elicit extra-ocular extension

Management

- Many factors must be taken into account – patient age, size of tumour, fellow eye, etc.
- Radiotherapy – can also be used in the form of a gamma knife or linear accelerator
- Transpupillary diode thermotherapy (TTT) – several sessions may be required
- Argon laser
- Local resection – use in combination with brachy therapy
- Enucleation – rarely used now

Treatment

- Small – plaque therapy (beta or gamma) + TTT (usually in combination), sometimes resection
- Medium – plaque therapy, sometimes external radiotherapy, sometimes resection
- Large – enucleation, no external radiotherapy

Criteria to be met if melanoma is to be left untreated

- Should be sufficient doubt about diagnosis
- Should be able to monitor ocular status adequately – baseline ultrasound, photograph, fluorescein angiography; reassess every 3 months
- Size of tumour and patient's life expectancy should indicate a low risk of metastatic disease
- Proximity to disc or fovea would compromise vision if treatment were given

Enucleation indications

- Patient unwilling or unable to attend for regular life long examinations
- Patient unhappy about possibility of local tumour recurrence
- Tumour cannot be destroyed because of excess involvement of disc, ciliary body, angle or orbit
- Eye will not be useful to the patient after treatment
- Large tumour (> 16 mm diameter or > 8 mm thick)

Enucleation – technique

- Radiation before enucleation is of no benefit
  Minimal manipulation, non-touch technique (cryo applied over tumour, globe removed with cryo)

Conservative treatment – indications

- Tumour medium or small
- Tumour does not involve more than one-third of ciliary body or optic disc
- Tumour > 3 mm from disc or fovea

Conservative treatment – modalities

- No difference in results following radiotherapy or resection or photocoagulation

- Plaque radiotherapy
  - I125 plaque
  - Sutured over the tumour for 5–7 days
  - I125 plaque can be shielded with 0.2 mm gold foil, but I125 has short half-life
  - Recurrence rate following I125 25%
- External beam radiotherapy – proton or helium ion beam from a cyclotron beam
- Transpupillary thermo therapy (TTT)
  - Argon laser to surface and surround of tumour
  - Then treat tumour with low energy krypton laser

Idiopathic multifocal white dot syndromes

Acute multifocal posterior placoid pigment epitheliopathy

- Uncommon

Aetiology

- ? Viral infection of RPE and choriocapillaris; often a preceding upper respiratory tract infection
- ? Due to a vasculitis

Features

- Young females, acute loss of vision, bilateral
- 50% have prodromal flu-like illness
- Yellowish white multifocal placoid lesions in posterior pole, resemble choroiditis
- One disc area or less in size; may be confluent
- Occasional vitreous cells, associated episcleritis, uveitis, optic neuritis, minimal anterior segment inflammation
- Fluorescein → early hypofluorescence → late hyperfluorescence due to staining
- Resolves after 1–2 weeks, takes 2–3 months; residual retinal pigment epithelial disturbance

Diagnosis

- Clinical; especially prodromal viral infection

Treatment

- ? Treat with steroids → better resolution; no evidence of benefit

Prognosis

- Good
- Most recover to 6/12 or better, unless fovea involved
- Can develop CNV

Multiple Evanescent White Dot Syndrome (MEWDS)

- Uncommon, idiopathic, self-limiting
- Acute decrease in vision, to about 6/12
- Usually unilateral, female > male, third decade
- ? Aetiology, ? viral
- 50% have flu-like symptoms
- Multiple white dots in posterior pole, hyperaemic disc, vitritis
- Enlarged blind spot
- Fluorescein angiography → early punctate hyperfluorescence, late staining
- ERG → decreased a and b wave on photopic and scotopic ERG
- No treatment; self-limiting, recovers

Serpiginous choroidopathy

- Uncommon, idiopathic, chronic, progressive, bilateral
- Male = female
- Fourth to sixth decades affected
- Loss of vision
- Indolent + prolonged course
- Active lesions cream coloured, start around optic disc, spread out
- As active areas become atrophic over weeks to months, new lesions can occur elsewhere or contiguously in a snake-like pattern
- May be associated with vitritis and anterior uveitis
- Successive attacks → outward spread of lesions

- Fluorescein → early hypofluorescence, late hyperfluorescence; early dark centre with hyperfluorescent border, late spotty hyperfluorescence
- Inactive lesions scarred and atrophic
- May be complicated by SRNV
- Treat with systemic steroids + systemic immunosuppressives → no evidence of benefit
- Poor prognosis

Birdshot choroidopathy

- Uncommon, bilateral, chronic with exacerbations and remissions
- Affects healthy middle-aged females
- ? Degenerative, ? inflammatory
- 50–80% are HLA A29 positive
- Decreased vision, nyctalopia, disturbance in colour vision
- Minimal or no anterior segment inflammation
- Multiple patches of choroiditis and RPE dropout, vitritis, retinal vasculopathy, optic disc oedema, cystoid macular oedema
- Slowly progressive, late narrowing of vessels and optic atrophy
- Fluorescein → early hypo + late hyper; early block and late staining
- ERG reduced
- Treat with steroids – a minority respond
- CSA shown better than steroids
- Poor prognosis

Punctate inner choroidopathy

- Uncommon, bilateral
- Affects young myopic females
- Small yellow choroidal spots at the posterior pole
- ± Serous retinal detachment
- Resolve with residual atrophic scars
- May be complicated by CNV
- No treatment
- Poor prognosis, unless macula spared

Multifocal choroiditis with panuveitis syndrome

- Uncommon, unilateral or bilateral, any age
- Multiple small discrete choroidal lesions
- Associated vitritis and anterior uveitis
- Crops of new lesions, old lesions atrophic
- Complications include cystoid macular oedema, subretinal fibrosis, choroidal neovascularistaion
- Treat with periocular and systemic steroids

Acute retinal pigment epitheliitis (Krill's disease)

- Rare, young adults
- Sudden decrease in vision
- 75% unilateral
- Two to 4 white dots surrounded by yellow-white haloes at the macula
- Spots may darken or lighten with resolution but the haloes remain
- Fluorescein: Active lesions – central hyperfluorescence
- Similar to central serous chorioretinopathy
- No treatment
- Resolves in 6–12 weeks

Steroids

Introduction

- Glucocorticoids → powerful anti-inflammatory + immunosuppressant
- Mainstay of treatment for ocular inflammation
- Side effects common
- Hydrocortisone is the body's natural glucocorticoid
- Adults normally produce 20 mg/day

Mode of action

- Cell-specific effects on lymphocytes, macrophages, polymorphs, fibroblasts + others

- Complicated mechanism of action
- Their effect appears to be on the efferent limb of the immune response
- The steroids penetrate cell membranes, bind to receptors, suppress mRNA → suppresses inflammation, regardless of cause, by an unknown mechanism
- Release of arachidonic acid is inhibited → inhibition of prostaglandin synthesis

Delivery

- Topical
- Oral
- Regional
  - Subconjunctival
  - Subtenon
  - Orbital floor
- Intravitreal
- Intravenous

Types of steroid

	Anti-inflammatory potency (1 = hydrocortisone)	Equivalent doses	Plasma half-life (hours)	Biological half-life (hours)
Short-acting				
Hydrocortisone (Solu-Cortef)	1	20 mg	1–2	8–12
Cortisone	0.8	25 mg	0.5–1.5	8–12
Intermediate acting				
Prednisolone	4	5 mg	2–3.5	18–36
Prednisone	4	5 mg	3.5	18–36
Methylprednisolone (Depo-medrol + Solu-medrol)	5	4 mg	3.5	18–36
Triamcinolone (Kenalog)	5	4 mg	2–5	18–36
Long-acting				
Dexamethasone (Decadron)	25	0.75 mg	3–4.5	36–54
Betamethasone (Celestone)	25	0.75 mg	3–5	36–54

7

Oral corticosteroids

Indications

- Non-infectious inflammatory diseases

Regimens

- Initial dose 1 mg/kg/day
- Maximum adult oral dose 80 mg/day
- Alternate day treatment can be used – less side effects; give 2 days' dose on 1 day
- 20 mg → anti-inflammatory
- 60 mg → anti-inflammatory + immunosuppressive

Tapering

- Prevents inflammation rebound + Addisonian crisis (hypothalamic-pituitary axis compromised after about 3 weeks on steroid)
- After a satisfactory anti-inflammatory response
- Try to discontinue if possible

Tapering schedule after chronic oral steroid use	
> 40 mg	Decrease by 10 mg every 1–2 weeks
20–40 mg	Decrease by 5 mg every 1–2 weeks
10–20 mg	Decrease by 2.5 mg every 1–2 weeks
0–10 mg	Decrease by 1–2.5 mg every 1–4 weeks

After acute use (up to 6 weeks)

- Taper as for chronic use but in days, not weeks
- Ten days to 2 weeks of high dose oral may not require a taper

Adverse effects

- Neurological side effects are almost universal
- Insomnia
- Euphoria
- Psychosis
- Hyperactivity
- Increased appetite
- Cushing's disease
- Muscle wasting
- Acne
- Adrenal insufficiency on withdrawal (hypothalamus-pituitary axis may not return for up to 1 year; at a prolonged dose of 20 mg/day 50% of patients have complete suppression)
- Infections
- Delayed puberty and growth in children
- Hypertension
- Diabetes mellitus
- Hyperlipidaemia
- Atherosclerosis
- Osteoporosis
- Glaucoma (topical, periocular, nasal, systemic – mechanism unknown)
- Scleral melting
- Mydriasis
- Eyelid skin atrophy
- Cataracts
- Bruising
- Delayed wound healing
- Idiopathic intracranial hypertension
- Insomnia – a near certainty
- Pancreatitis
- Aseptic bone necrosis of the hip (significant increase if > 60 mg for 1 month or > 20 mg for 6 months)
- Myopathy

Monitoring

- BP, weight and glucose (3-monthly)
- Bone density (yearly)
- Lipids (yearly)

High stress conditions

- Supplemental steroids are required before major surgery, after an accident or severe illness → otherwise severe hypotension or hypoglycaemia possible

When to change to immunomodulatory treatment

- High dose steroid required for > 1 month
- Disease worsens on high dose steroid
- No response after 2–4 weeks
- Disease not completely quiet after 4 weeks high dose
- Adverse effects
- Chronic prednisone requiring > 7.5 mg daily
- Two to 3 relapses/exacerbations while tapering

Osteoporosis prevention on prednisone

- A factor for all patients on > 7.5 mg for more than 6 months

- 7.5 mg for 1 year → 10–15% loss of lumbar spine bone density
- 30 mg for 1 year → 30–50% less of lumbar spine bone density
- All should have bone densitometry if steroid lasting > 3 months

When to treat osteoporosis		
For all patients ≥ 7.5 mg for ≥ 6 months		
If Or Or	≥ 15 mg/day > 65 years old Osteoporotic fracture	TREAT
Or	Bone density scan shows problem	
If Or	7.5–15 mg < 65 years	TREAT if more than 1 risk factor

Risk factors for osteoporosis

- Menopause < 45 years
- History of low trauma fractures
- Amenorrhoea
- Slender build
- Immobility

Treatment

- Stop smoking, regular exercise, high calcium diet
- Calcium 1 500 mg daily; 800 IU vitamin D daily
- Bisphosphonates
- ± Hormone replacement therapy if post-menopausal

Intravenous steroid

- Administer over at least 30 mins
- Rapid administration → arrhythmia, CVS collapse, MI, severe infection
- One injection of IVI MP lasts up to 2 weeks

Topical steroid

IOP elevation – steroid responsiveness

- IOP elevation most prominent in topical administration
- Much less prominent in systemic administration
- 31% > 20 mmHg, 4% > 31 mmHg after 6 weeks of topical dexamethasone
- Due to accumulation of glycosaminoglycans in the trabecular meshwork
- Depends on individual response, duration, strength, frequency, potency of agent
- Genetics → expression of myocillin very high in steroid responders
- Almost never occurs within 5 days, usually not within 2 weeks
- Usually reversible after 2 weeks; but use over 1 year often makes it irreversible on discontinuation

7

Topical steroid	Potency – in vivo	IOP rise (mmHg)
Dexamethasone 0.1%	24	22
Fluoromethalone 0.1%	21	6
Prednisolone 1%	2.3	10
Medrysone 1%	1.7	1
Triamcinolone 0.25%	1.4	2
Hydrocortisone 0.5%	1.0	3

Practical application

- Check IOP on starting steroid
- Check IOP at each visit
- Schedule a visit at 2–3 weeks after starting topicals to check IOP
- Extra attention to primary open angle glaucoma patients + family history of primary open angle glaucoma
- Consider low steroid response drugs – fluoromethulane, rimexolone, vexol (cause half the pressure rise of betamethasone)
- IOP elevation may not need active management – depends on pressure, the patients disc + condition, the duration the steroid is to be used for

Subconjunctival steroid

- A constant source of steroid lasting 2–4 weeks
- Can be removed if IOP a problem
- For anterior segment inflammation
- Triamcindone acetonide lasts up to 6 months
- Subtenon injection theoretically gives better penetration + is longer-lasting but this is unproven
- Given posteriorly for posterior segment inflammation

Orbital floor steroid

- High concentrations of steroid in optic nerve, sclera, choroid + retina for about 1 week
- Clinical efficacy for up to 3 weeks

Cataract surgery in uveitis

- Cataract is a common complication of any pattern of uveitis
- Frequently seen in patients with
    - Chronic anterior uveitis – 80%
    - Fuchs' cyclitis – 50%
    - Intermediate uveitis – 45%

Pre-operative management

- Uveitis controlled for 3 months
- Uveitis treatment stable
- Need for peri-operative steroid cover
- In some patients surgery is necessary in less than ideal conditions
- Patient made aware of increased risks of surgery and need for intensive follow-up

Peri-operative steroid regimens

- Steroids essential
    - Cataract + IOL
    - Vitrectomy + lensectomy
    - Cryotherapy
    - Retinal detachment
    - Some glaucoma surgery
- Steroids not necessary
    - Fuchs' cyclitis
    - Most glaucoma surgery
    - Laser photocoagulation
    - Peripheral iridectomy
- Prednisolone 40 mg/day for 14 days pre-operatively and taper by 5 mg/week post-op

- IVMP 500 mg at time of surgery and repeat between day 2–7 then weekly as necessary
- Topical non-steroid anti inflammatory agents
- No universally accepted regimen

Peri-operative steroid regimens – children

- Prednisolone 0.5 mg/kg daily for 14 days pre-op and taper by 2.5–5.0 mg/week post-op
- IV methylprednisdone 125–250 mg at time of surgery and repeat between days 2–7 then weekly as necessary
- Intensive topical therapy post-operatively

Intraocular lenses

- IOL safe in almost all forms of uveitis as long as there is meticulous control of uveitis
- Juvenile idiopathic arthritis has traditionally been a contraindication
- May be safe to use a lens if uveitis controlled
- Acrylic IOLs appear as safe as PMMA lenses
- Many surgeons avoid silicone IOLs and prolene haptics

Post-operative management

- Intensive topical steroids
- Topical non-steroid anti-inflammatory agents
- Taper systemic steroids to pre-operative dose
- Fibrin deposition treated with intensive topical steroids

Post-operative complications following cataract surgery in uveitis

Complication	
Severe uveitis	14%
CMO	5%
Elevated IOP	5%
PC opacification	45%

Posterior capsule opacification

- Very common
- More frequent than in other patient groups
- Some evidence that acrylic IOLs have lower incidence
- Edge design influences rate of capsule opacification
- Standard YAG capsulotomy technique
- Uveitis needs to be quiet to minimise CMO risk

Poor visual outcome

- More common in:
  - Posterior uveitis
  - Pre-existing pathology
  - Chronic maculopathy
  - Optic atrophy

Peri-operative management

- Pre-operative control of uveitis
- Standardised peri-operative steroid regimen
- Meticulous cataract surgery
- Close follow-up

Surgical technique

- Phacoemulsification
- Corneal incision
- Small pupil strategies
- Soft nucleus techniques
- Capsule polishing
- IOL in nearly all patients

Ciliochoroidal detachment

Pathogenesis

- Choroid elastic → negative pressure in suprachoroidal space cw IOP (2 mm less); therefore, there exists a tendency for the accumulation of fluid
- IOP → pressure gradient across sclera → fluid loss through sclera
- High blood flow in choroid, capillaries fenestrated; any fluid in suprachoroid removed by choroidal blood
- Decreased IOP → decreased pressure gradient across sclera → decreased fluid loss through sclera → accumulation of fluid in suprachoroid
- Inflammation → increased leakage into suprachoroid → fluid accumulation in suprachoroid
- Therefore, decreased IOP and inflammation are important
- Choroidal detachment
    - Ciliary body hyposecretion → decreased IOP
    - Increased uveoscleral outflow → decreased IOP
    - Low-grade iridocyclitis → decreased IOP

Aetiology

- Trauma
    - Surgical (lens extraction, glaucoma surgery); especially if hypotony is prolonged due to a leaking wound
    - Non-surgical
- Tumours
    - Primary
    - Metastatic
- Inflammation
    - Scleritis
    - VKH syndrome
    - Other uveitis
- Systemic disease
    - Hypertension, toxaemia of pregnancy
    - Disseminated intravascular coagulation
    - Carotid cavernous fistula
    - Chronic nephritis
- Local miscellaneous causes
    - Thickened sclera
    - Retinal detachment

Differential diagnosis

- Retinal detachment
    - Rhegmatogenous
    - Exudative
- Malignant melanoma

Features

- Fixed bullous detachment, usually inferotemporally
- May be annular, lobular or flat
- Shallow anterior chamber, hypotony, anterior chamber inflammation
- Forward movement of lens → myopia
- 'Kissing' detachment

Treatment

- Acetazolamide
    - Decreased aqueous leak through leaking wound
    - Decreased fluid extravasation from choroid; this may allow rapid absorption of suprachoroidal fluid
- Treat inflammation
- Cycloplegics → decreased ciliary muscle pull
- Repair any leaking wound
- Flat anterior chamber for > 1 week → peripheral anterior synechiae; therefore, drain suprachoroidal fluid after 1 week

Complications

- If prolonged may cause
    - Secondary glaucoma with peripheral anterior synechiae
    - Low-grade uveitis
    - Secondary cataract
    - Cyclitic membrane
    - Retinal detachment
    - Phthisis bulbi

8

Retina and vitreous

Congenital retinal pigment epithelium and vascular abnormalities 185
Retinopathy of prematurity 186
Retinoblastoma 190
Retinitis pigmentosa 196
Angioid streaks 199
Albanism 200
Phacomatoses 200
Age-related macular degeneration (ARMD) 203
Choroidal neovascularisation 207
Retinal vein occlusions 208
Retinal arterial occlusive disease . 211
Macular disease 214
Epiretinal membrane 214
Cystoid macular oedema 216
Central serous chorioretinopathy 217
Drug-induced maculopathies 218
Miscellaneous maculopathies 219
Hereditary fundal dystrophies 220
Vitreoretinal interface abnormalities 225
Diabetic retinopathy 227
Proliferative retinopathies 232
Eale's disease 233
Telangiectasias 234
Sickle cell retinopathy 235
Hypertensive retinopathy 236
Macroaneurysm 237
Vasculitis 237
Retinal detachment 238
Proliferative vitreoretinopathy 243
Peripheral retinal degenerations 244
Tears 245
Retinal pigment epithelium detachment 247
Retinoschisis 247
Myopia 248
Choroidal dystrophies 249
Choroidal folds 251
Vitreous disorders 251
Vitreous haemorrhage 253
Optic disc tumours 253
Fluorescein and ICG angiography . 254
Optical coherence tomography ... 256
Electrodiagnostics 256
The electro-oculogram 257
Trauma 258

Congenital retinal pigment epithelium and vascular abnormalities

Congenital hypertrophy of the RPE (CHRPE)

- Well circumscribed, benign; overlying photoreceptors degenerate → local field defect

Typical

- Solitary
  - Unilateral, flat, black/grey, well-circumscribed, round/oval, 1–3 disc areas, ± depigmented lacunae
- Grouped
  - Unilateral, organised in pattern resembling animal footprints

Atypical

- Multiple, bilateral, oval or spindle, varying size, haphazard distribution
- Associated with
  - Familial adenomatous polyposis coli – autosomal dominon; adenomatous polyps; carcinoma
  - Gardner syndrome – Bowel polyps, skull osteomas, cutaneous tumours
  - Turcot syndrome – Bowel polyps and central nervous system tumours

Cilioretinal artery

- Present in 30% of eyes; from posterior ciliary arteries
- Supplies fovea in 10% of eyes

Persistent hyaloid artery

- Involutes at 8 months of age, starting in middle and extending distally and proximally
- May persist in part or in toto
- Mittendorf's dot– anterior remnant of tunica vasculosa lentis on inferonasal posterior lens capsule
- Association with persistent hyperplastic primary virious (PHPV)
- May be complicated by vitreous haemorrhage

Bergmeister's papilla

- Glial sheath enveloping posterior one-third of the hyaloid artery
- May be associated persistent hyaloid artery, PHPV or prepapillary loops

Prepapillary loops

- Arterial usually, sometimes venous
- Extend into vitreous within Cloquet's canal
- Due to retinal vessels growing into Bergmeister's papilla
- May be complicated by retinal artery occlusion or vitreous haemorrhage

Retinal macrovessels

- Venous, large and tortuous, drain across horizontal raphe
- Graded I–III
- Racemose angioma – grades II and III
- Wyburn-Mason syndrome – racemose angioma associated with vascular malformations of skull and central nervous system

8

Retinopathy of prematurity

Embryology

- Retinal vascularisation from disc starts at 4 months, reaches nasal ora at 8 months and temporal ora at 9 months
- Temporal periphery, therefore, immature at birth and susceptible to high pO_2

Risk factors

- Preterm; gestational age < 32 weeks
- Birth weight < 1 500 g
- Ventilation > 1 week
- Hypotension

Pathogenesis

- High pO_2 in incubator → vasoconstriction of arterioles in (temporal) periphery
- Onset immediately, irreversible after 12–15 hours
- On restoration to atmospheric pO_2, retinal ischaemia → neovascularisation
- Spontaneous regression occurs in 85%

Incidence

- Second epidemic
- Decrease in 1950s, now increasing again
- A leading cause of childhood blindness in middle income countries
- 300 per million births have at least one blind eye from ROP
- Birth weight < 750 gm – 42% develop ROP
- Birth weight 1 000–1 200 gm – 10% develop ROP
- Birth weight < 1 500 gm
  - 20% develop ROP, most regress
  - 6.5% develop cicatricial ROP

Clinical classification of active ROP

■ Location	□ Zone 1 – within circle with a radius of twice the distance from disc to macula	
	□ Zone 2 – from edge of zone 1 to nasal ora serrata + temporal equator	
	□ Zone 3 – temporal crescent anterior to zone 2	
	□ Good prognosis in zone 3, worse in zone 2, worst in zone 1	
■ Extent	□ Number of clock hours involved	
■ Staging	□ Stage 1 (demarcation line)	– Thin, grey-white line – Separates avascular immature peripheral retina from vascularised posterior retina
	□ Stage 2 (mesenchymal ridge)	– Protruding from surface of retina – Blood vessels enter the ridge, small neovascular tufts ('popcorn') may occur posterior to it – Represents a mesenchymal shunt joining veins and arteries
	□ Stage 3 (ridge with extraretinal fibrovascular proliferation)	– Ridge becomes pink with development of fibrovascular proliferation along surface of retina into vitreous – Retinal and vitreous haemorrhage may occur; mild, moderate, severe
	□ Stage 4 (subtotal retinal detachment)	– Tractional retinal detachment, starts in periphery, spreads posteriorly – Extrafoveal – Including fovea
	□ Stage 5 (total retinal detachment)	– With a funnel
■ 'Plus' disease	□ Dilatation of veins and tortuosity of arterioles	
	□ An indicator of actively progressing disease	

	▫ Usually takes several weeks to develop, may progress within a few days ▫ Regress spontaneously in 80%	
▪ Pre-plus disease	▫ Abnormal dilatation of posterior pole vessels – but insufficient to diagnose full plus disease ▫ Preplus may progress to frank plus disease over time	
▪ Threshold disease	▫ More than 5 contiguous clock hours of extraretinal neovascularistation (stage 3) or 8 cumulative clock hours, in association with 'Plus' disease and location of vessels within zones 1 or 2	
▪ Aggressive posterior ROP	▫ Uncommon, rapidly progressive ▫ Progresses to stage 5 if untreated ▫ Posterior location, prominent plus disease, ill-defined retinopathy ▫ The diagnosis can be made on a single visit and does not require evaluation over time ▫ Occurs mostly in zone 1, but also in zone 2 ▫ Very tortuous vessels, cannot distinguish arteries + veins ▫ Does not progress from stage 1 through to stage 3	
▪ Cicatricial ROP	▫ 20% of cases of active ROP → cicatricial complications ▫ Stage 1	
	▫ Stage 2	– Myopia – Minimal peripheral RPE disturbance and haze at vitreous base – Temporal vitreoretinal fibrosis with dragging of disc and posterior retina

◻ Stage 3	– More severe peripheral fibrosis with contracture and falciform retinal fold
◻ Stage 4	– Partial ring of retrolental fibrovascular tissue with partial retinal detachment
◻ Stage 5	– Complete ring of retrolental fibrovascular tissue with total retinal detachment – May develop secondary angle closure glaucoma – Treat with lensectomy and anterior vitrectomy

Differential diagnosis of leukocoria in a neonate/infant

■ Congenital	◻ Persistent hyperplastic primary vitreous ◻ Posterior pole coloboma ◻ Myelinated nerve fibres ◻ Congenital retinal fold (13 and 15 trisomy) ◻ Massive retinal fibrosis
■ Traumatic	◻ Retinopathy of prematurity
■ Inflammatory	◻ Nematode endophthalmitis ◻ Vitreous abscess
■ Neoplastic	◻ Retinoblastoma ◻ Diktyoma ◻ Tuberous sclerosis
■ Other	◻ Congenital cataract ◻ Complete retinal detachment

Prevention

- Monitor pO2
- Screening
  - Retinal detachment rarely occurs before 32 weeks
  - ROP rarely starts after 36 weeks
  - If threshold disease found, cryo or laser within 72 hours

Screening

- At least two dilated indirect fundus exams for
  - < 1 500 g
  - Prems < 32 weeks
  - High risk cases 1 500–2 000 g
- Start within 31–33 weeks post conception or 6 weeks post-delivery – whichever comes first
- Examine every 1–2 weeks until vascularised

Weekly screening

- If ROP < threshold in zone 1
- If ROP in zone 2, including
  - Stage 3 ROP without plus disease
  - Stage 2 ROP with plus disease
  - Stage 3 ROP with plus disease not yet extensive enough to justify ablative therapy

1–2 weekly screening

- If less severe ROP in zone 2
- If No ROP but incomplete retinal vascularisation in zone 1

8

Mydriasis for screening

- 0.5% tropicamide
- 0.5% cyclopentolate
- 2.5% phenylephrine

Treatment of active ROP

Ablation of avascular immature retina

- With either cryotherapy or laser photocoagulation
- Laser can be done in the nursery under fentanyl anaesthesia or in theatre under GA
- If there is threshold disease
  - Five contiguous clock hours or 8 non-contiguous clock hours
  - Of stage 3 disease
  - In zone 1 or zone 2
  - Associated with plus disease
- Halves the incidence of unfavourable outcome
- 25% progress to retinal detachment in spite of treatment
- Cryo can cause cardiorespiratory arrest in 5%

Vitreoretinal surgery for tractional retinal detachment

- Poor prognosis
- Only 25% remain attached at 5 years

Prognosis

- Complications can cause problems throughout the patient's life
- Associated conditions
  - Significant refractive error + anisometropia
  - Strabismus 12%
  - Cortical blindness 1%
  - Amblyopia
  - Cataract
  - Glaucoma → angle closure
  - Retinal detachment

Retinoblastoma

Incidence

- One in 15 to 20 000 live births, increasing in incidence
- Male = female, no racial difference
- Bilateral in 25–30%
- Accounts for 4% of childhood tumours
- Most common intraocular tumour of childhood
- Average age of diagnosis 18 months; varies birth to adulthood; 80% < 5 years

Genetics and heredity

- 6% inherited (familial) – autosomal dominant with high (80%) penetrance
- 94% sporadic – 80% somatic mutation, 20% germinal mutation
- Heritable (germline) → 40%
- Non-heritable (somatic) → 60%
- Inherited and germinal mutation forms are usually unilateral and multifocal, or bilateral
- The *RBL* gene is located on 13q14 – protects against the expression of retinablastoma (RB) (it is a recessive suppressor gene)
- Both copies of the 13q14 locus must be inactive for tumour expression (Knudson's 2-hit hypothesis)
- May be associated with trisomy 21 and deletion of long arm of chromosome 13 (13q deletion syndrome → craniofacial dysmorphism and other systemic manifestations)
- Gene responsible is RB1 locus on 13q14 chromosome; intact gene suppresses development of retinoblastoma

Genetic classification

- RB can be classified as
  - Familial or sporadic
  - Bilateral or unilateral
  - Heritable or non-heritable
- Generally familial or sporadic and bilateral or unilateral used clinically e.g. unilateral sporadic, bilateral sporadic, unilateral familial, bilateral familial
- Unilateral – two-thirds, bilateral – one-third
- 10–15% with a unilateral sporadic have a germline mutation → do DNA testing

Aetiology

- Hereditary predisposition
- External stimulus e.g. virus
- 15% chance of developing other neoplasms (osteogenic sarcoma); due to deletion of antioncogene
- Pinealoblastoma may be associated in 5–15% of germline RB (3% in total)
- Spontaneous regression occurs in 1% → retinoma

Life-threatening problems

Retinoblastoma metastases

- Usually within 1 year of RB diagnosis
- Risks – RB invasion
  - Extension beyond the lamina cribrosa in the optic nerve
  - Choroid
  - Sclera
  - Orbit
  - Anterior chamber
- Treat invasive RB with chemotherapy for 4 to 6 months
- Reduce incidence of metastasts from 24% to 4%

Trilateral retinoblastoma/ intracranial neuroblastic malignancy/pineoblastoma/ other parasellar tumours

- Invariably fatal
- Chemotherapy in germline RB may prevent trilateral RB

Secondary tumours

- 5% get a tumour in the first 10 years; 18% in the first 20 years; 26% within 30 years of age
- The 30 year cumulative incidence in those receiving radiation is 35%, only 6% in those who avoided external beam radiation
- Mean latency 13 years
- Osteogenic sarcoma – mostly in the femur
- Also spindle cell sarcoma, chondrosarcoma, rhabdomyosarcoma, neuroblastoma, glioma, leukaemia, sebaceous cell carcinoma, squamous cell carcinoma, malignant melanoma
- Patients who survive a second tumour are at risk of developing more tumours

Clinical features

- Presentation – leucocoria (50–62%), strabismus (20%), dilated pupil, proptosis, discovery on routine exam (3%), iris heterochromia (rubeosis), hyphaema or pseudohypopyon, vitreous haemorrhage, distant metastases
- Early lesions – flat, creamy-pink lesion in sensory retina
- Later lesions
  - Exophytic or endophytic growth
  - Exophytic arise from outer nuclear layer, growth into subretinal space → exudative retinal detachment → can resemble Coat's disease; often multicentric; yellow/white, large overlying vessels
  - Endophytic arise from inner nuclear layer, grow into vitreous; cream/ white, small or no vessels; vitreous seeding occurs → can even form an endophthalmitis-like picture or pseudohypopyon
- Advanced lesions
  - Optic nerve extension → central nervous system involvement
  - Orbital extension
  - Distant metastases (bone and elsewhere)
  - Choroidal invasion is associated with increased risk of metastatic disease
- Optic nerve extension for 10–12mm → reaching of point where central retinal artery and vein exit through subarachnoid space → gain access to subarachnoid space

Pathology

- Gross
  - White and friable, with foci of calcification
  - Endophytic or exophytic, ± multifocal, rarely diffuse
- Microscopic
  - Arises from primitive photoreceptor, varies from well-differentiated → poorly-differentiated
- Well-differentiated
  - Flexner-Wintersteiner rosettes – columnar cells around a central clear lumen
  - Homer-Wright rosettes – columnar cells around a central tangle of neural fibres; seen also in neuroblastoma and medulloblastoma
  - Fleurettes – groups of tumour cells containing eosinophilic processes
- Poorly-differentiated
  - Small round cells, large nuclei, numerous mitotic figures
  - Areas of necrosis and calcification may be seen
- Histology outside eye – rosettes rare, necrosis and calcification absent, cells larger
- Very rarely (1%) the retinoblastoma may spontaneously regress → retinoma/retinocytoma

Differential diagnosis of leukocoria

- Retinoblastoma
- PHPV (19–28%)
- ROP (4–13.5%)
- Cataract (7–13.5%)
- Coloboma of choroid or disc (10%)
- Uveitis (3–10%)
- Toxocariasis (6.5–20%)
- Congenital retinal fold (5%)
- Coat's disease (4–16%)
- Organised vitreous haemorrhage (4%)
- Retinal dysplasia (2.5%)
- Astrocytic hamartoma, haemangioblastoma
- Corneal opacity
- Familial exudative vitreoretinopathy
- High myopia/anisometropia
- Myelinated nerve fibres
- Norrie disease
- Retinal detachment
- Rhegmatogenous retinal detachment
- Retinoschisis
- Toxoplasmosis
- Incontinentia pigmenti

8

Differential diagnosis of retinoblastoma

- Persistent hyperplastic primary vitreous
- Retinal dysplasia
- Congenital retinal fold
- Ocular toxocara/toxoplasmosis
- Metastatic endophthalmitis
- Retinal hamartoma
- Coat's disease
- Retinopathy of prematurity
- Retinal detachment

Diagnostic approach

- History
- Physical exam
- External ocular exam
- Slip lamp exam
- Indirect fundoscopy
- Fluorescein → numerous vessels filled in arterial phase, leak profusely
- X-ray – calcification visible in 70% of cases
- CT scan – to detect calcification and optic nerve enlargement (5–10% show no calcification)

- MRI – does not detect calcification but very good for optic nerve invasium and pinealoblastoma
- Ultrasound – high reflectivity, persists after soft tissue echoes disappeared on lowering sensitivity
- Aqueous enzymes – increased LDH + increased phosphaglucose isomerase (normal LDH < 200 u; >1 000 u diagnostic)
- Aqueous cytology
- Serum esterase D absent in deletion of long arm of chromosome 13
- Lumbar puncture
- Bone marrow biopsy
- Examine parents and siblings
- Genetic counselling

Differential diagnosis of intraocular calcification

- Retinoblastoma
- Retinal astrocytoma
- Coat's disease
- Angiomatosis
- Nematode
- Endophthalmitis

Classification and staging

1. **Reese-Ellsworth:** (A classification for conservative globe salvaging)

Group	A	B
I – very favourable	Solitary tumour, ← 4 DD size, at/behind the equator	Multiple tumours, ← 4 DD, at/behind the equator
II – favourable	Solitary tumour 4-10 DD at/behind the equator	Multiple tumours 4-10 DD at/behind the equator
III – doubtful	Any lesion anterior to the equator	Solitary tumour 10DD posterior to the equator
IV – unfavourable	Multiple tumours some larger than 10 DD	Any lesion anterior to the ora serrata
V – very unfavourable	Massive tumour occupying half or more of the retina	Vitreous seeding

Reese-Ellsworth no longer widely used in a clinical setting

2. **Murphree classification:**

Group A – very low risk	Eyes with small discrete tumours away from critical structures All tumours are 3 mm or smaller, confined to the retina, and located at least 3 mm from the foveola and 11.5 mm from the optic nerve. No vitreous or subretinal seeding is allowed

8

Group B – low risk	Eyes with no vitreous or subretinal seeding and discrete retinal tumour of any size or location Retinal tumours may be of any size or location not in Group A. No vitreous or subretinal seeding allowed, A small cuff of subretinal fluid extending no more than 5 mm from the base of the tumour is allowed.
Group C – moderate risk	Eyes with only focal vitreous or subretinal seeding and discrete retinal tumours of any size and location. Any seeding must be local, fine, and limited so as to be theoretically treatable with a radioactive plaque. Retinal tumours are discrete and of any size and location. Up to one quadrant of subretinal fluid may be present.
Group D – high risk	Eyes withy diffuse vitreous or subretinal seeding an/or massive, nondiscrete endophytic or exophytic disease Eyes with more extensive seeding than Group C. Massive and/or diffuse intraocular disseminated disease may consist of fine or "greasy" vitreous seeding or avascular masses. Subretinal seeding may be plaque-like. Includes exophytic disease and more than one quadrant of retinal detachment.
Group E – very high risk eyes	Eyes that have been destroyed anatomically or functionally by the tumour. Eyes with one or more of the following: Irreversible neovascular glaucoma, massive intraocular haemorrhage, aseptic orbital cellulitis, tumour anterior to the anterior vitreous face, tumour touching the lens, diffuse infiltrating retinoblastoma, phthisis and pre-phthisis.

8

3. **Surgical staging**

Stage 0	Patient treated conservatively – no enucleation done
Stage I	Eye was enucleated, no residual tumour histologically
Stage II	Eye was enucleated, residual tumour microscopically
Stage III	Regional extension a. Overt orbital disease b. Preauricular or cervical lymph node extension
Stage IV	Metastatic disease a. Haematogenous metastasis (without central nervous system involvement) 1. Single lesion 2. Multiple lesions b. Central nervous system extension (with or without any other site of regional or metastatic disease)

1. Prechiasmatic lesion
2. Central nervous system mass
3. Leptomenigeal and CSF disease

Management

South African Children's Cancer Study Group – retinoblastoma treatment protocol

- **Group A:**
  Focal therapy:
  If using TTT, combine with IVI.
  Carboplatin* 2-3 hours before TTT.
  Repeat Carboplatin one week later for larger tumours.
  *Dosage: Carboplatin 20 mg per kg under 2 years. Run in a 50 ml saline solution over ½ hour, and use Navopan as anti-emetic
- **Group B:**
  Focal therapy or
  Shrink with chemotherapy (Carboplatin and Etoposide) in order to apply focal therapy.
  Expect maximal response to chemotherapy after first cycle.
  EUA monthly and apply TTT or Cryotherapy
  Consider plaque therapy or 'claws' after 2 cycles.
  Macular tumours can be treated as above
- **Group C:**
  Aim to shrink the tumour with chemotherapy prior to consolidating with radiotherapy.
  2 Cycles of chemotherapy is usually adequate.
  EUA monthly and apply TTT or Cryotherapy during the chemotherapy.
- **Group D:**
  Poor prognosis but 50% can be saved.
  Attempted conservative treatment in unilateral disease is not always in the patient's best interest.
  Vincristine, Etoposide and Carboplatin (VEC) for 1-2 cycles flattens the retina and shrinks the tumours.
  EUA monthly and apply TTT where possible.
  The whole eye will require RT and this can be given with 'claws' 6 weeks[4] after the last chemotherapy, or earlier if the tumours have not shrunk at the last EUA.
  Further chemotherapy may be necessary after RT.
- **Groups E:**
  Enucleation
  (Focal therapy – includes cryotherapy, argon laser or transpupillary thermotherapy, radioactive plaque therapy)

Enucleation

Aim to get a long segment of optic nerve
In Stage 3 with frank orbital tumour, obvious orbital tumour preoperatively that would interfere with the enucleation, give VEC chemotherapy first ± 10 Gy external beam radiation to facilitate enucleation
Exenteration should be avoided if at all possible.
Volume replacement – Aim to put in a ball implant unless there is obvious orbital tumour. Long-term appearance and quality of life is much better with ball implants

Chemoreduction

To reduce tumour volume thus allowing more focussed therapy
Attempt to save globe + avoid external beam radiation
VEC (Vincristine, Etoposide, Carboplatin) protocol used most widely
Generally 6 cycles of 1 month used
Mean reduction: 35% tumour base, 50% thickness
24% develop new tumours during or after chemo
Some use a sub-conjunctival boost of carboplatin → penetrates sclera

8

Retinitis pigmentosa

Definition

- Group of hereditary dystrophies of the photoreceptors characterised by progressive loss of photoreceptors and RPE
- Over 80 responsible genes have been identified, distributed randomly over the genome
- Primary confined to the eyes
- Secondary pigmentary retinopathy → RP associated with single or multiple organ system disease

Incidence

- One in 4 000 live births

Heredity

- Spontaneous – 40%
- Autosomal recessive – 20% (15 forms)
- Autosomal dominant – 10–20% (12 forms)
- Sex-linked recessive – 10–20%; female carriers have perimacular tapetal sheen and peripheral pigment atrophy

Pathogenesis

- Primary abnormality in rods and cones
- Disordered vitamin A metabolism
- Some primarily affect rods, some affect both rods and cones → secondary retinal pigment epithelium disorder, with disordered phagocytic activity

Pathology

- Starts peripherally, extends posteriorly
- Atrophy of rods and cones, replaced by glial tissue
- Secondary retinal pigment epithelial atrophy, with pigment migration and proliferation
- Pigment accumulates around veins → corpuscles
- Glial proliferation → vessel constriction with attenuation
- Gliosis in front of disc

Symptoms

- Nyctalopia, poor dark adaptation
- Poor vision
- Constricted field
- Photoaversion; ? due to decreased contrast sensitivity → photopsia, headaches

Signs

- Pale waxy disc, narrowed arteries, pigment disturbance (clumping, bone spicules/corpuscles)
- Posterior subcapsular lens opacities, myopia, chronic open angle glaucoma, ophthalmoplegia, keratoconus, cystoid macular oedema, Coat's disease, vitreous cells, disc drusen

Special investigations

- Visual field – annular scotoma between 30° and 50°, extends in and out
- ERG and EOG – decreased, especially rod loss
- Colour vision – blue defect

Variants

Leber's congenital amaurosis

- Accounts for 18% of congenital blindness
- Autosomal recessive, some may be autosomal dominant
- Blindness, sensory nystagmus, sunken eyeballs, photophobia, oculodigital reflex (? phosphene production)
- Fundus normal → full-blown retinitis pigmentosa
- Progressive with age, though blindness is not
- Ocular associations are keratoconus, cataract, glaucoma
- ERG and EOG decreased/absent
- Systemic associations are mental retardation (most have normal intelligence), musculoskeletal abnormalities, renal disease, deafness and cardiomyopathy

Sector retinitis pigmentosa

- Usually inferonasal and bilateral; stationary or progressive

Unilateral retinitis pigmentosa

- May be secondary to posterior ciliary artery occlusion, syphilis, infection, uveitis, settled retinal detachment no evidence that it is genetic

Retinitis pigments sine pigmenti

- May be early retinitis pigmentosa

Inverse retinitis pigmentosa

- Changes occur in macular and paramacular area
- Autosomal dominant
- Black patients are more likely to be affected

Retinitis punctata albescens

- Stationary or progressive
- May be early retinitis pigmentosa

Retinitis pigmentosa with exudative vasculopathy

- Coat's-like appearance

Associated systemic diseases

- Metabolic
- Neurologic
- Miscellaneous

Metabolic

Bassen-Kornzweig syndrome (abetalipoproteinemia)

- Associated with decreased vitamin A
- Treatment with vitamin A → recovery of ERG

Refsum's disease

- Autosomal recessive
- Phytanic acid in serum
- Atypical retinitis pigmentosa, chronic polyneuritis, ataxia, increased CSF protein, cataract, anosmia deafness, myopia, iccthyosis, skeletal abnormalities, cardiac arrythmias
- Retinal changes precede biochemical changes by several years, by which time the retina is permanently damaged

Amaurotic familial idiocy (ceroid lipofuscinosis)

- Infantile, late infantile, juvenile, adult
- Lipid accumulation in ganglion cells and destruction of photoreceptors
- Decreased vision, cherry-red spot, optic atrophy, peripheral retinal pigment degeneration

Mucopolysaccharidoses

- Types I II III V
- Corneal clouding, mental retardation, tapetoretinal degeneration

Neurologic

Lawrence-Moon-Biedl syndrome

- Autosomal recessive
- Obesity, polydactyly, hypogonadism, mental retardation, deafness, retinitis pigmentosa

Cockayne's syndrome

- Autosomal recessive
- Dwarfism, progeria, deafness, oligophrenia, retinitis pigmentosa, band-shaped keratopathy

Kearns-Sayre-Daroff syndrome

- Autosomal dominant
- Progressive external ophthalmoplegia, retinitis pigmentosa, heart block, cerebellar deficit, muscle weakness

Usher's syndrome

- Congenital deafness occurring with retinitis pigmentosa
- Occurs together in 20% of cases
- Autosomal recessive
- Profound (type I)
- Partial (type II)

Pseudoretinitis pigmentosa

- Trauma
- Chorioretinitis – syphilis, rubella, other viruses, Vogt-Koyanagi-Harada syndrome
- Drugs – phenothiazines, chloroquine
- Vascular – ophthalmic artery occlusion
- Resolution of detachment
- Paraneoplastic syndromes

Treatment

- CMO → acetazolamide
- Bassen-Kornzweig – vitamin A
- Refsum's – low phytanic acid
- Genetic counselling
- Low vision aids
- Cataract extraction, refractive correction
- Occlusion with opaque contact lens or red filter
- One study showed a modest decrease in RP progression by supplementing with 3 times the normal daily dose of vitamin A, but this can cause liver toxicity and teratogenicity
- Use of antioxidants may be helpful
- Probable benefit in protection from high levels of light exposure

Prognosis

- Total blindness is an infrequent endpoint
- Deafness in Usher's is congenital; if patients are not born deaf then they are unlikely to become deaf
- Autosomal recessive – blind at 20 years of age
- X-linked recessive – blind at 30 years of age
- Autosomal dominant – blind at 50 years of age

Systemic diseases associated with pigmentary retinopathy

- Autosomal dominant
  - Arteriohepatic dysplasia
  - Charcot-Marie-Tooth
  - Myotonic dystrophy
  - Oculodentodigital dysplasia syndrome
  - Olivopontocerebellar atrophy
  - Stickler syndrome
  - Wagner's hereditary vitreoretinal degeneration
  - Waardenburg syndrome
- Autosomal recessive
  - Bardet-Biedel
  - Bietti's crystalline retinopathy
  - Friedreichs ataxia
  - Homocystinurea
  - Mannosidiosis
  - Hurler's syndrome (mucopolysaccaridosis)
  - Scheie syndrome (mucopolysaccaridosis)
  - Sanfilipino syndrome – (mucopolysaccaridosis)
  - Neonatal adrenoleukodystrophy
  - Refsum's disease
  - Usher's syndrome
  - Zellweger syndrome
- X-linked recessive
  - Incontinentia pigmenti (Bloch-Sulzberger syndrome)
  - Mucopolysaccaridosis II (Hunter's syndrome)
  - Pelizaeus-Merzbacher disease

Angioid streaks

Associations

- No association in 50%
- Common associations
  - Pseudoxanthoma elasticum (80%) – calcium deposition in Bruch's membrane
  - Paget's disease (8%) – calcium deposition in Bruch's membrane
  - Sickle cell haemaglobinopathy – ? iron deposition in Bruch's membrane
- Other associations
  - Marfan's syndrome
  - Ehlers-Danlos syndrome
  - Aging
  - Dwarfism
  - Acromegally
  - Lead poisoning
  - Systemic lupus erythematosis
  - Diabetes
  - Myopia
  - Senile elastosis
  - Neurofibromatosis
  - Tuberous sclerosis

Pathogenesis

- Crack-like dehiscences in elastic layer of Bruch's membrane caused by degenerative process
- Brittle Bruch's membrane, from calcium or iron deposition
- Traction by extraocular muscles → cracks

Pathology

- Linear breaks in Bruch's membrane
- Adjacent choroid and RPE degeneration
- Fibrovascular ingrowth from choriocapillaris → disciform maculopathy

Clinical features

- Usually bilateral, male > female
- Radiate from disc, may form incomplete ring around disc
- Beneath normal retinal vessels
- May be red (whites) or grey (blacks), vary in distribution, localised or widespread
- Salmon spots – focal peripheral chorioretinal lesions
- Peau d'orange – due to RPE mottling posterior pole; lighter orange appearance
- Disc associations – disc drusen, vascular loops
- Usually asymptomatic, visual loss may follow minor trauma
- Visual loss due to subretinal neovascular membrane in macula; macular degeneration may be non-exudative or exudative

Fluorescein angiogram

- May show either hypo or hyperfluorescence – RPE atrophy
- Subretinal neovascular membrane → early hyperfluorescence and late staining

Differential diagnosis

- Macular degeneration
- Choroidal sclerosis
- Myopic degeneration

Diagnostic work up

- Skin biopsy (pseudoxanthoma elasticum)
- X-ray skull, abdomen, legs (Paget's)
- Haemaglobin electrophoresis (haemaglobinopathies)

Treatment

- Prophylactic photocoagulation contraindicated – may stimulate subretinal neovascularisation
- Photocoagulate subretinal neovascular membrane; repeat angiogram after 1 week
- Physician referral for heart valves + vessels
- Avoid blunt eye trauma e.g. contact sport

8

Prognosis

- Visual impairment in 70%
- Due to exudative maculopathy, choroidal haemorrhage, foveal streaks

Pseudoxanthoma elasticum

- Inherited, 4 types, 2 recessive, 2 dominant
- Degenerative condition of elastic fibres
- Characteristic skin changes in the face, neck and flexures
- Cardiovascular and gastrointestinal features
- Angioid streaks occur in 80–90% (Groenblad-Strandberg syndrome)

Paget's disease

- Due to a slow virus
- Increased bone resorption + increased formation of defective, enlarged bone → pain, deformities
- Angioid streaks occur in 8–15%

Ehlers-Danlos syndrome

- Autosomal dominant
- Disorder of collagen (deficiency of hydroxylysine)
- Characteristic skin changes
- Hyperextensible joints
- Cardiovascular features
- Ocular features – angioid streaks, epicanthic folds, keratoconus, high myopia, retinal detachment, blue sclera, lens subluxation

Albinism

- Genetically determined disorder of hereditary fundus dystrophy and hypopigmentation
- Deficiency of tyrosinase and inability to convert tyrosine to melanin

Oculocutaneous

Tyrosinase-negative

- Can synthesise no melanin
- Blond hair, pale skin
- Translucent iris, no fundal pigment, prominent choroidal vessels, foveal and optic nerve hypoplasia, refractive errors, VA <6/60, pendular horizontal nystagmus, abnormal visual pathways from lateral geniculate nucleus to visual cortex

Tyrosinase-positive

- Can synthesise some melanin
- Near normal complexion
- Normal iris, variable fundal hypopigmentation, foveal hypoplasia
- Associated syndromes: Chediak-Higashi, Hermansky-Pudlak

Ocular

- Predominantly eye involvement
- X-linked recessive inheritance (autosomal recessive less common)
- Asymptomatic female carriers – may have iris translucency, macular stippling, midperipheral depigmentation and granularity
- Males – hypopigmented irises and fundi

Phacomatoses

- Characterised by disseminated hamartomas of the eye, skin and brain (hamartoma = a benign tumour-like nodule composed of an overgrowth of mature tissues and cells normally present there but with one element predominating)
- Most, not all, hereditary

Von Hippel-Lindau disease

- Capillary haemangiomas of retina + disc
- Hereditary or sporadic
- Automomal dominant, incomplete penetrance
- Von Hippel-Lindau = retinal angiomatosis + central nervous system involvement + visceral involvement

- Early lesions small, easily overlooked, seen on fluorescein
- Later, large, spherical, orange-red tumour
- Multiple tumours in one eye
- 50% bilateral
- Large feeding + draining vessels
- Surrounding exudate + serous detachment +– exudate at macula
- Vitreous haemorrhage, tractional retinal detachment
- Central nervous system tumours in 20% (haemangioblastomas of cerebellum, medulla, pons, spinal cord)
- Visceral lesions – cysts of kidney, pancreas, liver, epididymis, ovary
- Associations: Renal cell carcinoma, meningiomas, phaeochromocytomas
- Leading cause of death → cerebellar haemangioblastoma + renal cell ca
- Rx: cryopexy, laser, (PDT)
- Treatment early
- Rarely involutes spontaneously

Wyburn-Mason syndrome

- Congenital arteriovenous malformations, racemose haemangioma
- Congenital retinal AV communication with no intervening capillary bed
- Unilateral, non-hereditary, retina or optic nerve
- Associated with intracranial, face and orbital haemangiomas ipsilaterally
- Retinal malformations mostly asymptomatic unless very large → subretinal fluid (SRF) + exudate
- Usually unilateral

Retinal cavernous haemangioma

- Mostly sporadic, may be autogomal dominant
- Mostly restricted to retina, may involve skin and brain
- Grape-like clusters of thin-walled saccular angiomatous lesions in the inner retina or on the optic nerve head
- Blood from normal retinal circulation → stagnant → characteristic fluorescein angiogram pattern
- No SRF or exudates (cf telangiectasis, von Hippel, racemose)
- Mostly asymptomatic, may cause vitreous haemorrhage
- Laser or cryo if recurrent vitreous haemorrhage, otherwise leave

Neurofibromatosis

- The most common
- Type 1 (peripheral) more common (1 in 3 000). Type 2 (central) less common (1 in 1 million)

Type 1 (peripheral, von Recklinghausen's disease)

- Autosomal dominent, 100% penetrance, variable expressivity
- Gene 17q11.2, product is neurofibromin → acts as a tumour suppressor normally

8

Diagnosis 2 or more

- ≥ Six café au lait spots ≥ 5 mm before puberty, ≥ 15 mm after puberty
- Twp neurofibromas or one plexiform neuroma
- Axillary or inguinal freckling
- Optic nerve glioma
- Lisch nodules
- An osseous lesion or first degree relative with one

Ocular features

- Plexiform neuromas or neurfibromas of the lids
- Prominent corneal nerves
- Lisch nodules (melanocytic hamartomas) → 95% of cases
- Glaucoma
- Retinal hamartomas (rare)
- Optic nerve or chiasmal gliomas – 15%
- Optic nerve meningiomas (uncommon – may be multiple)
- Papilloedema – following aqueductal stenosis

- Diplopia – neurilemomas + schwannomas of cranial nerves
- Orbital asymmetry – sphenoid wing dysplasia with pulsatile proptosis
- Proptosis – orbital fibroma, or plexiform neuroma

Type 2 (central, bilateral acoustic neurofibromatosis)

- Autosomal dominent, 95% penetrance, variable expressivity
- Gene 22q11.2, product is Merlin or Schwannomin → defect linked to vestibular schwannomas and meningiomas

Diagnosis

- Bilateral VIII nerve neuromas
- Or unilateral VIII neuroma, first degree relative with one
- Or two of neurofibromas, meningiomas, gliomas, schwannomas, juvenile PSCLO

Ocular features

- Posterior subcapsular lens opacities
- Retinal membranes
- Hamartomas
- RPE abnormalities
- Optic nerve meningiomas

Management

- Genetic counselling
- Screening of family
- Bilateral optic gliomas are occasionally progressive, may require chemo therapy
- Surgery for acoustic neuromas often followed by ipsilateral facial palsy

Tuberous sclerosis

- Autosomal dominent, high penetrance, variable expressivity, 50% new mutations
- 1 : 10 000
- Genes: TSC1 at 9q34 → hamartin, or TSC2 at 16p13 → tuberin (both tumour suppressors
- Clinically: Epilepsy (90%), mental retardation (65%), adenoma sebaceum (80%) – highly vascular angiofibroma in malar distribution, vitiligo, intracranial astrocytomas and gliomas, renal tumours, myocardial rhabdos, pulmonary fibrosis

Ocular features

- Retinal astrocytic hamartoma (50%) → confusion with retinoblastoma
- Can increase in size with age and calcify
- Hypopigmented iris spots
- Papilloedema due to gliomas
- VI palsy due to raised ICP

Sturge-Weber syndrome (encephalotrigeminal angiomatosis)

- Non-heritable
- Port wine stain – one or more divisions of the trigeminal nerve
- Can cross midline and affect trunk
- Bilateral in 10% → increased central nervous system involvement + risk of glaucoma
- Skin + hemiface hypertrophy unless early laser
- Meningeal angiomas ipsilateral to port wine stain → calcification + railroad track sign on CT scan
- Epilepsy, ± mental impairment

Ocular features

- Ipsilateral glaucoma – 50%, especially if upper lid involved in port wine stain
- Glaucoma – infantile, mid-childhood (episcleral venous pressure), adulthood (idiopathic open angle)
- Choroidal cavernous haemangiomas 40% (if present 90% chance of glaucoma)
- Retinal vascular tortuosity ± leakage, cystic degeneration of retina, exudative detachment
- Iris heterochromia – prominent iris vascularisation
- Field defects → compression of visual pathway by meningeal angiomas

Treatment

- Careful with all intraocular surgery – prone to expulsive haemorrhage
- Post-op choroidal effusions after anterior segment surgery

Louis-Bar syndrome (ataxia telangiectasia)

- Autosomal recessive
- Gene: ATM gene, 11q23
- Progressive cerebellar ataxia, oculocutaneous telangiectasia, immunodeficiency, chromosomal instability, predisposition to malignancy, early death
- Ataxia soon after child starts walking
- Conjunctival telangiectatic vessels early
- Frequent sinus and lung infections
- Lymphoma + leukaemia
- Mental and growth retardation, choreoathetosis, dysarthria, dry skin + hair

Ocular features

- Inability to initiate saccades and, later, pursuit
- Total supranuclear ophthalmoplegia late
- Conjunctival telangiectasia
- Cerebellar oculomotor signs

Kleppel-Trenaunay-Weber syndrome

- Capillary haemangiomas → retina + disc
- Hereditary or sporadic
- Autosomal dominent, incomplete penetrance
- Von Hippel-Lindau = retinal angiomatosis + central nervous system involvement + visceral involvement
- Early lesions small, easily overlooked, seen on fluorescein
- Later, large, spherical, orange-red tumour
- Multiple tumours in one eye
- 50% bilateral
- Large feeding + draining vessels
- Surrounding exudate + serous detachment ± exudate at macula
- Vitreous haemorrhage, TRD
- Central nervous system tumours in 20% (haemangioblastomas of cerebellum, medulla, pons, spinal cord)
- Visceral lesions – cysts of kidney, pancreas, liver, epididymis, ovary
- Associations: Renal cell carcinoma, meningiomas, phaeochromocytomas
- Leading cause of death → cerebellar haemangioblastoma + renal cell carcinoma

Cutis marmarata telangiectasia congenita

- Non-heritable
- A vascular disorder associated with brain + eye involvement

Age related macular degeneration (ARMD)

Definition

- Dystrophic disease of choriocapillaris, Bruch's membrane and RPE

Normal age-related changes

- Photoreceptors – decreased density
- RPE – loss of melanin, increased lipofuscin formation, residual body accumulation
- Basal lamina – between RPE + Bruch's membrane → deposits of granular, lipid-rich material + collagen fibres
- Choriocapillaris – involutional changes

Epidemiology

- The major cause of blindness in white people over 60 years of age, rare in black people
- Bilateral; 12% chance per year of the second eye being involved
- Risk increases with age
- Affects
    - 2% of people from 52–64 years of age

    - 10% of people from 65–74 years of age
    - 30% of people from 75–85 years of age

Risk factors for ARMD

- Family history
- Smoking
- Hypermetropia
- Light iris
- Hypertension
- Hypercholesterolaemia
- Female gender
- Cardiovascular disease
- UV light exposure (unproven)

Pathophysiology

- Normal senescence
- Pre-disciform ARMD
- Disciform ARMD

8

Normal senescence

- ARMD is merely an exaggeration of the normal process of senescence of the RPE and Bruch's membrane
- RPE degeneration is the primary change
- RPE cells continually degrade their own structural components + material from the photoreceptors
- UV light + oxygen metabolism → alteration in the structure of substrate molecules → incomplete digestion → accumulation of residual bodies; start accumulating from 16 months of age
- RPE cells are eventually damaged by these
- Basal laminar deposits are formed from RPE secretions between basal folds of RPE and basement membrane
- Drusen are formed as extracellular masses between RPE basal lamina and inner layer of Bruch's membrane
- Bruch's membrane undergoes thickening, hyalinisation, debris deposition, aberrant collagen, cracks and gaps
- New vessels penetrate Bruch's membrane from choriocapillaris

Pre-disciform ARMD

- RPE – atrophy, proliferation, hypertrophy
- Rods + cones – loss of some cells, adjacent become shorter and broader
- Drusen
    - Small and hard early, large and soft later
    - May calcify
    - Small drusen are benign, large drusen → subretinal neovascularisation in 56% of cases
    - If they stain in the late phase of the angiogram, they tend to progress to subretinal neovascularisation

Disciform ARMD

- Choroidal vessels are attracted by substances released by degenerating RPE
- Invade Bruch's membrane, spread laterally beneath RPE
- Leak and bleed → RPE detachment ± sensory detachment
- Fibrosis healing → scar

Non-neovascular abnormalities (dry/atrophic ARMD)

- 85–90% of cases
- Atrophy of neurosensory retina, RPE and choriocapillaris
- Slowly progressive, mild, bilateral decreased visual acuity
- Focal RPE clumping + atrophy
- Sharply circumscribed RPE atrophy
- Choriocapillaris atrophy
- Fluorescein – window defects and scleral staining

Drusen

- Small, round, yellow lesions, RPE level
- Largely asymptomatic but can cause photoreceptor loss with decreased VA + poor dark adaptation
- Histologically

- Abnormal thickening of Bruch's
  - Basal laminar deposits (granular lipid-rich material + widely spaced collagen)
  - Basal linear deposits (phospholipids vesicles + electron-dense granules within the inner aspect of Bruch's)
- RPE detachment – thickened inner aspect of Bruch's separates from rest of Bruch's
- Small RPE detachment → small druse
- Larger area → RPE detachment
- Most people > 50 have drusen
- Most will not lead to geographic atrophy or CNV
- Small drusen
  - < 64 μ – may lead to ARMD but not enough alone to make a diagnosis of AMD
  - Risk of progression to advanced ARMD = 1.3% in 5 years
- Intermediate drusen
  - 64–124 μ – 18% risk of progression over 5 years
- Large
  - > 125 μ – 18% risk of progression over 5 years as well
- Hard drusen – focal and smaller
- Soft drusen
  - Diffuse thickening of the inner aspect of Bruch's
  - May be confluent
  - Greater risk of CNV or geographic than hard drusen
- Fluorescein stains drusen late and may cause pooling

RPE abnormalities

- Geographic atrophy
- Non-geographic atrophy
- Focal hyperpigmentation
- Spontaneous flattening of RPE detachment + regression of soft, confluent drusen → RPE geographic atrophy if contiguous
- Non-geographic if the area is not contiguous
- Corresponding photoreceptor loss
- Incidence of legal blindness with central geographic → 12–20%
- Focal hyperpigmentation – increases risk of progression to advanced AMD
- Drusen may regress or calcify as atrophy develops
- Differential diagnosis for geographic
  - CSCR
  - Pattern dystrophy
  - Drug toxicity e.g. chloroquine
  - Basal laminar drusen syndrome

Management of non-neovascular abnormalities

- Test for metamorphopsia, scotomas + visual change with Amsler
- Low vision clinic
- Treat other diseases e.g. cataract
- Micronutrients

Neovascular abnormalities (wet/exudative ARMD)

8

- 10–15% of cases; 90% of cases with severe visual loss
- Subretinal neovascularisation → serous or haemorrhagic RPE detachment, serous or haemorrhagic detachment of sensory retina, cystoid degeneration of sensory retina, organised disciform scar
- More severe loss of vision, poorer prognosis
- Fluorescein → early lacy hyperfluorescence, later leak
- Clinical features suggestive of wet/exudative include
  - Haemorrhage in macular area
  - Macular oedema
  - Dirty grey membrane
- Presence of CNV
- Disturbance in Bruch's → neovascular tissue from choroid into the sub-RPE space → accompanied by fibroblasts → fibrovascular complex → photoreceptor and outer retinal destruction → disciform scar

Clinical

- Symptoms – sudden loss of vision, metamorphopsia, paracentral scotomas
- Signs
  - RPE elevation, subretinal/intraretinal lipid/fluid/blood
  - PED, RPE tears, green-grey lesion, subretinal pigment ring, CMO, sea-fan pattern of subretinal small vessels
- Fluorescein: patterns vary because the CNV may be a complex of several lesion components
- Classic CNV – bright, uniform hyperfluorescence early, lacy pattern, progressively intensifies, late leakage obscuring the boundaries
- Predominantly classic – the CNV occupies > 50% of the lesion, including all components (pigment, scar and staining) and the classic part of the CNV is > 50% of the CNV component
- Minimally classic – < 50% of entire lesion classic
- Extrafoveal – CNV > 200 μ from centre of foveal avascular zone
- Subfoveal – centre of FAZ involved
- Juxtafoveal – CNV closer than 200 μ from centre of FAZ but does not involve it
- Occult CNV – poorly defined membrane, starts to fluoresce + leak later ± at 1–2 mins
- Fibrovascular PED
  - A combination of CNV + PED
  - Granular, irregular fluorescence ± 1–3 mins
  - Progressive leakage, but not as diffuse as classic
- Benefits of PDT are for predominantly classic or purely occult
- Serous PED vs occult CNV
  - Serous PED – smooth RPE elevation, rapid early homogenous intense hyperfluorescence at 20–60 secs; retaining same boundaries and intensity
  - Occult CNV – irregular topography, non-homogenous, stippled hyperfluorescence, slow filling at 1–3 mins; leaking or staining late

Differential diagnosis of neovascular AMD

- Macroaneurysm
- Vitelliform dystrophy with RPE detachments
- Polypoidal choroidal vasculopathy
- CSCR
- Inflammatory conditions
- Small tumour e.g. choroidal melanoma

Management

- Laser
- Photodynamic therapy
- Other modalities

Laser

- For classic CNV with well-demarcated borders
- For classic/occult component lesions with well-demarcated borders
- For extrafoveal, juxtafoveal lesions where fovea will not be damaged by the laser
- Decreases chance of severe visual loss
- Must cover the whole lesion and be intensely white

Photodynamic therapy

- Visudyne IVI over 10 mins
- Systemic photosensitising drug complexes with low density lipoprotems, taken up by vascular endothelium of CNV which has high density lipoproteins receptor concentration → photosensitised by light of a specific wavelength (red 689 nm, started 15 mins after start of infusion, for 1.5 mins) → local reaction → reactive oxygen → capillary endothelial cell and vessel damage/occlusion
- Vision usually stabilises 6–12 months after treatment has started

- Must follow 3-monthly for 2 years
- Then 6-monthly if no leakage
- No need for follow-up if becomes disciform and endstage

Other modalities

Thermotherapy

- Transpupillary thermotherapy (TTT)
- For occult subfoveal CNV
- Heat-induced damage to CNV

Radiotherapy

- So far studies have failed to show benefit
- Ongoing study

Submacular surgery

- PPV, small retinotomy, subfoveal blister of BSS, CNV pulled out with forceps

Macular translocation

- Relocating undamaged neurosensory retina to another location
- Giant retinotomy or limited retinotomy with scleral shortening

Pneumatic displacement of haemorrhage

- Thick blood damages photoreceptors with fibrin clots + oxygen radicals
- Haemorrhage displaced with gas

Anti-angiogenesis

- **Bevacizumab**
  - A humanised monoclonal antibody
  - FDA approved as chemotherapy for metastatic colon and non-small cell lung carcinomas
  - Widely used off-label as an intravitreal injection for choroidal neovascularisation in ARMD
  - Dosage – 1.25mg in 0.05ml
  - One 1.25mg injection once a month for 3 months and then 1-3 monthly depending on individual response
- **Ranibizumab**
  - Derived from the bevacizumab molecule
  - Delivered as an intravitreal injection
  - FDA approved for treatment of choroidal neovascularisation in wet ARMD
  - Dosage – 0.5mg in 0.05ml
  - One 0.5mg injection once a month for 3 months and then 1-3 monthly depending on individual response
- **Pegaptanib sodium**
  - A pegylated anti-VEGF aptamer
  - Binds to VEGF 165 which is important in angiogenesis
  - FDA approved for treatment of choroidal neovascularisation in wet ARMD
  - Intravitreal injection, 0.3mg every 6 weeks
- Anecortave acetate
  - A steroid-like molecule with minimal glucocorticoid effects like raised IOP
  - For the treatment of choroidal neovascularisation in wet ARMD
  - Delivered as a sub-Tenon capsule injection

8

Choroidal neovascularisation

Degenerative

- ARMD
- Myopic degeneration
- Angioid streaks

Hereodegenerative

- Vitelliform macular dystrophy
- Fundus flavimaculatus
- Optic nerve head drusen

Inflammatory

- Ocular histoplasmosis syndrome
- Multifocal choroiditis
- Serpiginous choroiditis
- Toxoplasmosis
- Toxocariasis
- Rubella
- VKH syndrome

- Behçet's syndrome
- Sympathetic ophthalmia

Tumour

- Choroidal naevus
- Choroidal haemangioma
- Metastatic choroidal tumours
- Hamartoma of the RPE

Traumatic

- Choroidal rupture
- Intense photocoagulation

Idiopathic

Retinal vein occlusions

Central retinal vein occlusion (CRVO)

Classification

- Ischaemic – 25%
- Non-ischaemic – 75%

Aetiology and pathogenesis

- Younger patients (< 50 years of age)
  - May be vasculitis in common fibroelastic arterovenous sheath at lamina cribrosa → thrombus formation
  - No evidence of vasculitis in most; probably due to a congenital abnormality of central retinal vein
- Older patients (> 50 years of age)
  - Arteriosclerosis in central retinal artery + decreased BP at night → vein obstruction → thrombus formation
  - Predispositions – hypertension (60%), arteriosclerosis, diabetes, glaucoma (30%), oral contraceptives, smoking, dehydration, vasculitis, blood dyscrasias, congestive cardiac failure, chronic obstructive airways disease, hypercoagulable states

Pathology

- Block at lamina cribrosa → few collaterals → ischaemic
- Block behind lamina cribrosa → more collaterals → non-ischaemic
- Haemorrhagic infarction of inner retinal layers, oedema of all layers, later atrophy and glial replacement

Features

- Non-ischaemic
  - Minimal decrease in visual acuity
  - Few haemorrhages, mild macular oedema, ± evidence of vasculitis, venous engorgement
  - Intact perifoveal capillary arcade
- Ischaemic
  - Ten disc areas of ischaemia
  - Painless profound loss of vision, afferent pupil defect
  - Extensive haemorrhages, macular and disc oedema, soft exudates, venous engorgement
  - Capillary dropout
  - Decreased b wave on ERG, decreased light peak on EOG
- Distinction between ischaemic and non-ischaemic
  - Ischemic → Afferent pupil defect, >10 cotton wool spots, capillary dropout on fluorescein angiogram, decreased b wave on ERG, decreased light peak on EOG

Special investigations

- Check blood pressure
- Blood sugar
- FBC + ESR, if ESR elevated, find cause and treat
- Lipid profile
- Syphilis serology
- Chest xray
- ECG
- Serum protein profile
- Antinuclear antibody
- Serum uric acid
- Protein C + S

Treatment

- Medical
  - Treat any underlying cause found
  - Treat glaucoma if present; NB other eye

  - ± Aspirin for the other eye; efficacy unproven, typically not recommended
- Laser
  - Non-ischaemic – ? treat macular oedema with gentle grid
  - Ischaemic – PRP to prevent rubeotic glaucoma (before 90 days)
  - Wait 6–8 weeks for haemorrhage to clear, do fluorescein; if area of capillary non-perfusion is > 10 disc areas, this confirms ischaemic
- Surgery
  - Radial optic neurotomy
  - Sectioning the posterior scleral ring to relieve neurovascular compression at the optic nerve head
  - To allow retinal reperfusion

Complications

- Non-ischaemic
  - May become ischaemic; risk 15% within 4 months, 30% within 3 years
  - Intractable macular oedema → macular hole and preretinal fibrosis
- Ischaemic
  - Intractable macular oedema → macular hole and preretinal fibrosis
  - Retinal neovascularisation → vitreous haemorrhage and traction retinal detachment
  - Iris rubeosis after 1 month, neovascular glaucoma after 3 months (in 50% cases)

Prognosis

- Non-ischaemic – good for recovery of vision; 50% return to normal vision
- Ischaemic – poor for recovery of vision
- Risk of involvement of second eye – 15%
- Risk of second episode in same eye – 5%
- Life expectancy
  - Ischaemic – 7 years
  - Non-ischaemic – 11–13 years
  - Bilateral – 6 years

Branch retinal vein occlusion (BRVO)

Incidence

- Three times more common than CRVO

Aetiology

- Increased blood viscosity and hypercoagulability – blood dyscrasias, oral contraceptives
- Pressure from outside
  - Arteriosclerotic artery + decreased BP at night
  - Increased IOP
- Diseases of vessel wall
  - Retinal vascular malformations – von Hippel-Lindau, Coat's
  - Retinal vasculitis (Eale's, Behçet's, toxoplasmosis, sarcoid)

Risk factors

- Systemic arterial hypertension
- Chronic open angle glaucoma
- Hypermetropia – ? mechanism
- Old age
- Obesity
- Diabetes found to not be a major risk factor

8

Systemic diseases associated with pigmentary retinopathy

- Shilling and Kohner
  - Hemisphere occlusion; at edge of optic cup
  - A-V crossing occlusion; involving superotemporal branch in 60–70%, most common type, usually associated hypertension
  - Peripheral occlusion; in retinal vasculitis
  - Nasal vein occlusion; in diabetic retinopathy

- Orth and Patz
  - Main vein occlusion at disc margin – without macular oedema, with macular oedema
  - Major BVO away from disc – without macular oedema, with macular oedemaV
  - Macular BVO – superior, inferior
  - Peripheral BVO
  - BVO with disc neovascularisation
  - BVO with neovascularisation elsewhere

Clinical features

- Variable loss of vision, depending on site
- Sectoral involvement, fundoscopic features as for CRVO
- Usually superotemporal, nasal occlusions rarely detected

Fluorescein angiogram features

- Acute
  - Increased venous circulation time
  - Masking defects of haemorrhage
  - Areas of non-perfusion
  - Fluorescein leakage
- Chronic
  - Collaterals and shunt vessels
  - Microaneurysms and telangiectatic vessels
  - Capillary non-perfusion
  - Persisting macular oedema
  - Fluorescein leakage from new vessels
  - Serous detachment of sensory retina

Complications

- Chronic macular oedema
  - 60–100% have macular oedema at some time
  - 33% have macular oedema after 1 year
  - Integrity of perifoveal capillary arcade on angiogram at 6 weeks important
- Neovascularisation
  - Occurs in 10–30% of cases
  - If capillary non-perfusion on angiogram is > 5 disc diameters, risk of neovascularisation is high (40%)
  - Iris rubeosis occurs in 1–3% only
- Vitreous haemorrhage
  - Risk is greatest with partial posterior vitreous detachment causing traction on new vessels
  - 10% of spontaneous vitreous haemorrhage is due to BRVO
- Retinal detachment
- Internal limiting membrane contraction
- Hard exudate formation

Treatment

- Medical – of underlying disorder
- Prophylactic sectoral PRP prevents neovascularisation and vitreous haemorrhage
  - If the area of retina involved is < 5DD – no treatment
  - If the area of retina involved is > 5DD – wait 6 weeks for haemorrhage to clear
  - Do fluorescein angiogram
  - If capillary non-perfusion is > 5DD, follow up 4 monthly for the development of neovascularisation
  - Do sector PRP if neovascularisation occurs
  - If the capillary arcade is intact, no treatment and good prognosis
  - If the capillary arcade is not intact, treat with sector PRP and visual prognosis is poor
- Macular oedema present after 6 months
  - Treat with macular grid laser
- Vitrectomy and retinal detachment surgery if required
- IVT triamcinolone
- PPV + AV sheathotomy

Prognosis

- 50% will maintain a VA of 6/12 or better after 1 year

Thrombophilia

- Genetic and acquired predisposition to venous thrombosis

Genetic risk factors for thrombophilia

Activated protein C resistance

- Protein C → inactivates procoagulant factors V + VIII → limiting thrombin production
- Factor V Leiden → a point mutation at the factor V gene
- Causes 80% of protein C resistance + the most common genetic predisposition to venous thrombosis

Prothrombin variant 20210A

- Mutation of nucleotide 20210 → associated with thrombophilia, mechanism unknown

Antithrombin III deficiency

- AT-III → an endogenous inhibitor of thrombin
- Deficiency associated with CRVO + Cilioretinal artery occlusion

Protein C deficiency

- Activated protein C + S inactivate factors V + VIII
- BRVO

Protein S deficiency

- Retinal artery occlusions

Antiphospholipid syndromes

- Antiphospholipid antibodies → immunoglobulins associated with thrombosis in connective tissue disorders
- Hyperhomocystinaemia
- Defects of fibrinoloysis

Screening for thrombophilia

- Family history of venous thrombo-embolism → strongest reason for screening
- Recurrent, young, bilateral retinal vein occlusions
- Factor V Leiden
- Prothrombin variant 20210A → CRVO + BRVO
- Antithrombin III → CRVO + cilioretinal occlusion
- Protein C → BRVO
- Protein S → arteriolar occlusion
- Antiphospholipid testing – lupus anticoagulant + anticardiolipin
- Hyperhomocystinaemia

Retinal arterial occlusive disease

Carotid artery occlusion and stenosis (Ocular ischaemic syndrome)

Aetiology

- Carotid artery occlusion – atherosclerosis
- Aortic arch syndrome
  - 1° – Takayasu's disease
  - 2° – syphilis, dissecting aneurysm; bilateral, more severe
  - Eisenmenger syndrome
  - Giant cell arteritis

Pathogenesis

- Slow occlusion → compromised blood supply
- Emboli break off – fibrin, platelets, cholesterol

Clinical Pictures

- Amaurosis fugax
  - Transient monocular blindness
  - Recovers in seconds to minutes, no sequelae
  - Due to emboli from carotid or heart
  - Treatment with aspirin may prevent further attacks

8

  - Differential diagnosis includes carotid artery occlusion, temporal arteritis, Raynaud's disease, migraine, glaucoma, papilloedema, impending central retinal vein occlusion
- Gradual loss of union, weeks, months
- Venous dilatation, tortuosity, microaneurysms, cotton wool spots, macular oedema
- Central/branch retinal artery occlusion
- Ischaemic papillitis/AION
- Retinopathy from capillary occlusion – venous dilatation, microaneurysms, haemorrhages, soft and hard exudates, neovascularisation
- Peripheral retinal neovascularisation
- Anterior segment ischaemia – injection, corneal oedema, cells + flare, sluggish pupil, cataract, rubeosis + glaucoma
- Normal pressure glaucoma (IOP can be normal or reduced because ciliary body non-perfusion)
- Horner's syndrome

8

Special investigations

- Ausculate/palpate carotids
- Doppler ultrasound of carotids
- Ophthalmodynamometry – > 20% difference in diastolic pressure is significant
- Fluorescein angiogram
  - Delayed choroidal filling
  - Prolonged arterovenous filling
  - Capillary non-perfusion
  - Late leakage
  - Arterial staining

Treatment

- General measures – exclude associated risk factors (hypertension, diabetes, hypercholesterolaemia, smoking)
- Antiplatelet therapy
- Carotid endarterectomy (can cause severe rise in IOP because reperfusion of ciliary body)

Giant cell/temporal arteritis

- An enigmatic granulomatous, necrotising arteritis with predilection for medium and large arteries
- Predominantly cranial branches of aortic arch (especially superficial temporal, ophthalmic, posterior ciliary, vertebral)
- Medical emergency

Aetiology

- Unknown – may be autoimmune

Pathology

- Chronic full thickness inflammatory infiltrate in artery walls
- Internal elastic lamina injury, giant cells present in inflammatory infiltrate

Features

- Occurs in old age, rare in Blacks
- 9% old persons subclinically involved
- Anorexia, loss of weight, fever, fatigue, depression, dementia, anaemia, polymyalgia rheumatica
- Headache, tongue + jaw claudication, scalp tenderness; involved arteries thickened, tortuous, pulseless, scalp necrosis
- Ophthalmic artery involved in 50%
- Both eyes involved in 33%
- Eye features – arteritic anterior ischaemic optic neuropathy due to occlusive inflammation of posterior ciliary arteries
- Transient obscuration of vision, diplopia (III, IV, VI palsies), central retinal artery occlusion, anterior segment ischaemia (rare)

Diagnosis

- Four most important criteria
  - Jaw claudication
  - Neck pain
  - CRP > 2.45
  - ESR > 47

Special investigations

- ESR > 60, normal in 20% normal ESR: male – age /2, female – (age+10)/2)
- Temporal artery biopsy
  - If ESR > 20, remove 2.5 cm, do serial sections ('skip lesions')
  - If negative, repeat on other side
  - Do not withhold steroids pending biopsy
- IgG anticardiolipin antibodies – 50–100%

Treatment

- High dose steroids
  - Methylprednisolone 1g daily IVI × 3 days
  - Or hydrocortisone 300 mg daily IVI + oral prednisolone 1.5–2 mg/kg/day, then taper to 100 mg or less orally daily to protect fellow eye
- Keep ESR normal for 4–6 months
- In ischaemic optic neuropathy, acetazolomide and timolol to decrease IOP
- Disease self-limiting to 2 years

Retinal artery occlusion

Classification

- CRAO
- BRAO
- Cilioretinal artery occlusion

Aetiology

- Atherosclerosis-related thrombus – 80%
- Embolic – carotid (bifurcation of common carotid), myocardial disease – thrombus, cholesterol (Hollenhorst plaque– usually asymptomatic), fibrinoplatelet or calcific (dangerous)
- Retinal migraine – young; diagnosis of exclusion
- Periarteritis – polyarteritis nodosu, Weger's, dermatomyositis, plasmosis lupus, Behçet's, toxo
- Giant cell arteritis (1–2% of CRAO)
- Thrombophilic disorders – hyperhomocysteinaemia, antiphospholipid antibody syndrome, oral contraceptive pill
- Trauma
- Sickle Cell
- Diabetes, hypertension, glaucoma predispose

Features

- Male > female
- CRAO > BRAO; BRAO usually upper temporal
- Sudden painless loss of vision
- Afferent pupil defect
- Retina pale, cloudy swelling, cherry red spot at macula; arteries attenuated, cattle trucking in veins
- Later fundus returns to normal appearance, optic atrophy develops, 2–17% to develop rubeosis
- 20% of people have cilioretinal artery supplying papillomacular bundle → sparing of central vision

8

Pathology

- Intracellular oedema of ganglion cells → irreversible coagulative necrosis → glial replacement
- Ischaemic infarction of inner two-thirds of retina; cells undergo cloudy swelling and necrosis, later disintegrate and phagocytosed by macrophages; retina is left thin and shrunken

Special investigations

- Cardiac consult
- FBC, ESR, collagen screen, haemoglobin electrophoresis, lipid screen
- Carotid ultrasound

Treatment

- Emergency – treat within 48 hours; damage starts after 90 mins
- Initial
  - Ocular massage
  - Lower IOP – IV diamox 500 mg, IV mannitol 20% 1 g/kg, glycerol 50% 1g/kg orally

- Subsequent
  - If circulation not re-established in 20 mins
  - AC paracentesis
  - IV streptokinase

Macular disease

Symptoms of macular disease

- Impairment of central vision
  - Positive scotoma (something obstructing vision), cw negative scotoma in optic nerve disease (hole in visual field)
  - Metamorphopsia – image distortion
  - Micropsia – due to cones spreading apart
  - Macropsia – due to cones compressing together
- Impairment of colour vision
  - Occurs later than in optic nerve disease

Signs of macular disease

- Subjective
  - Visual acuity
  - Colour discrimination/identification
  - Photostress testing – to detect maculopathy when fundoscopy equivocal + to differentiate macular and optic nerve disease
  - Best control VA determined
  - Fix on light 3 cm away for 10 secs
  - Photostress recovery time is the time taken to read any 3 letters in the pre-test Best corrected VA line
  - 15–30 secs normal; prolonged in macular disease, normal in optic nerve
  - Amsler grid – evaluates the 10 degrees surrounding fixation; 7 charts
  - Pupillary reactions – normal in macular disease
- Objective
  - Pupillary response; normal, compared to optic nerve disease
  - Fundoscopy – red-free helpful for looking for superficial lesions e.g. internal limiting membrane (ILM) wrinkling or CMO or outline of serous elevations
  - Fluorescein angiography + ICG
  - Ultrasound
  - OCT

Epiretinal membrane

- Macular epiretinal membrane, epiretinal gliosis
- Proliferation of retinal glial cells that have gained access to the retinal surface through breaks in the ILM
- A vitreoretinal interface abnormality

Incidence

- Found in 20% of eyes at autopsy, usually have evidence of arteriosclerosis

Aetiology

- Idiopathic (usually idiopathic in patients > 50 years), male = female
- Associated with retinal holes and tears (trauma, surgery, primary degeneration)
- Associated with retinal vascular disease(CRVO + BRVO)
- Associated with vitreous inflammatory disease

Pathogenesis

- Cells implicated are
  - Vitreous hyalocyte – posterior vitreous detachment → remnants attached to internal limiting membrane containing hyalocytes
  - Retinal astrocytes – migrate through internal limiting membrane
  - Retinal pigment epithelium – migrate through retinal breaks, undergo metaplasia to fibroblasts; may → proliferative vitreoretinopathy
  - Macrophages – in vitreous inflammation

- Simple epiretinal membranes contain only hyalocytes, asymptomatic
- Complex epiretinal membranes contain also astrocytes; astrocytes contain contractile filaments → contraction and surface wrinkling

Classification of retinal traction
- Perpendicular/vitreoretinal – induced by hypocellular gel contraction of vitreous
- Tangential – induced by contraction of epiretinal and subretinal membranes

Idiopathic
- Most common, unilateral, associated with posterior vitreous detachment in 80%
- 10–20% bilateral

Symptoms
- Poor vision
- Metamorphopsia
- Micropsia

Signs
- Almost all have a posterior vitreous detachment (PVD)
- Grade 0 – cellophane maculopathy, best seen with red-free light, asymptomatic
- Grade I – crinkled cellophane maculopathy; wrinkling, distorted vessels, mild symptoms
- Grade II – semi translucent membrane, severe visual loss
- Complications – cystoid macular oedema (traction on retinal vessels), intraretinal haemorrhages, localised serous retinal detachment, pseudo macular hole, macular hole
- Vision may recover due to resolution of cystoid macular oedema, peeling or sliding

Macular pucker

- Caused by thickening and contraction of the epiretinal membrane (ERM)
- Retinal wrinkling, CMO, pseudoholes

Associated with retinal breaks

- Migration of retinal pigment epithelium and astrocytes
- Membrane formation occurs after 2–4 months
- Occurs independent of retinal surgery

Associated with vitreous inflammatory disease

- Post-uveitis
- Vitreous haemorrhage
- Ocular tumours

Associated with vascular disease

- Causing intraretinal exudation
- Diabetic retinopathy, hypertension, venous occlusion, telangiectasia, angiomatosis, pseudophakic cystoid macular oedema, photocoagulation

Prognosis
- VA very stable, 75% maintain 6/12 or better
- Partial visual recovery occurs following resolution of cystoid macular oedema or membrane sliding
- Total visual recovery occurs following peeling

Treatment
- Vitrectomy + membrane peel, segmentation and delamination
- Guideline: VA 6/18 or worse, marked metamorphopsia
- 60–80% improve by two or more lines
- VA continues to improve for 6–12 months post-surgery
- Complications: Tear, detachment

Secondary premacular gliosis

- Retinal detachment surgery
- Photocoagulation
- Cryotherapy
- Retinal vascular diseases
- Intraocular inflammation
- Ocular trauma

Cystoid macular oedema

Causes of cystoid macular oedema

Leakage of perifoveal capillaries

- Post-op
  - Lens extraction (Irvine Gass Norton syndrome), 6–10 weeks post-op
  - Other (cryo, PRP, retinal detachment surgery, vitrectomy)
- Retinal vascular disease
  - Diabetic retinopathy, hypertension, CRVO/BRVO, hyperviscosity, Coat's, macroaneurysm, telangiectasia
- Intraocular inflammation
  - Pars planitis, Behçet's, sarcoid, retinal vasculitis, birdshot, multifocal choroiditis, toxo, CMV retinitis, scleritis
- Miscellaneous
  - Retinitis pigmentosa
  - Drugs (epinephrine in aphakia, thiazides, oral contraceptives, prostaglandins, nicotinic acid)

Subretinal leakage

- Central serous retinopathy
- Subretinal neovascularisation
- Trauma
- Uveal tumours

No vascular leakage

- Retinitis pigmentosa
- Juvenile retinoschisis
- Optic pit
- Trauma
- Myopia
- Dominantly inherited CMO
- Gyrate atrophy
- Juvenile retinoschisis
- Goldman-Favre disease

Vitreoretinal interface disorders

- Vitreomacular traction syndrome
- ERM
- CMO is non-specific and may occur with any kind of macular oedema

Pathogenesis

- Final common pathway of a multifactorial syndrome
- Vitreous traction
  - Traction on Muller cells → damage to Muller cells
  - Become oedematous, fail to clear extracellular proteins
- Vascular dysfunction – increased blood retinal barrier permeability with leakage
- Inflammation – ? Mediated by prostaglandin E2 → isruption of blood retinal barrier
- Altered tissue compliance
- Ischaemia

Pathology

- Underlying inflammatory + vascular factors
- Early intracytoplasmic swelling of Muller cells
- Later pseudocysts in outer plexiform layer, RPE generation
- Peak prevalence 6 weeks post-surgery

Course

- Irvine-Gass – 95% resolve spontaneously within 6 months
- Chronic → pseudohole formation, true hole formation
- Better prognosis if – young, black, milder, no ischaemia, intact capillaries + RPE
- 2% of clinical CMO still present after 1 year

Incidence

- Difficult to determine
- Using fluorescein angiogram criteria – 40–70% post-lens extraction (ICLE 60%, ECLE 30%)
- Clinically significant CMO – 0–20% (probably 2–4%) post-lens extraction

Risk factors

- AC IOL
- Cardiovascular disease, DM

- PC rupture – vitreous loss, touch, manipulation, late rupture of face
- Ocular inflammation
- CMO in first eye; 50% chance in second eye
- Secondary implant – decreased risk with increased interval; usually advisable to wait 1 year
- YAG capsulotomy – usually advisable to wait 6 months
- Very young or very old patient
- ICLE cw ECLE cw phaco; there is increased risk of transient CMO, due to vitreous traction, loss of barrier to prostaglandin, and vitreous touch on iris; but long-term CMO is equal
- UV light from operating microscope → photochemical injury

Clinical features

- Two types
    - Early post-op (within 3 months); inflammatory, good prognosis
    - Late post-op (up to 10 years); vascular, poor prognosis
- Symptoms – red uncomfortable eye with photophobia, late (3 months) decrease in vision
- Signs – sensory retina elevated, foveal reflex lost, honey comb radial cysts, splinter haemorrhages, no exudates, even disc oedema
- Photostress test abnormal
- Fluorescein – late (10–15 minutes) leakage in rosette/stellate/petalloid pattern (Henle's layer)
- OCT

Prophylaxis

- Pre-op control of hypertension, diabetes, uveitis
- Role of steroids – probably not
- Topical + systemic indomethacin
    - Use for 3 months post-op
    - Decreases the incidence of angiographic CMO, not clinical CMO
    - Decreases inflammatory CMO, which is less significant
- UV filter on microscope and decreased exposure duration and intensity

Treatment

- Treat accompanying systemic disease; cardiovascular, renal, diabetes
- Steroids; periocular + topical; some cases respond
- Topical indomethacin; not shown to have any effect (studies have shown prevention of angiographic CMO with topical and systemic administration)
- Vitrectomy; lysis of strands to wound, ? role of total vitrectomy in all cases
- Photocoagulation of focal leakage
- Remove I0L as a last resort; ? effectiveness
- Acetazolamide; some cases respond, ? acts by restoring normal cell ph and polarity → increased outward movement of water from RPE
- Ketorolac tromethamine 0.5%; cyclooxygenase inhibitor, non-steroidal anti-inflammatory

Central serious choroidopathy

- A sensory retinal detachment due to fluid leakage at the RPE level

Aetiology

- Unknown
- May be RPE dysfunction or choriocapillaris dysfunction
- Sporadic and self-limiting
- May be induced by stress, hypertension, lupus, systemic steroids, pregnancy, solid organ transplantation

Pathology

- Abnormality at Bruch's membrane → leak through RPE → sensory retinal detachment

Features

- Male : female = 8 : 1, 25–40 years of age, type A personality
- Bilateral in 10–20%, recurrent in 40%

- Lasts days to months
- VA: 6/9–6/12, acquired hypermetropia correctable with weak +lens
- Acutely decreased central vision, metamorphopsia, micropsia, positive relative central scotoma (Amsler), decreased colour vision
- Sensory retinal detachment with clear or turbid subretiral fluid; ± PED, RPE disturbance, 'lemon drop' (focal yellow nodular swelling at level of RPE)
- Occasional multiple small serous detachments in midperiphery
- OCT findings: Fluid between RPE + sensory retina (also good for monitoring resolution)

Angiogram

- Most commonly – early pinpoint RPE leak, ± RPE detachment, slow filling of sensory retinal detachment – mushroom/umbrella configuration
- RPE leak is in upper third of sensory retinal detachment
- Filling of sensory retinal detachment may be inkblot or smokestack (10%)
- Diffuse retinal pigment epitheliopathy
- 20% show two sites of leakage

Differential diagnosis

- Optic disc pit
- Choroidal tumours – metastases, haemangiomas
- Unilateral acute idiopathic maculopathy
- CNV
- Harada
- Malignant hypertension + eclampsia

Treatment

- Most recover spontaneously; 40% within 1 month, 80% within 6 months
- If it persists for more than 3 months, permanent loss of central vision occurs in 50%
- Treat with local photocoagulation or PDT
    - Persistence beyond 3–4/12
    - Recurrence in eyes with visual deficit from previous episodes
    - Permanent visual deficit from previous episode in fellow eye
    - Development of chronic signs e.g. sensory retinal cysts, retinal pigment epitheliopathy
    - Prompt restoration of vision important
- PDT – half normal strength: For leakage near the fovea
- Argon: For leakage away from the fovea
- May be complicated by haemorrhage, subretinal neovascularisation (Risk of causing CNV 2–5% with argon – but may rarely get CNV even without laser)
- Resolution of fluid occurs after 1–3 weeks, visual acuity improves after 1–3 months
- Use of acetazolamide + B-blockers not convincing

Secondary central serous detachment

- Associated with subretinal leaks – VKH syndrome, malignant hypertension, subretinal neovascularisation, choroidal tumours, trauma
- No subretinal leaks – retinal detachment, macular hole, optic pit, trauma, myopia, juvenile retinoschisis

Drug-induced maculopathies

Chloroquine

- Chloroquine
    - Melanotropic, concentrates in RPE and choroid
    - Retinotoxicity + corneal deposits (vortex keratopathy)
    - Retinotoxicity related to a total accumulative dose, cumulative dose < 100 g or treatment < 1year rarely produces damage
    - 300 g (250 mg daily for 3 years) significantly increased risk

- Hydroxychloroquine
  - Safer as long as daily dose does not exceed 400 mg
  - Screening unnecessary

Chloroquine maculopathy

- Premaculopathy
  - Normal VA, loss of foveal reflex, fine macular granular changes, mild colour vision abnormality
  - Reversible
- Early maculopathy
  - Mild VA loss, paracentral scotomas, central foveolar pigmentation surrounded by a depigmented zone of RPE atrophy and another hyperpigmented zone
  - Irreversible
- Established maculopathy
  - Moderate VA loss
  - Bull's eye maculopathy
- Severe maculopathy – marked VA loss, ++RPE atrophy at fovea
- End-stage maculopathy – severe loss of VA, arteriolar attenuation, pigment clumping in peripheral retina
- Screening
  - No standard method
  - Weekly Amsler, VA + fundoscopy by physician, refer if problem
  - High dose or lengthy duration of treatment – annual examination

Phenothiazines

- No screening at standard doses required
- Thioridazine
  - For schizophrenia + psychosis
  - Normal dose 150–600 mg, > 800 mg/day causes VA + dark adaptation loss
  - Salt and pepper retinopathy, plaque-like pigmentation + RPE loss
  - RPE + choriocapillaris atrophy
- Chlorpromazine (Largactil)
  - For schizophrenia
  - Normal dose 75–300 mg
  - Retinotoxic in much larger doses over long periods – very rare
  - Pigmentary granularity and clumping
  - Yellow-brown granules on anterior lens capsule, corneal endothelial deposits, eyelid pigmentation

Tamoxifen

- Anti-oestrogen for breast carcinoma
- Normal dose 20–40 mg
- Higher doses may produce retinotoxicity
- Bilateral, multiple, yellow, crystalline, ring deposits at maculae
- Vortex keratopathy, optic neuritis
- No screening required

Methoxyflurane

- Inhaled anaesthetic agent
- Deposits in RPE
- Retinal vascular crystal deposits

Canthaxanthin

- To enhance sun tanning
- Innocuous superficial retinal deposits, posterior pole

Isotretinoin

- Nyctalopia
- Patients undergoing repetitive courses
- Reversible

Miscellaneous maculopathies

- Idiopathic polypoidal choroidal vasculopathy
- Maculopathy in optic disc pit
- Solar maculopathy
- Valsalva maculopathy

Idiopathic polypoidal choroidal vasculopathy

- Posterior uveal bleeding syndrome
- Multiple serosanguinous RPE detachment syndrome

Pathogenesis

- Abnormal inner choroidal vessels
- A dilated network, multiple terminal aneurysmal protruberances in polypoidal configuration
- Macular + parapapillary distribution
- Episodic leakage + bleeding beneath retina

Clinically

- Mostly non-whites
- Sudden unilateral loss of vision
- Serosanguinous RPE detachments
- Bullous retinal detachment, vitreous haemorrhage

ICG

- Large choroidal vascular complexes, fill slowly, leak intensely

Treatment

- Argon laser

Prognosis

- Good, spontaneous resolution

Maculopathy in optic disc pit

- Rare, congenital, unilateral
- Large disc, oval or round pit, usually temporal
- Glaucoma-like field defects
- Fluorescein angiogram:Early hypofluorescence, late hyperfluorescence
- Maculopathy in 45%
- Subretinal fluid from vitreous or subarachnoid space
- Schisis-like separation inner retinal layers, followed by detachment of outer retinal layers from RPE
- Treatment: 25% resolve spontaneously, therefore, watch at 3-monthly intervals
- Laser: If VA dropping; temporal aspect of disc; 30% success
- PPV – 65% success
- C3F8 gas without PPV

Solar maculopathy

- Solar effects of radiation from looking into sun
- 1–4 hours after exposure
- Central scotomas or metamorphopsia
- Yellow foveolar spots with grey margin
- Two weeks later, RPE mottling or lamellar hole
- Good prognosis – near normal within 6 months

Valsalva maculopathy

- Sudden increase in intrathoracic or intraabdominal pressure resulting in intraocular bleeding
- Mostly premacular haemorrhages
- Prognosis excellent

Hereditary fundal dystrophies

Photoreceptor dystrophies

- Retinitis pigmentosa
- Congenital stationary night blindness
- Progressive cone dystrophy
- Leber's congenital amaurosis
- Congenital monochromatism

RPE dystrophies

- Best vitelliform macular dystrophy
- Stargaardt macular dystrophy
- Fundus flavimaculatus
- Familial dominant drusen
- Sorsby pseudo-inflammatory macular dystrophy
- North Carolina macular dystrophy
- Pattern dystrophies
- Butterfly macular dystrophy
- Dominant cystoid macular oedema
- Bietti's crystalline dystrophy
- Alport syndrome
- Benign familial fleck retina

Choroidal dystrophies

- Choroideremia
- Gyrate atrophy

- Central areolar choroidal dystrophy
- Diffuse choroidal atrophy
- Helicoidal parapapillary chorioretinal degeneration
- Pigmented paravenous retinochoroidal atrophy

Hereditary vitreoretinal degenerations

- Stickler syndrome
- Congenital retinoschisis
- Favre-Goldmann syndrome
- Familial exudative vitreoretinopathy
- Erosive vitreoretinopathy
- Dominant neovascular inflammatory vitreochoroidopathy
- Dominant vitreoretinochoroidopathy

Albinism

- Oculocutaneous albinism
- Ocular albinism

Cherry red spot at macula syndromes

General features of hereditary macular dystrophies

- Familial, bilateral, symmetric
- Early age of onset, slowly progressive course
- Predominantly posterior pole changes, marked loss of vision
- No other abnormalities

Photoreceptor dystrophies

Congenital stationary night blindness

- Six forms
- Autosomal dominant congenital nyctalopia (Nougaret type)
- Autosomal dominant stationary nyctalopia without myopia (Riggs type)
- Autosomal recessive stationary nyctalopia
- Autosomal recessive or XL congenital nyctalopia with myopia (Schubert-Bornschein type)
- Oguchi disease
    - Autosomal recessive, 2–12 hour delay in attaining normal dark-adapted thresholds
    - Mizuo phenomenon – fundus colour changes from golden brown in light-adapted state to normal in dark-adapted
- Fundus albipunctatus – autosomal recessive, tiny white-yellow spots posterior pole sparing fovea

Progressive cone dystrophy (progressive rod-cone dystrophy)

- Usually autosomal dominant, rarely autosomal recessive, XL
- Onset first to second decade, progressive
- Can have pure cone or rod-cone dystrophy, many start with pure cone and get rod later
- Degeneration of photoreceptors in posterior pole, secondary degeneration of RPE
- Decreased central vision, defective colour vision, photophobia (play at dusk), pendular nystagmus
- Fundus usually normal, ± bull's eye maculopathy, optic pallor, arteriolar attenuation, midperipheral bone spicules, progressive macular RPE atrophy, eventually geographic atrophy
- ERG photopic absent, scotopic reduced; EOG normal or reduced
- Dark adaptation – cone abnormal, rod initially normal becoming abnormal later
- Colour vision – severe deuteron-tritan defect
- Fluorescein – bull's eye
- Prognosis varies depending on severity of rod involvement

Leber's congenital amaurosis

- Autosomal recessive
- Blind at birth or within a few years
- Fundus may be normal initially
- Patches of peripheral chorioretinal atrophy and granularity

- Disc oedema, salt and pepper fundus, diffuse white spots, macular coloboma, bull's eye maculopathy
- Optic disc pallor and attenuation of retinal arterioles
- Other ocular features – hypermetropia, keratoconus, keratoglobus, cataracts, nystagmus, strabismus, oculodigital syndrome
- Mental handicap, deafness, epilepsy, central nervous system and renal abnormalities, skeletal malformations, endocrine dysfunction

Congenital monochromatism

- Complete rod monochromatism – autosomal recessive, absent colour vision, VA 6/60, nystagmus + photophobia
- Incomplete rod monochromatism – autosomal recessive or XL, some colour vision, VA 6/18, ± nystagmus + photophobia
- Cone monochromatism – uncertain inheritance, absent colour vision, VA 6/9, no nystagmus + photophobia

8

Dystrophies of the RPE

Best vitelliform dystrophy (juvenile Best)

- Autosomal dominant, gene 11q13, onset first decade
- Mild decrease in central vision, slowly progressive to moderate to severe decrease in central vision
- Lesions may be unilateral or bilateral, single or multiple, macular or eccentric
- Evolves gradually through 5 stages
    - Stage 1 – Previtelliform – abnormal EOG, no symptoms, normal fundus
    - Stage 2 – Vitelliform – egg yolk appearance, visual acuity normal or slightly decreased
    - Stage 3 – Pseudohypopyon – lesion partially absorbs
    - Stage 4 – Vitelliruptive – scrambled egg appearance, visual acuity decreased
    - Stage 5 – End stage – macular scarring and atrophy, moderate to severe decrease in visual acuity
- ERG normal, EOG decreased
- Histology → generalised RPE abnormality with lipofuscin accumulation, macrophages in subretinal space

Adult vitelliform foveomacular dystrophy (adult Best disease)

- Considered a 'pattern dystrophy'
- Autosomal dominant, gene 6p21–22, onset fourth to sixth decade
- Minimal symptoms, mild metamorphopsia
- Macular lesion as in Best's, but smaller
- ERG + EOG – normal, colour vision tritan defect
- Prognosis good

Multifocal Best disease

- Presents in adulthood, very rare

Stargardt disease (juvenile macular dystrophy)

- Autosomal recessive, onset first and second decades
- Most common dystrophy
- Decreased central vision, out of proportion to macular changes (children suspected of malingering), defective colour vision
- Fundus normal early, later beaten bronze macula from RPE atrophy, later choricapillaris atrophy, bull's eye; ± pisciform flecks, ± retinitis pigmentosa – like picture in periphery
- FA: Dark choroid (lipofuscin deposits), geographic atrophy at macula
- ERG + EOG: Decreased if periphery involved, VER decreased
- Colour vision – deuteran-tritan defects
- Histology → complete disappearance of visual elements within macular area

Fundus flavimaculatus

- Variant of Stargardt's
- Autosomal recessive, onset first and second decades

- Asymptomatic → slow decrease in central vision; colour vision normal
- Pisciform yellow-white flecks in posterior pole and midperiphery; consist of enlarged RPE cells packed with lipofuscin
- ERG normal, EOG decreased
- Fluorescein → RPE blockage + transmission by flecks; later choriocapillaris non-perfusion ('silent fluorescein')
- Differential diagnosis, other causes of flecked retinal syndrome – drusen, fundus albipunctatus, fundus albescens
- 50% associated with Stargardt-like changes at the macula

Familial dominant drusen

- Autosomal dominant, onset in second to fourth decades
- Histology → hyaline material under RPE, breaks in Bruch's membrane, subretinal neovascularisation, disciform scar
- Pathonogmonic feature is its occurrence on nasal side of disc
- Mild – a few innocuous hard drusen at meacula
- Moderate – large, soft drusen at macula and disc; mild loss of VA
- Advanced – uncommon; CNV, geographic atrophy
- Malattia leventinese – hundreds of small drusen in a radial distribution centred on fovea
- If extensive, RPE rip may occur with exposure of choroid and sclera; ERG normal, EOG decreased late

Sorsby pseudo inflammatory macular dystrophy (hereditary haemorrhagic inflammatory dystrophy)

- Autosomal dominant, onset in second to fourth decades
- Yellow-white confluent spots along arcades and nasal to disc
- Later development of choroidal neovascularisation and exudative maculopathy
- ERG normal
- Prognosis poor

North Carolina macular dystrophy

- Autosomal dominant, onset during second decade
- Drusen-like flecks in the periphery and at the macula
- Macular lesions become confluent, develop atrophic or exudative maculopathy
- ERG normal
- Prognosis variable

Pattern dystrophy

Butterfly dystrophy

- Autosomal dominant
- Yellow pigment in macula in triradiate pattern
- Prognosis good

Dominant cystoid macular oedema

- Autosomal dominant
- First and second decades
- Gradual visual impairment
- CMO does not respond to diamox
- Prognosis poor – eventual geographic atrophy

Bietti's crystalline dystrophy

- XL or autosomal recessive
- Presents in third decade, progressive visual loss
- Yellow-white crystals throughout posterior pole
- Localised macular RPE and choriocapillaris atrophy
- ERG, EOG subnormal
- Prognosis variable

Alport syndrome

- XL dominant
- Rare collagen abnormality of glomerular basement membrane
- CRF and sensorineural deafness

- Scattered, perimacular punctuate flecks, sparing fovea, normal VA
- ERG normal
- Prognosis excellent

Benign familial fleck retina

- Autosomal recessive
- Asymptomatic
- Widespread flecks at RPE level, fovea spared

Hereditary vitreoretinal degenerations

Stickler syndrome (hereditary arthro-ophthalmopathy)

- Autosomal dominant collagen disease

Ocular features

- Vitreous – syneresis and liquefaction ('empty vitreous')
- Retina
    - Large areas of radial lattice like degeneration with associated RPE hyperplasia
    - Sheathing and sclerosis of retinal vessels
    - Retinal detachment in 30% of cases – multiple breaks or giant tears (prophylactic laser)
    - High myopia
    - Presenile cataract in 50% of cases
    - Ectopia lentis in 10% of cases
    - Chronic glaucoma in 10% of cases

Systemic features

- Facial anomalies – flattened nasal bridge, maxillary hypoplasia
- Skeletal anomalies – premature degenerative changes of articular cartilage
- Robin sequence – micrognathia, glossoptosis, cleft soft palate
- Deafness, mitral valve prolapse

Congenital retinoschisis

- XL recessive
- Onset 5–10 years of age
- Maculopathy – cystoid spaces in bicycle wheel pattern → non-specific atrophy
- Retinoschisis – in 50% of cases
- Defect at Muller cell level, splitting nerve fibre layer from rest of sensory retina
- Inner wall very thin, may develop large defects
- Can be complicated vitreous haemorrhage and RD
- Poor prognosis due to progressive maculopathy

Favre-Goldmann syndrome

- Autosomal recessive
- Features of retinoschisis and primary pigmentary retinopathy
- Presents in childhood with nyctalopia
- Vitreous syneresis
- Retinal changes similar to congenital retinoschisis + pigmentary changes similar to retinitis pigmentosa + peripheral dendritiform lesions of retinal blood vessels

Familial exudative vitreoretinopathy (Criswick-Schepens syndrome)

- Autosomal dominant
- Vitreous membranes, prominent vitreoretinal attachments
- Abrupt cessation of retinal capillary network at equator, similar to ROP; fibrovascular proliferation with temporal dragging of macula, retinal exudation
- Complications include retinal detachment, vitreous haemorrhage and cataract

Erosive vitreoretinopathy

- Autosomal dominant
- Vitreous syneresis, multiple foci of vitreoretinal traction
- RPE thinning, progressive choroidal atrophy
- Complicated by giant tears and detachment

8

Dominant neovascular inflammatory vitreochoroidopathy

- Autosomal dominant
- Presents in second and third decades with floaters
- Uveitis, RPE detachment, peripheral vascular closure + neovascularisation
- Complicated by vitreous haemorrhage, tractional retinal detachment, CMO

Dominant vitreoretinochoroidopathy

- Autosomal dominant
- Presents in adulthood
- Encircling band of pigmentary disturbance between ora and equator with a sharply defined posterior border
- Neovascularisation, arteriolar attenuation, white opacities and chorioretinal atrophy within the band
- Good prognosis

Cherry red spot at the macula syndromes

Sphingolipidoses

- Progressive intracellular storage of excessive quantities of glycolipids and phospholipids in retina and body
- Lipid stored in ganglion cell layer → white retina + red macula (ganglion cells absent at fovea)
- Late stage: Retinal nerve fibre layer and optic atrophy

Tay-Sachs disease

- Autosomal recessive, Ashkenazi Jews
- Death at 2 years of age
- Progressive neurological disease + blindness

Niemann-Pick disease

- Autosomal recessive, Ashkenazi Jews
- Sphingomyelin accumulation in reticuloendothelial cells
- Death in second decade

Sandhoff disease

- Almost identical to Tay-Sachs

Generalised gangliosidosis

- Hypoactivity and oedema of the face + extremities
- Skeletal anomalies

Sialidosis (cherry red spot myoclonus syndrome)

- Myoclonus

Vitreoretinal interface abnormalities

- Idiopathic macular hole
- Idiopathic premacular gliosis
- Vitreomacular traction syndrome

Idiopathic macular hole

Pathogenesis

- Spontaneous focal contraction of perifoveal vitreous cortex + tangential vitreomacular traction

Classification of idiopathic macular hole (Gass)

■ Stage 1A – Impending hole	□ Vitreous contraction with foveal detachment □ May see a central yellow spot at foveola (an intrafoveal cyst)
■ Stage 1B – Occult hole	□ Further vitreous contraction with dehiscence of photoreceptors □ Decreased visual acuity mild; metamorphopsia

	▫ 50% of stage 1 holes undergo spontaneous resolution following PVD ▫ Progression from stage 1 to 2 takes between 1 week + several months
▪ Stage 2 – Early full thickness macular hole	▫ Separation of prefoveolar cortical vitreous from retina to form a pseudo operculum ▫ < 400 μm in size ▫ Retinal defect seen on fundoscopy
▪ Stage 3 – Macular hole	▫ Separation of pseudo operculum from edge of hole ▫ > 400 μm in size
▪ Stage 4 – Macular hole	▫ Complete separation of posterior vitreous ▫ VA stable at 6/60

Clinical features
- Elderly females
- Fellow eye affected – 15% in 5 years
- Decreased visual acuity
- Round punched-out defect one third of disc diameter, surrounding halo of sensory retinal detachment
- Watzke-Allen test positive in full thickness hole (interrupted slit beam) cw pseudo hole
- Fluorescein: Window defect
- Laser aiming beam test
- OCT

Differential diagnosis
- Full thickness – window defect on fluorescein
- Lamellar – no window defect on fluorescein
- Macular cyst
- Pseudohole in preretinal membrane

Treatment
- Indication – full thickness hole up to stage 3, visual acuity < 6/18, duration < 1 year
- Technique – vitrectomy and fluid – gas exchange; ± internal limiting membrane peel
- Results – improvement in > 90%; 65% 6/12 or better

Macular hole – aetiology
- Idiopathic
- Trauma
- Chronic cystoid macular oedema
- Solar burn (foveamacular retinitis)
- Severe intraocular inflammation
- High myopia + posterior staphyloma

Idiopathic premacular gliosis

Synonyms
- Cellophane maculopathy, surface wrinkling retinopathy, preretinal fibrosis, premacular gliosis, macular pucker

Pathology
- Proliferation of retinal ganglion cells
- Gain access to retinal surface through break in internal limiting membrane, ? with posterior vitreous detachment

Clinical features
- Otherwise healthy elderly individuals
- Bilateral in 10%
- Mild cellophane maculopathy; visual acuity normal or minimally reduced; irregular light reflex at macula
- More serious macular pucker; metamorphopsia, decreased vision, distortion of blood vessels, retinal wrinkling

8

Vitreomacular traction syndrome

- Partial vitreous separation, traction on macula and disc
- Affects elderly individuals
- Abnormal opacities in the vitreous overlying the macula
- Causes chronic cystoid macular oedema, retinal striae

Diabetic retinopathy

Incidence

- Incidence of diabetes increasing
- Retinopathy – 40–60% of diabetics
- Risk increases with time after 5 years, to a maximum at 10 years, thereafter, it is stable
- 100% of people with diabetes for 20–25 years develop non-proliferative retinopathy
- 60% of people with diabetes for 30 years develop proliferative retinopathy
- Type 2 diabetes well controlled
  - 25% develop retinopathy after 5 years
  - 50% develop retinopathy after 10 years
  - 75% develop retinopathy after 15 years
- Type 1 diabetes well controlled – 50% develop retinopathy after 15 years
- Proliferative retinopathy occurs in 10% of all patients with retinopathy
- Blindness – 2% of diabetic population is blind
- Diabetics 25 times more likely to be blind than non-diabetics
- Blindness results from maculopathy, vitreous haemorrhage or traction retinal detachment
- Blind patients have a life expectancy of less than 6 years
- Disc new vessels untreated → 25% blind after 1 year
- Other new vessels untreated → 25% blind after 5 years

Risk factors

- Duration of diabetes – as above
- Poor diabetes control
- Pregnancy – occasional rapid progression; pre-eclampsia + fluid imbalance bad
- Hypertension
- Nephropathy – treatment of renal dysfunction improves PDR
- Other – smoking, obesity, hyperlipidemia

Benefits of intensive metabolic control

- Delays onset of DBR
- Slows progression of NPDBR
- Decreases conversion to proliferative diabetic retinopathy (PDR)
- Decreases incidence of macular oedema
- Decreases need for PRP

Natural history

- Preclinical retinopathy
  - Decreased retinal blood flow
  - Increased capillary permeability
  - Basement membrane thickening
  - Loss of pericytes
- Early clinical retinopathy
  - Microaneurysms
  - Capillary hyperpermeability (oedema, exudates, maculopathy) – more common in type 2
  - Capillary obliteration (soft exudates, haemorrhage) – more common in type 1
- Proliferative retinopathy
- Late proliferative changes
  - Vitreous membranes
  - Retinal detachment
  - Neovascular glaucoma

Pathogenesis

- Hyperglycaemia leads to tissue protein glycosylation + endothelial damage
- Microangiopathy affecting precapillary arterioles, capillaries and post-capillary venules
- Microvascular occlusion and leakage

8

Microvascular occlusion

- Capillary changes
  - Pericyte loss
  - Basement membrane thickening
  - Endothelial cell damage + proliferation
- Haematological changes
  - RBC deformation
  - Platelet stickiness → decreased oxygen transport
  - Leads to retinal ischaemia (initially in midperiphery) → this causes AV shunts
- AV shunts
  - Arterioles to venules
  - IRMA
- Neovascularisation
  - Vasoendothelial growth factor (VEGF) is NB (there are others) → new vessels at eh disc (NVD), new vessles elsewhere (NVE), rubeosis

Microvascular leakage

- BRB breakdown; capillary wall weakening, microaneurysms + oedema
- Diffuse oedema
- Localised oedema
  - Hard exudates (lipoprotein and lipid-filled macrophages) at junction of normal and oedematous tissue
  - Takes months to years to resorb when oedema resolves
  - Can lead to cholesterol deposition
- Impaired oxygen transfer to the retina occurs due to:
  - Hyperglycaemia → increased growth hormone → hepatic synthesis of large plasma proteins → red blood cell aggregation
  - Increased platelet adhesiveness + increased plasma proteins → increased blood viscosity
  - Decreased 2, 3 diphosphoglycerate in red blood cells
  - Accumulation of abnormal haemoglobin
  - Sorbitol accumulation in endothelial cells → oedema
  - Basement membrane thickening
- All lead to hypoxia → loss of pericytes → leakage → haemorrhages + hard exudates and oedema occlusion → soft exudates, microaneurysms, intraretinal microvascular anomalies (arterio venous shunts), new vessels
- Deep capillary net more affected than superficial capillary net

Pathology

- Background DR
  - Microaneurysms – inner nuclear layer
  - Hard exudates – outer plexiform layer
  - Retinal oedema – between outer plexiform and inner nuclear layers
- Preproliferative DR
  - Cotton wool spots – focal infarcts of nerve fibre layor
  - Interrupted axoplasmic flow with build-up of material gives white appearance
  - IRMA – do not cross major blood vessels, do not leak on angrogram
  - Venous changes – dilatation, beading, looping, segmentation
- Diabetic maculopathy
  - Most common cause of visual impairment, especially type 2
  - Focal exudative
  - Diffuse exudative ± CMO
  - Ischaemic

Clinically significant macular oedema

- Retinal oedema within 500 μm of centre of fovea
- Hard exudates within 500 μm of centre of fovea if associated with oedema
- Retinal oedema ≥ or =1 500 μm area if any part of it is within 1 disc diameter of the centre of the fovea
- Requires laser; reduces risk of visual loss by 50%; improved VA uncommon
- 70% stabilise VA, 15% improve, 15% deteriorate

- Takes up to 4 months for oedema to resolve
- Proliferative DR
  - Neovascularisation + fibrous tissue proliferation; intraretinal, on retinal surface, on disc surface, into vitreous; 25% at disc, 25% superior temporal vein
  - Vitreous alterations and haemorrhage
  - Macular disease – oedema, ischaemia, surface wrinkling retinopathy, traction detachment
  - Retinal detachment – due to anteroposterior and tangential traction, initially without holes (75%), later with posteriorly situated holes (25%)
- 25% of retina non-perfused for PDR to develop
- NVD common because of lack of internal limiting membrane here
- Arise mostly from veins; use vitreous as a scaffold for growth
- Mild NVD < one-third of disc area, severe > one-third
- Mild NVE < half of disc area, severe > half
- Elevated new vessels less responsive to PRP
- Subhyaloid or vitreous haemorrhage important risk factor for visual loss

Effects of diabetes on other ocular tissues

- Conjunctiva – microaneurysms
- Iris
  - Rubeosis
  - Ectropion
  - Vacuolation of pigment epithelium from glycogen accumulation
  - Anterior uveitis (? on an ischaemic basis)
- Cornea
  - Decreased sensitivity
  - Decreased epithelial adhesion
  - Endothelial cell dysfunction
  - Polymegathism of endothelial cells
  - Due to sorbitol accumulation
  - Treat with topical aldose reductase inhibitor
- Glaucoma – neovascular glaucoma, increased incidence chronic glaucoma
  - Lens
  - Transient myopia
  - Juvenile subcapsular snowflake lens opacities
  - Age-related cataract
  - Following cataract extraction, 40% of cases of retinopathy show progression
- Optic nerve
  - Ischaemic optic neuropathy
  - Acute disc swelling (type 1)
  - Optic atrophy (type 1)
- Vitreous – asteriod hyalosis
- Orbit – mucormycosis
- Cranial nerves
  - III, IV, VI palsies, due to localised demyelination secondary to focal ischemia
  - Pupil sparing III
  - Argyll-Robertson pupil

Factors aggravating retinopathy

- Pregnancy
- Hypertension
- Renal decompensation
- Abnormal blood coagulability
- Poor diabetic control
- Alcohol, smoking
- Obesity
- Hyperlipidemia

Factors reducing severity of retinopathy

- Axial myopia
- Increased IOP
- Optic atrophy
- Chorioretinal scarring
- Reduced central retinal artery diastolic pressure
- Central retinal artery occlusion
- Carotid artery disease
- PVD

Clinical classification of diabetic retinopathy	
■ Mild NPDR	
■ Moderate NPDR	
■ Severe NPDR	□ 15% chance of progression to high risk PDR in 1 year □ One of the following: Diffuse intraretinal haemorrhages and micro-aneurysms in 4 quadrants; venous beading in 2 quadrants; IRMA in 1 quadrant
■ Very severe NPDR	□ 45% chance of progression to high risk PDR in 1 year □ Any 2 of the 4:2:1 rule
■ Proliferative DR – low risk	
■ Proliferative DR – high risk	□ Risk of visual loss within 2 years □ Mild NVD with haemorrhage → 26% risk visual loss, reduced to 4% with PRP □ Severe NVD, no haemorrhage → 26% risk visual loss, reduced to 9% with PRP □ Severe NVD with haemorrhage → 37% risk visual loss, reduced to 20% with PRP □ Severe NVE with haemorrhage → 30% risk visual loss, reduced to 7% with PRP
■ Maculopathy	□ Dry □ Focal exudative □ Diffuse exudative □ Ischaemic □ Mixed

8

Causes of visual loss in diabetic retinopathy

- Vitreous haemorrhage
- Retinal detachment
- Macular oedema
- Rubeotic glaucoma
- AION
- Masular ischaemia

Management of diabetic retinopathy

- Early detection
- Follow-up
- Management of maculopathy
- Management of retinopathy
- Vitrectomy

Early detection

- SACE elevated; (? released by damaged endothelial cells)
- ERG decreased
- Screening; all diabetics over the age of 12; very rare under the age of 10

Follow-up

- Type 1 – every year for 10 years, then every 6 months
- Type 2 – every 6 months ab initio
- Screening can be by fundus photo with non-mydriatic camera at physician's office, reviewed by ophthalmologist

Management of maculopathy

- Correct contributory cardiac failure, hypertension, renal failure, diabetes control
- Ischaemic – untreatable
- Focal exudative – focal photocoagulation to centres of circinate exudates and individual IRMA
- Diffuse exudative
  - Use either gentle grid sparing fovea or horseshoe photocoagulation from disc along arcades and joined temporally
  - Give 150–200 small light burns
- Intravitreals – triamcinolone, ranibizumab, bevacizumalo
- Vitrectomy – if post-hyaloid attached with tangential traction

Management of retinopathy

- Correct contributing cardiac failure, hypertension, renal failure, diabetes control; sustained good diabetic control → reversal of retinopathy
- Mild NPDR – no treatment, annual review
- Moderate NPDR – regular follow-up
- Severe NPDR – no PRP unless poor follow-up, poor fellow eye natural history
- PRP
- Mechanism of action
  - Destruction of hypoxic retina
  - Closer apposition between retina and choroid → increased oxygen delivery
  - Destruction of unhealthy retina → oxygen diversion
  - Destruction of leaking vessels
  - Breakdown of blood retinal barrier → facilitation of outward diffusion of angiogenic factor into choroid or inward diffusion of plasma constituents having an inhibitory effect on angiogenesis
- When to treat:
  - Preproliferative – 20% will develop proliferative retinopathy within 1–2 years, therefore, follow regularly but only treat if other eye has shown a volatile progression
  - Proliferative – allocate points on risk factors and treat with 3 or 4 points
  - 1 Point – only eye, vitreous haemorrhage, moderate to severe new vessels
  - 2 Points – disc new vessels, new vessels away from disc
  - 1 Point → 7% chance of visual loss after 2 years
  - 2 points → 10% chance of visual loss after 2 years
  - 3 points → 25% chance of visual loss after 2 years
  - 4 points → 40% chance of visual loss after 2 years
  - Treat eyes with 3 or 4 points
  - Review in 4–6 weeks; if vessels are not regressing, fill in

Vitrectomy

Indications

- Persistent vitreous haemorrhage
  - No time parameters; tailor to patient
  - Type 1 is more likely to have severe proliferative retinopathy
- Tractional retinal detachment, threatening macula
  - Complication rate of vitrectomy 20%
  - Macular detachment rate14% per year
- Combined tractional and rhegmatogenous retinal detachment
  - Urgent treatment because fluid spreads with macular involvement
- Premacular subhyaloid haemorrhage
- Macular oedema may benefit
  - 70% get visual improvement, 10% worse, 20% no change
  - Pre-op retinal assessment – macular and retinal function tests
  - ERG → normal a + decreased b with inner layer ischaemia, decreased a + b with retinal detachment

- Contraindications
  - Corneal opacity
  - Rubeosis
  - Long-standing total retinal detachment
  - Decreased ERG
  - NPL eye
  - Extra macular traction retinal detachment
- Specific complications
  - Increased proliferative retinopathy and rubeosis ? due to removal of angiogenic inhibitor
  - Prevent with pre-op cryo or PRP
  - Anterior hyaloidal fibrovascular proliferation
  - Cataract
  - Glaucoma
  - Retinal detachment
- Results
  - 70% success for vitreous haemorrhage
  - 40% success for traction detachment

8

Suggested follow-up

- Normal or rare microaneurysms → annually
- Mild NPDR → 9 months
- Moderate NPDR → 6 months
- Severe NPDR → 4 months
- CSMO → 2–3 months
- PDR → 2–3 months

Important studies

Early Treatment Diabetic Retinopathy Study (ETDRS)

- Randomised, prospective study evaluating PRP and asprin treatment of patients with less than high risk PDR
- Studied efficacy of laser for CSMO (50% reduction in major loss of vision)
- Studied optimal timing for PRP

Diabetic Retinopathy Study (DRS)

- Randomised prospective clinical trial evaluating PRP in one eye in PDR or advanced NPDR
- Defined high risk PDR
- 50% reduction in severe visual loss up to 5 years

Diabetic Retinopathy Vitrectomy Study (DRVS)

- Prospective evaluation of PPV for very severe PDR
- Outcome – VA
- Early PPV in type 1 DM with severe vitreous haemorrhage very beneficial; no advantage in type 2
- Early PPV advantageous in very severe PDR

Diabetes Control and Complications Trial (DCCT)

- To evaluate the connection between metabolic control and retinal/renal/neurological complications in type 1
- Intensive insulin delays onset and slows progression of retinopathy/nephropathy/ neuropathy

Proliferative retinopathies

- Preretinal neovascularisation peripheral to the major vascular arcades

Causes

- Vascular disease with ischaemia
- Inflammatory diseases with possible ischaemia
- Miscellaneous

Vascular disease with ischaemia

- Sickling haemaglobinopathies (prototype)
- Other haemaglobinopathies
- Eale's disease (diagnosis by exclusion)
- Diabetes
- Hypertensive retinopathy
- Branch retinal vein occlusion (25% → peripheral neovascularisation)
- Retinal embolisation (talc in IVI drug abusers)
- Retinopathy of prematurity

- Hyperviscosity syndromes (leukaemia, polycythaemia, dysproteinemia)
- Aortic arch syndrome (Takayasu's, syphilis, arteriosclerosis)
- Carotid – cavernous fistula

Inflammatory diseases with possible ischaemia

- Sarcoidosis
- Retinal vasculitis (syphilis, collagen diseases)
- Uveitis (pars planitis, Behçet's)

Miscellaneous

- Incontinentia pigmenti
- Familial exudative vitreoretinopathy
- Long-standing retinal detachment
- Multiple sclerosis

Angiogenesis

- Angiogenic factor produced by – ischaemic retina, inflammatory cells
- Vitreous normally contains an angiogenic inhibitory factor, as it has a low pO2

Diagnostic work-up

- Full blood count
- Haemoglobin electrophoresis
- Chest x ray
- SACE
- Gallium scan
- Glucose tolerance test
- Collagen screen

Management

- Fluorescein angiogram
- Systemic steroids in the inflammatory conditions
- Local photocoagulation – photocoagulate feeder arterioles and drainage venules
- If local photocoagulation not possible – single freeze cryotherapy of retinal periphery
- PRP → regression of neovascularisation

Complications

- Vitreous haemorrhage
- Retinal detachment – traction and rhegmatogenous
- Rubeotic glaucoma
- Cataract
- Phthisis bulbi

Eale's disease

- Primary idiopathic retinal vasculitis

Aetiology

- Unknown
- Peripheral proliferative retinopathy, diagnosis by exclusion
- May subsequently develop features of other peripheral proliferative retinopathies
- Inflammatory basis; ? ischaemic basis
- Thought to be due to reaction to tuberculin
- Recurrent microemboli (e.g. talc), focal infections (e.g. dental) may be important

Pathology

- Obliterative periphlebitis – lymphocyte infiltration in peripheral vein walls
- Endothelial proliferation, lumen obliteration, ischaemia, neovascularisation
- May also occur centrally

Clinical features

- Typically occurs in young adult males, bilateral in > 90%
- Stage 1 – perivascular sheathing of peripheral veins, adjacent haemorrhage and capillary non-perfusion
- Stage 2 – larger vessels affected
- Stage 3 – neovascularisation + vitreous haemorrhage
- Stage 4 – retinal detachment – tractional; rhegmatogenous
- Complications: Rubeotic glaucoma, cataract, phthisis bulbi

Treatment

- Steroids – systemic and periorbital

- Photocoagulation – new vessels + PRP
- Vitrectomy – vitreous haemorrhage

Differential diagnosis
- Other causes of retinal periphlebitis – TB, sarcoid, syphilis, acute frosted retinal periphlebitis

Telangiectasias

- Group of rare, idiopathic, congenital, retinal vascular anomalies
- Characterised by:
  - Dilatation and tortuosity of retinal vessels
  - Formation of multiple aneurysms
  - Varying degrees of leakage and deposition of lipid exudates
- Always involve capillary bed
- Arterioles and venules may also be affected
- May progress and become symptomatic later in life
- Idiopathic juxtafoveolar retinal telangiectasia is least severe form
- Leber's miliary aneurysm is of intermediate severity
- Coat's disease is most severe form

Idiopathic juxtafoveolar retinal telangiectasia

Group 1
- Unilateral parafoveal telangiectasias, congenital or acquired
- One eye of a middle-aged male
- Resembles a localised variant of Coat's

Group 1a
- Parafoveal telangiectasis, involving a small area of temporal area of macula
- Treat by photocoagulation

Group 1b
- Area of capillary telangiectasis of one clock hour at the edge of the foveal avascular zone

Group 2
- Bilateral parafoveal telangiectasias
- Affects both eyes of elderly person, male or female
- May develop CNV
- Symmetrical capillary dilatation, one disc area or less, involving all or part of parafoveal retina
- Guarded long-term prognosis, laser unsuccessful, except for CNV

Group 3
- Bilateral perifoveal telangiectasis and capillary occlusion
- Sixth decade
- No response to photocoagulation
- Changes more severe than other types, visual prognosis is worse

Leber's miliary aneurysms

- A localised + milder form of Coat's?
- Present in adult life → unilateral impairment of vision
- Fusiform and saccular dilatation of venules and arterioles, most commonly involving temporal retinal periphery
- Chronic leakage → intraretinal hard exudates
- Treat with cryo or photocoagulation

Coat's disease

Pathogenesis
- Primary arteriolar disturbance → capillary closure → disturbed blood-retinal barrier , incompetent vessels → exudates and haemorrhages
- Neovascularisation very uncommon
- Congenital, ? post-inflammatory (TB, syphilis), ? post-hypoxia

Pathology
- 'Early'/Leber's disease – multiple miliary aneurysms of arterioles
- 'Late'/Coat's disease – telangiectasia in inner retinal layers; subretinal exudate of lipid, accumulation of lipid laden macrophages (bladder cells), glial proliferation
- Not hereditary but can be associated with retinitis pigmentosa

Clinical features

- General – juvenile form usual, adult form sometimes
- Presents in first decade (average 5 years of age)
- Healthy young males, usually unilateral; males 85%, unilateral in 80–90%
- Initially asymptomatic → loss of vision, leukocoria (may simulate retinoblastoma), squint
- Fundoscopy – raised yellow subretinal exudates in posterior pole, cystoid macular oedema may occur
- Macular vessels normal but exudate can accumulate at macula
- Large range in clinical findings from very mild telangiectasia to massive exudation and RD
- Light bulb telangiectasia with haemorrhages, mainly in supertemporal quadrant
- Fluorescein: Telangiectasia and leakage
- Aqueous LDH – elevated

Differential diagnosis

- Dominant (familial) exudative vitreoretinopathy
- Fascioscapulohumeral muscular dystrophy
- ROP

Complications/natural history

- Usually progressive → retinal detachment, secondary glaucoma, cataract, phthisis
- Sometimes stationary → massive retinal fibrosis
- Rarely that spontaneous remissions occur

Treatment

- Document progression with colour photos + fluorescein
- Observe if mild and non-sight threatening
- Eliminate vascular anomalies → photocoagulation + cryopexy
- PPV if retinal detachment deep and not suitable for cryo
- If effective, → resorbtion of exudate over 2–12 months
- Follow every 6 months

Sickle Cell retinopathy

Aetiology and pathology

- Mendelian inheritance
- AS (Sickle Cell trait) – 8% of African-Americans; mildest; severe hypoxia needed to produce sickling
- SS (Sickle Cell disease/Sickle Cell anaemia) – 0.4% of African-Americans; systemic → severe, ocular → mild
- SC (Sickle Cell C disease) – 0.2% of African-Americans; severe ocular complications
- Sthal (Sickle Cell thalassaemia) – severe ocular complications
- Mutant haemoglobins S and C, normal Hb A
- Valine replaces glutamic acid in position 6 of B chain of haemoglobin → decreased haemoglobin stability → rbc's rigid and crescentic-shaped when haemoglobin reduced and there is hypoxia or acidosis
- Rigidity → red cell impaction → ischaemia,
  hypoxia, necrosis → more sickling
- Ocular complications most severe in SC + SThal, systemic in SS

Conjunctiva and iris

- Corkscrew capillaries in lower bulbar conjunctiva
- Focal iris atrophy

Non-proliferative retinopathy

Asymptomatic lesions

- Venous tortuosity
- Black sunbursts – equatorial, resemble chorioretinal scars, ? result from arteriolar occlusion → blowout haemorrhage → accumulation of melanin and hemosiderin

8

- Refractile deposits – ? hemosiderin in schisis cavities, from haemorrhage
- Silver wire arterioles – occluded vessels
- Salmon patch haemorrhage – blowout haemorrhage from arteriolar occlusion
- Retinal holes – equatorial or pre-equatorial
- Macular depression sign – oval depression of macular reflex due to atrophy of sensory retina

Symptomatic lesions

- Central retinal artery occlusion
- Macular arteriole occlusions
- Branch/central retinal vein occlusion
- Choroidal vascular occlusion
- Angioid streaks – ? Iron deposition in Bruch's membrane → increased brittleness

Proliferative retinopathy

- Stage 1 – Peripheral arteriolar occlusion
- Stage 2 – Peripheral arteriovenous anastamosis, ischaemic retina beyond
- Stage 3 – Peripheral neovascularisation, typical sea-fan configuration, flat; spontaneous involution → grey, fibrovascular tufts → may continue to proliferate + bleed
- Stage 4 – Vitreous haemorrhage
- Stage 5 – Retinal detachment
  - Tractional
  - Rhegmatogenous – tear formation adjacent to fibrovascular tissue

Treatment

- Post-traumatic hyphaema → screen for sickling in African-Americans
- Fluorescein angiograms every 6–12 months, to pick up early neovascularisation
- Local photocoagulation of neovascularisation – arteriole feeder + venous drainer → no longer recommended → may cause retinal + choroidal haemorrhages, breaks in Bruch's membrane, CNV, retinal breaks and detachments
- Peripheral cryopexy if local laser not possible
- Vitrectomy for vitreous haemorrhage
- Retinal detachment surgery – anterior segment ischaemia reported with 360 buckles

Hypertensive retinopathy

- Hypertensive narrowing is seen in its pure form only in young individuals because they do not have much existing replacement fibrosis/sclerosis of vessels
- The main role of fundoscopy is to establish target organ damage

Pathology

- Benign → reactive hypertonus, medial and intimal hyperplasia, replacement fibrosis
- Malignant → medial and intimal fibrinoid necrosis
- Capillary ischaemia → retinopathy

Classification

- Keith Wagener
  - Narrowing of vessels and sclerosis (spasm) – Grade 1
  - Calibre variation and AV nipping (hypertrophy → copper wiring, etc.) – Grade 2
  - Haemorrhages and exudates – Grade 3
  - Neuroretinal oedema – Grade 4

OR

- Grade A: Non-accelerated hypertension – generalised arteriolar narrowing + focal constriction
- Grade B: Accelerated hypertension – haemorrhages, exudates, cotton wool spots, ± disc swelling; Grade B necessitates investigation of cause; 5 year survival only 20%

Features

- Narrowing; normal A : V = 2 : 3
- Sclerosis
  - Grade increases lustre, copper

  - wiring, silver wiring, no visible bloodstream
  - Straightening of vessels due to sclerosis behind the disc
- AV crossings
  - Gunn sign (compression/tapering of vein)
  - Salus sign (deflexion of vein at AV crossing)
  - Bonnet sign – banking of blood in vein
  - AV nipping is not a sign of severity but only of long-standing disease
- Haemorrhages – flame-shaped, in nerve fibre layer
- Exudates
  - Hard – protein > lipid; in outer plexiform layer; macrophages also present
  - Soft – infarcts in nerve fibre layer
- Optic nerve oedema – obstructed axoplasmic flow, ? due to ischemia, ? due to raised intracranial pressure – malignant hypertension
- Focal choroidal infarcts
  - Elschnig spots – small black spots surrounded by yellow haloes
  - Siegrist streaks – flecks arranged linearly along choroidal vessels – fibrinoid necrosis in malignant hpypertension
  - Serous retinal detachment – due to choriocapillaris occlusion
- Retinal oedema – due to ischemia
- Retinal macroaneurysms
- Central/branch vein/arterial occlusion

Other ocular manifestations of hypertension

- Retinal vein occlusion
- Retinal artery occlusion
- Retinal artery macroaneurysm
- Anterior ischaemic optic neuropathy
- Ocular motor nerve palsies
- Ischaemic choroidal infarcts
- Serous retinal detachment (in acute hypertension)
- Worsening of diabetic retinopathy

Macroaneurysm

- Unilateral, single or multiple, within three orders of retinal arterial bifurcations
- Most frequently at an AV crossing

Incidence

- Sixty years, female > male
- Unilateral in 90%
- Hypertension and arteriosclerosis associated
- Retinal vein occlusion associated; ? share systemic risk factors; ? macroaneurysm → vein occlusion, ? vein occlusion → macroaneurysm
- Leakage → exudate, vitreous haemorrhage, oedema, cystoid macular oedema, macular hole. (bleeding rarely occurs more than once)
- 30% of untreated → permanent loss of vision

Management

- Observe – good VA, macula not threatened, mild retinal haemorrhage, no significant oedema
- Treat with photocoagulation – large spot, long burns, low intensity, treat lesion, surrounding area or both
- May take months for exudates and oedema to clear

Vasculitis

Signs

- Perivascular infiltrates
- Vessel sheathing (vascular wall thickening with vessel involution)
- Distinct vein or artery involvement uncommon → usually both

Aetiology

- Giant cell artentis
- Polyarteritis
- SLE
- Behçet's
- Inflammatory bowel disease
- Multiple sclerosis

- Pars planitis
- Sarcoidosis
- Syphilis
- Toxoplasmosis
- Viral retinitis
- Lyme disease
- Cat scratch disease
- Primary idiopathic retinal vasculitis → Eale's disease

Retinal detachment

Incidence

- One per 10 000 per year
- Bilateral in 10–15% eventually
- General population – 0.01%
- Aphakia – 1–3%
- Phaco – 0.1%
- Myopia – 1%
- YAG increases detachment 3–5 times

Pathogenesis

- Hole formation
  - Vitreous traction
  - Retinal weakness
- Detachment
  - Hole formation
  - Subretinal fluid accumulation, from choroid and vitreous
- Spread of subretinal fluid – Linkoff's scheme
  - Upper temporal and nasal holes: Does not cross midline; lower than other side; inferior bullae often occur
  - Superior midline holes: Fluid spreads down symmetrically
  - Inferior holes: Higher on side of hole; seldom bullous; seldom total
  - Total detachments: Usually due to holes close to the midline, in the superior position
- Natural history untreated → proliferative vitreoretinopathy, uveitis, cataract, glaucoma or phtisis bulbi
- Predispositions
  - Myopia – 8 times increased risk; 3–5D 1–1.5 times, 5–10D 7–10 times, >10 D 20 times
  - Pseudophakia – 1–2% incidence; usually in the first 3 months to 1 year
  - Lattice degeneration
  - Retinal coloboma
  - Familial tendency
  - Vitreoretinal syndromes – Stickler syndrome, Marfan's
  - Trauma
  - Retinal neovascularisation

Vitreoretinal adhesions

- Normal – vitreous base, disc margin, fovea, blood vessels
- Abnormal – posterior border of lattice, RPE clumps, white without-pressure, vitreous base anomalies e.g. isolated islands, peripheral paravascular condensations, congenital cystic retinal tufts

Symptoms

- Classical
  - Posterior vitreous detachment → photopsia from traction
  - Weiss ring, visible detached posterior hyaloid face
  - Hole formation occurs in 10–15% of posterior vitreous detachment → floaters from haemorrhage, pigment in vitreous
  - Retinal detachment occurs within a few weeks → field defect
- Other – insidious deterioration in visual acuity, asymptomatic

Signs

- Afferent pupil defect
- Decreased IOP
- Iritis
- Tobacco dusting in anterior vitreous
- Typical fundal appearance of hole and detachment

Vitreoretinal traction

Dynamic

- Rapid eye movements
- Centripetal, towards vitreous cavity → retinal tear → retinal detachment

Static

- Independent of eye movements
- Tractional retinal detachment
  - Tangential – surface, due to contraction of epiretinal or subretinal membranes
  - Anteroposterior – towards vitreous base
  - Bridging – from one part of the retina to another, usually along the posterior hyaloid surface

Holes in retinal detachment

- 60% in upper temporal quadrant
- 15% in upper nasal quadrant
- 15% in lower temporal quadrant
- 10% in lower nasal quadrant

> One hole in 60% of detachments

- Dialysis in 10% of detachments
- Giant tears in 1–2% of detachments (= > 90°/posterior flap mobile)
- Macular holes in 1–2% of detachments

Signs of long-standing retinal detachment

- Retina transparent and cystic
- Pigment tidemarks
- Subretinal glial membranes

Differential diagnosis of rhegmatogenous retinal detachment

- Retinoschisis
- Exudative retinal detachment → VKH syndrome or other exudative uveitis
- Retinal detachment secondary to choroidal tumour

Pseudophakic retinal detachment

- Often associated with small atrophic vitreous base holes
- Bilateral in 25%, tends to be total rather than partial
- Occurs in 2–4% of pseudophakes, within 3 months to 1 year
- Increased tendency to develop proliferative vitreoretinopathy
- IOL insertion does not affect retinal detachment rate
- Prophylaxis – 360° cryopexy, with encircling band

Principles of treatment

- Break closure
  - Ab externo → buckle
  - Ab interno → gases, oil
- Break seal
  - Cryo
  - Laser – endolaser; indirect
- Relief of traction (at break and elsewhere)
  - Ab externo – buckle
  - Ab interno – gases, oil
  - Surgical dissection – pars plana vitrectomy, membrane dissection, retinotomy

Planning of surgery

- Pre-op assessment; choice of operation
  - Conventional/external; with prophylaxis of second eye
  - Vitrectomy
- Examination
  - Indirect with scleral indentation (both eyes)
  - Three mirror
  - Ultrasound
  - X-rays
- Choice of surgery determined by:
  - Break details – detection of breaks; site, size, number, relationship to one another of breaks
  - Assessment of traction

Cryopexy

- Around break
- Creates adhesion
- Achieves maximal strength after 11 days
- With cryo, exo laser, endo laser
- Complications of cryo – scleral rupture, vitreous and choroidal haemorrhage, serous choroidal detachment, pigment fallout

Scleral buckle

- Silastic sponge plomb
  - Radial
  - Circumferential
  - To close hole; sponge creates a high profile indent → decrease vitreous traction; radial sponge better

8

- Silastic band encirclement
  - To decrease vitreous traction
  - Close hole; must use if holes separated by < 8 mm
  - Usually at 12 mm
  - May be complicated by anterior segment ischaemia, glaucoma, choroidal detachment, enophthalmos

Subretinal fluid drainage

Indications

- If adequate scleral buckling cannot be achieved without subretinal fluid drainage
- Superior and posterior break usually creates a bullous detachment, therefore subretinal fluid drainage is necessary
- Inferior and anterior breaksw 'never' create bullous detachments, therefore subretinal fluid drainage is unnecessary

8

Technique

- 25 or 27 gauge needle prick
- Over deepest subretinal fluid
- With digital pressure and constant indirect control

Complications

- Intraocular haemorrhage – choroidal, subretinal, intravitreal, intracorneal
- Avoid by raising IOP, diathermy, drainage before cryo, avoid previous cryo'ed site, beware of diabetics
- Vitreoretinal incarceration – can lead to haemorrhage, new break, proliferative vitreoretinopathy, break distortion, prevention of closure
- Avoid by draining over deepest subretinal fluid, small hole, indirect ophthalmoscopy, avoid breaks

Non-drainage conventional explant operations

Rationale

- Break closure → absorption of subretinal fluid across retinal pigment epithelium; takes 2–3 days

Pre-op assessment

- Assess whether or not break can be closed with a scleral depressor
- Only necessary to drain subretinal fluid if there is inadequate apposition

Technique

- Use silastic sponge radial explant

Disadvantages

- Buckle localisation difficult, cryo heavy

Pneumoretinopexy

Indications

- For superior tear, either single or close together, and no proliferative vitreoretinopathy

Technique

- Inject C3F8 (perfluoro propane) → tamponade and break of dynamic vitreoretinal traction
- Combine with cryo or argon laser

Complications

- Increased risk of proliferative vitreoretinopathy
- Increased risk of other breaks
- Endophthalmitis

D-ACE procedure

Indications

- Upper breaks

Advantages

- Aids localisation of breaks
- Less cryopexy
- Low buckles

Disadvantages

- Drain subretinal fluid
- Multiple bubbles
- Minifies breaks
- High intraocular pressure

Contraindications

- Multiple complex breaks
- Little subretinal fluid
- Pars plana vitrectomy indicated

Technique

- Sequence of: drain subretinal fluid, air injection, cryotherapy, explant

Intraocular injection

Indications

- For internal tamponade or hypotony

Technique

- Using 27 gauge needle
- 5 mm from limbus, in superonasal quadrant
- Ensure needle is in centre of vitreous, then withdraw to keep tip in high position

Gases

- Air – absorbs rapidly
- Sulphahexafluoride (SF6) – absorbs nitrogen, expands to 2 × volume; may cause posterior subcapsular lens opacities; lasts 10–14 days
- Perfluoropropane (C3F8) – expands to 4 × volume; lasts 55–65 days
- Perfluoroethane (C2F6) – expands to 3 × volume; lasts 30–35 days

Heavy liquids

- Perfluorocarbons – high specific gravity, not resorbed, need removal
- Silicone – low specific gravity, not resorbed, needs removal
- May cause cataract, glaucoma, keratopathy, retinopathy

Pars plana vitrectomy

Indications

- Advanced proliferative vitreoretinopathy
- Awkward breaks
    - Unseen
    - Site e.g. macula
    - Size e.g. giant tears (> one clock hour in width)
    - Arrangement – multiple breaks at widely disparate a–p locations, posterior breaks (posterior to equator)
- Other
    - Macular pucker
    - Foreign bodies
    - Choroidal detachment

Technique

- Remove opacities in media
- Identify breaks
- Gas tamponade

Disadvantages

- Cataract; nuclear sclerosis rate increased
- Missed break → rapid retinal detachment
- Increase in proliferative vitreoretinopathy

Complications

- Subretinal infusion
- Lens touch
- Entry site tears
- Retinotomy
- Hypotony
- Haemorrhage

Results

- 90% success with 1 or more operations
- 10% failure → most common cause is unsealed break

Complications of conventional explant surgery

Early

- Sudden blindness – central retinal artery occlusion, optic nerve injury
- Infection – extraocular, intraocular
- Anterior segment ischaemia
- Sterile uveitis
- Glaucoma
- Choroidal detachment
- Vitreous haemorrhage
- Exudative detachment

Late

- Implant extrusion and infection
- Intraocular erosion of implant
- Choroidal folds
- Pain, diplopia, refractive changes
- Macular pucker

Post-operative course

- Visual recovery noticed immediately, may take 2–3 years

Posterior retinotomy

Indications

- For severe traction retinal detachment, with anterior retinal shortening, intraretinal fibrosis, subretinal fibrosis, retinal incarceration, chorioretinal adhesions

Technique

- Posterior vitrectomy with removal of epiretinal membrane
- Endophotocoagulation around limit of retinotomy
- Cut retina
- Remove anterior retina
- Silicone oil

Retinal detachment surgery on long-standing detachment

- Rapid drop-off in macular function (post-op) from onset of detachment
- Detachment duration
  - 1/52 → 6/12 vision
  - 9/52 → 6/60
  - 6/12 → most < 6/60, some achieve 6/12

Rhegmatogenous retinal detachment following trauma in Caucasians

- Occurs in 4.6% of blunt injuries in Caucasians
- 63% occur at ora, most inferotemporally
- May also occur at site of contusion, due to retinal necrosis

Rhegmatogenous retinal detachment following trauma in Blacks

Incidence

- 10–12% of retinal detachments in Blacks are due to blunt trauma

Morphology of retinal breaks

- Large posterior retinal slits
- Large posterior holes
- Retinal dialyses are less common
- Most have macular holes
- Most have multiple holes

Epidemiology

- 90% are males < 40 years
- Assault is the most common cause
- Often a delay in presentation
- May have other signs of trauma – lens dislocation, vitreous haemorrhage, and angle recession

Rhegmatogenous retinal detachment without preceding trauma in blacks

- Incidence less than in whites (0.46 per 100 000 cw 10 per 100 000)
- Due to:
  - Strong adherence of retinal pigment epithelium to sensory retina
  - Firmer adherence of posterior hyaloid face to retina decreased syneresis

Tractional retinal detachment

Causes

- Proliferative diabetic retinopathy
- Penetrating posterior segment trauma
- Retinopathy of prematurity
- Sickle cell retinopathy

Exudative retinal detachment

Causes

- Choroidal tumour
- Intraocular inflammation
  - VKH syndrome
  - Posterior scleritis
- Subretinal neovascularisation
- Iatrogenic
  - Panretinal photocoagulation
  - Retinal detachment surgery
- Systemic causes
  - Hypertension
  - Toxaemia of pregnancy

Proliferative vitreoretinopathy

- Preretinal neovascularisation peripheral to the major vascular arcades

Causes of proliferative vitreoretinopathy

- Vascular disease with ischaemia
  - Sickling haemaglobinopathies (prototype)
  - Other haemaglobinopathies
  - Eale's disease (diagnosis by exclusion)
  - Diabetes
  - Hypertensive retinopathy
  - Branch retinal vein occlusion (25% → peripheral neovascularisation)
  - Retinal embolisation (talc in IVI drug abusers)
  - Retinopathy of prematurity
  - Hyperviscosity syndromes (leukaemia, polycythaemia, dysproteinaemia)
  - Aortic arch syndrome (Takayasu's, syphilis, arteriosclerosis)
  - Carotid – cavernous fistula
- Inflammatory diseases with possible ischaemia
  - Sarcoidosis
  - Retinal vasculitis (syphilis, collagen diseases)
  - Uveitis (pars planitis, Behçet's)
- Miscellaneous
  - Incontinentia pigmenti
  - Familial exudative vitreoretinopathy
  - Long-standing retinal detachment
  - Multiple sclerosis

Angiogenesis

- Angiogenic factor produced by – ischaemic retina, inflammatory cells
- Vitreous normally contains an angiogenic inhibitory factor, as it has a low pO2

Diagnostic work-up

- Full blood count
- Haemoglobin electrophoresis
- CXR
- SACE
- Gallium scan
- Glucose tolerance test
- Collagen screen

Management

- Fluorescein angiogram
- Systemic steroids in the inflammatory conditions
- Local photocoagulation – photocoagulate feeder arterioles and drainage venules
- If local photocoagulation not possible – single freeze cryotherapy of retinal periphery
- PRP → regression of neovascularisation

Complications

- Vitreous haemorrhage
- Retinal detachment – traction and rhegmatogenous
- Rubeotic glaucoma
- Cataract
- Phthisis bulbi

Peripheral retinal degenerations

Developmental variations

- Most common in superonasal quadrant, may occur in up to 20% of eyes
- Meridional fold – from ora, extending 6 mm into retina
- Meridional complex – fold connecting to a large ciliary process
- Enclosed ora bay – island of pars plana epithelium posterior to ora
- Peripheral retinal excavation – near ora, oval depression in retina

Classification of retinal degenerations

- Predisposing peripheral retinal degenerations
  - Lattice degeneration
  - Snailtrack degeneration
  - Degenerative retinoschisis
  - White without pressure
- Lesions not requiring prophylaxis
  - Microcystoid degeneration – tiny vesicles, indistinct boundaries, grey-white background, retina appears thickened, less transparent
  - Snowflakes – often associated with lattice, snailtrack, acquired retinoschisis; minute, glistening yellow-white dots, diffuse in peripheral fundus
  - Pavingstone degeneration – in 25%; discrete, yellow-white patches of focal chorioretinal atrophy
  - Honeycomb (reticular) degeneration – age-related change, fine network of perivascular pigmentation
  - Drusen – small pale lesions with hyperpigmented borders
  - Oral pigmentary degeneration – age-related change, hyperpigmented band adjacent to ora

8

Microcystoid degeneration

- Spaces develop in outer plexiform and inner nuclear layers
- No significance, no treatment required

Retinoschisis

- 5% of the population over 50
- Retinal splitting in outer plexiform layer, from coalescence of cysts
- May spread posteriorly, may develop holes, may require treatment

Pavingstone degeneration

- Discrete yellow foci of depigmentation and thinning/atrophy between ora and equator
- Overlying vitreous normal
- Of no significance, no treatment required

Tapetochoroidal degeneration

- As for pavingstone, but in a continuous band

Retinal hole (trophic)

- Round, full thickness, within vitreous base, more common superotemporally
- No treatment required

Lattice degeneration

- Demarcated circumferential retinal thinning, round atrophic hole formation,

sclerosis of vessels → 'lattice' and adjacent vitreous liquefaction; vitreous firmly adherent along posterior margin; horseshoe tears with traction may occur along posterior margin
- Associated with local RPE hyperplasia
- Radially orientated tears may extend to the equator
- Trophic or tractional breaks associated
- Occurs anterior to equator, more common superotemporally
- Snailtrack degeneration is a variant
  - Present in 8% of adult eyes; → retinal detachment in 2% of cases, contributes to retinal detachment in 30% of cases
  - Present in 33% of myopic eyes, more common in moderate myopia rather than severe myopia
  - Indications for treatment – hole with traction or subretinal fluid, retinal detachment in other eye, young patient, only eyes, pseudophakia
  - Treat with cryo or photocoagulation

Retinal tuft

- May be non-cystic, cystic, or zonular traction
- Cystic may → retinal tear
- Zonular traction may → round atrophic intrabasal holes; traction may occur following lens extraction → retinal detachment

White without pressure

- Giant tears may form along the posterior border of such lesions

Diffuse chorioretinal atrophy

- May give rise to small round holes in highly myopic eyes

Paravascular vitreoretinal attachments

- May predispose to tears in acute PVD

Tears

Incidence

- In adults 6%
- But only 0.07% of all people will develop a detachment
- If a retinal detachment develops, it does so within 6 weeks of break

Classification

- Flap/horseshoe tear – a strip of retina pulled anteriorly by vitreoretinal traction
- Giant retinal tear – extends ≥ 90 degrees circumferentially
- Operculated hole – traction pulls a piece of retina completely free
- Dialysis – circumferential, linear breaks along the ora serrata (often due to blunt trauma)
- Atrophic retinal hole – not associated with traction, no risk of retinal detachment
- Macular hole
- Tear
  - Oral (dialysis)
  - Intrabasal
  - Juxtabasal
  - Extrabasal/equatorial
- Vitreous base seen as white with/without pressure, adjacent to ora

Prophylactic treatment of retinal breaks

- Vast majority of tears do not lead to detachment
- Laser to reduce risk of detachment (controversial as to which tears to laser)
- Old tears – criteria for prophylactic treatment
  - Symptoms of tear – photopsia, floaters
  - Myopia
  - Vitreoretinal syndromes (Marfan's, Ehlers-Danlos, Stickler syndrome)
  - Cataract surgery
  - Retinoschisis
  - Posterior vitreous detachment

8

  - Lattice degeneration
  - Miotic treatment
  - Contralateral detachment
- New tears– acute breaks are more dangerous than old; criteria for prophyloctic treatment
  - Most retinal breaks
  - Lattice or snailtrack degeneration
  - other eye of detachment
  - myopia
  - young patient
- Other eye of non-traumatic giant tears

Pathogenesis

- Retinal weakness – ? abnormal glycosaminoglycan in RPE cement
- Vitreous traction – ? abnormal vitreous collagen or matrix

Oral tears (dialysis)

- Trauma → avulsion of vitreous base
- Developmental, rarely
- Younger patients
- Common inferotemporally or superonasally (because inferonasal protection of the globe by the orbit is the poorest and the superonasal area gets the cotracoup injury)
- Seen in 10% of detachments
- < 90°–360°, insidious progression → macular detachment
- Must be differentiated from a giant tear: no anterior flap, elevated and posterior rolled posterior flap
- Management – prophylactic buckle and cryo

Intrabasal tears

- From zonuloretinal traction
- No surrounding retinal traction, no treatment necessary
- Traction may occur in aphakia, therefore watch carefully

Juxtabasal tears

- Posterior vitreous detachment → increased juxtabasal traction → horseshoe or giant tear with traction
- High risk of retinal detachment, therefore treat with cryo or photocoagulation

Extrabasal tears

- Posterior vitreous detachment → traction on pre-existing cystic retinal tuft
- Usually operculated, no treatment required; if operculum is still attached, watch carefully

Giant tears

- Tear extending for > 90°; posterior flap has independent mobility and tears posteriorly
- 40% are bilateral and non-traumatic
- 50% in 5 years incidence in second eye
- May develop along posterior border of white without pressure
- 70% are idiopathic
- 20% are traumatic
- 10% occur in vitreoretinal syndromes (e.g. Stickler syndrome)

Treatment

- Pars plana vitrectomy
- Perfluoropropane injection
- Buckle

Traumatic retinal breaks

- Open or closed ocular trauma
- Blunt trauma: caused by coup or contracoup injury → eye deforms → traction on vitreous base
- Contusion injury → large equatorial breaks, dialysis, macular hole → inferotemporal (poor orbit protection here) + superonasal (because of the contracoup injury)
- Dialyses: small or large. Usually posterior border of vitreous base, may be anterior border
- Less commonly – horseshoe tears, operculated holes
- Young eyes: rarely develop acute detachments because vitreous not syneretic

- May develop later, when gel liquefies
- Detachments may be shallow and show signs of chronicity (demarcation lines, subretinal deposits, intraretinal cysts)

Retinal pigment epithelium detachment

Pathogenesis

- Due to break in Bruch's membrane → collection of fluid under RPE from choroid
- Due to subretinal neovascular membrane
- Due to accumulation of fluid pumped from RPE, due to decreased conductivity of Bruch's membrane from lipid accumulation on its inner surface

Aetiology

- In isolation
- Component of central serous retinopathy
- Component of age related macular degeneretaion
- Secondary to – choroidal tumour, subretinal neovascular membrane, inflammation

Classification

- Type 1 – localised, < 1 disc area, no enlarge-ment, slow focal RPE degeneration
- Type II – generalised, > 1 disc area, progressive, generalised RPE degeneration
- Stage 1 – drusen
- Stage 2 – new vessels under RPE
- Stage 3 – serous RPE detachment
- Stage 4 – atrophic
- Stage 5 – exudative
- Stage 6 – haemorrhagic

Clinical features

- Decreased vision, metamorphopsia, scotoma
- Dome-shaped elevation
- ± Lipofuscin accumulation in a ring or across dome (hot cross bun, wheel spoke; = long-standing detachment)
- RPE changes
- ± Subretinal neovascularisation, ± haemorrhage

Fluorescein

- Early hyperfluorescence, increase in intensity not in size, well-defined
- Leakage → subsensory space occurs near margin of detachment
- Subretinal neovascularisation may → hot spot, nodular beading on edge, or subretinal haemorrhage

Natural course

- May be static
- May resolve with no sequelae
- May resolve with RPE atrophy
- May → central serous retinopathy; may → subretinal neovascularisation → haemorrhage → disciform scar
- May → RPE tear

Treatment

- RPE alone – no treatment; photocoagulation may make it worse
- RPE and CSR – treat as for CSR
- RPE and SRNV – photocoagulate SRNV membrane, green, 250 U, 0.5 secs, 100–150 mw

RPE tear

- Occurs in 10% of RPE detachments
- 30% are bilateral
- At junction of attached and detached RPE
- May occur after laser to RPE detachment, may occur spontaneously
- Poor prognosis

Retinoschisis

Classification

- Degenerative
- X-linked juvenile
- Secondary (traction in diabetic retinopathy)

8

Degenerative

- Split in sensory retina
- Peripheral cystoid degeneration (present in all adult eyes) → cavities coalesce and progress to a typical degenerative retinoschisis
- Occurs in 5% of adults
- More common in hypermetropes
- Nearly always asymptomatic
- Occurs initially inferotemporally, bilateral
- May be typical → split in outer plexiform layer
- May be reticular → split in nerve fibre layer, with more extensive tissue loss and hole formation
- Difficult to make the distinction clinically
- Inner layer holes may occur, of no consequence
- Outer layer holes may occur → retinal detachment
- May extend to involve posterior pole

Treatment

- Outer layer holes – photocoagulate around the margins
- Retinal detachment – conventional treatment
- Posterior extension – delineating photocoagulation

X-linked juvenile

- X-linked recessive, rare, gene RS 1
- Bilateral maculopathy + peripheral retinoschisis in 50%
- Schisis occurs in nerve fibre layer, problem with Muller cells
- Foveal schisis – occurs in 100%; tiny cystoid spaces, bicycle wheel pattern of radial striae
- Peripheral schisis occurs in 50%, initially inferotemporally
- Foveal schisis is initially a cystoid maculopathy → hole formation
- Inner wall of schisis may show glial proliferation → retrolental membrane and leucocoria
- Deterioration in visual acuity → blind at 60 years of age

Treatment

- Unsatisfactory
- ± Photocoagulation, ± retinal detachment surgery

Differential diagnosis of schisis and detachment

- Schisis morphology
  - Taut, smooth, thin, immobile, domed; detachment undulating
  - Snowflaking on schisis (remnants of Muller cells that formally bridged the cavity)
- Laser → white burn with schisis, no visible burn with detachment
- Visual field → schisis causes an absolute scotoma, retinal detachment causes a relative scotoma
- Tobacco dust + haemorrhage → rare in schisis, common in detachment
- Schisis → smooth surface, dome-shaped, detachment → corrugated, irregular surface (although it may look like schisis if long-standing)
- Shifting fluid – schisis → absent, RRD → variable

Myopia

- High myopia often associated with progressive, excessive elongation of the globe often followed by degenerative changes involving sclera and choroid

Incidence

- 5–20% of the general population
- 4th – 7th leading cause of permanent blindness

Classification

- Low < 8D simple
- High > 8D degenerative

Pathogenesis of degenerative myopia

- Early degeneration due to increased axial length

- Late degeneration due to ? vascular insufficiency
- Fundus changes usually occur when myopia measures 6D or more

Features of degenerative myopia
- Sclera – thinning → posterior staphyloma
- Choroid – atrophy of choriocapillaris, atrophy of stroma, decreased melanocytes, choroidal sclerosis
- Bruch's membrane
    - Breaks → lacquer cracks (yellow-white lines), CNV
    - Subretinal coin haemorrhages – transient, not related to CNV
- RPE – atrophy → tigroid fundus, pigment migration and proliferation
- Neuroretina – rods and cones degenerate; peripheral degeneration (pavingstone + lattice), holes, and tears
- Vitreous – liquefaction + posterior vitreous detachment; Weiss ring
- Disc
    - Tilted, crescent of chorioretinal atrophy, usually temporal, may encircle disc, choroidal or scleral
    - Nasal supertraction, shallow cup
- Macula
    - Degenerative macular changes associated with refractive error > 6D + axial length > 26 mm
    - Degeneration, resembling age related macular degeneration– better prognosis
- Foster-Fuchs' spot = pigment accumulation in deep retina (RPE hyperplasia) – following haemorrhage or CNV that does not lead to disciform
- Macular cyst and hole – may lead to detachment
- Associations – retinal detachment; 8 times higher than in non-myopic population; incidence following uncomplicated cataract extraction 7%, following complicated cataract extraction 15%
- Primary chronic open angle glaucoma, pigmentary glaucoma, steroid responsiveness
- Posterior subcapsular lens opacities
- ROP may be associated with subsequent onset of myopia

Treatment
- Argon laser for extra-foveal CNV
- PDT for juxtafoveal + subfoveal

Choroidal dystrophies

Classification
- Choroideremia
- Gyrate atrophy
- Central areolar choroidal dystrophy
- Diffuse choroidal atrophy
- Helicoidal parapapillary chorioretinal degeneration
- Pigmented paravenous retinochoroidal atrophy
- Choroidal sclerosis

Choroideraemia

Inheritance
- Sex-linked recessive – only males affected (gene locus Xq21)
- All daughters of affected fathers carry
- Half sons of female carriers develop disease
- Half daughters of female carriers also carriers
- Affected male cannot transmit gene to sons

Female carriers
- Salt and pepper fundus
- Patchy peripheral atrophy + RPE mottling
- Normal VA, fields, ERG

Pathology
- Choroidal atrophy + secondary retinal atrophy → baring of sclera

Signs
- Presents with nyctalopia in first decade

- Affected males → choroidal atrophy in mid periphery, spreads out, spares area around disc and macula until late
- Arterioles thin and disc pale.
- Intermediate and large choroidal vessels preserved
- Posterior subcapsular lens opacities and myopia may be associated
- Loss of peripheral field, late loss of central vision (50–60 years)

ERG
- Decreased or absent
- Scotopic adaptation absent

Angiogram
- Filling of retinal + large choroidal vessels but not choriocapillaris

Treatment
- Genetic counselling
- Protect from light; light → rhodopsin breakdown → toxic effects

Prognosis
- Poor
- Useful vision until sixth decade, severe loss thereafter

Gyrate atrophy

Types
- Congenital – stationary
- Associated with high myopia
- Associated with hyperornithinemia – autosomal recessive, due to deficiency of ornithine ketoacid aminotransferase; progressive + starts in midperiphery

Inheritance
- Autosomal recessive

Features
- Presents in second decade with axial myopia
- Large areas of bare sclera in periphery and midperiphery, with scalloped border causes by confluence of lesions
- Fovea spared until late
- Field constricted

ERG
- Decreased, later extinguished

Associations
- Retinitis pigmentosa features (attenuated arterioles and pale waxy disc)
- Posterior sub-capsular lens opacities in 50%, CMO, epiretinal membrane, myopia, iris heterochromia

Differential diagnosis
- Choroideremia
- Retinitis pigmentosa

Treatment
- Genetic counselling
- Limit ornithine intake (arginine restriction)
- Pyridoxine (B6) – decreases plasma ornithine

Prognosis
- Poor
- Legal blindness by fourth to sixth decades

Central areolar choroidal dystrophy

Inheritance
- Autosomal dominant, locus 17p

Clinical
- Presents in third to fourth decade, bilateral central visual impairment
- Initial central oedematous exudative change → bilateral symmetric sharply defined oval area of atrophy; central scotoma; foveal granularity

ERG
- Normal

Prognosis
- Poor
- Severe loss of vision by sixth to seventh decades

Diffuse choroidal dystrophy

Inheritance
- Autosomal dominant

8

Clinical

- Presents in fourth to fifth decade – impaired central vision, nyctalopia
- Parapapillary and pericentral RPE and choriocapillaris atrophy
- Gradual spread until entire fundus affected
- Baring of sclera

ERG

- Subnormal

Prognosis

- Poor, early macular involvement

Helicoidal parapapillary choroidal degeneration

Inheritance

- autosomal dominant

Clinical

- Presents in childhood
- Bilateral, slowly enlarging, tongue-like, well-defined strips of chorioretinal atrophy radiating from the optic nerve head

ERG

- Normal to severely subnormal

Prognosis

- Variable
- Young – severe, old – mild

Pigmented paravenous retinochoroidal atrophy

Inheritance

- Unknown

Clinical

- Bone spicules and chorioretinal atrophy along major retinal veins

ERG

- Normal

Prognosis

- Excellent – macular involvement rare

Choroidal folds

- Parallel grooves or striae involving inner choroid, Bruch's, RPE, ± sensory retina

Aetiology

- Congenital + idiopathic
- Orbital disease – dysthyroid eye disease, orbital tumours
- Choroidal tumours e.g. melanomas
- Hypotony – post-glaucoma surgery
- Other – posterior scleritis, chronic papilloedema, scleral buckling in retinal detachment surgery

Clinical

- Asymptomatic, metamorphopsia, permanent RPE and sensory changes
- Seen as alternating light and dark lines; usually horizontal
- Fluorescein → alternating hypo(troughs) and hyper (crests) lines (cw retinal striae)

Vitreous disorders

Persistent primary hyperplastic vitreous (persistent foetal vasculature)

- May be anterior, posterior or a combination
- Unilateral in 90%
- Microphthalmos, shallow anterior chamber, elongated ciliary processes
- Varies Mittendorf's dot → dense retrolental mass; may have congenital retinal fold
- Posterior lens capsule dehiscence → swelling of lens, cataract, 2° angle closure
- May develop 2° retinal detachment, 2° glaucoma (incomplete development of anterior chamber angle), amblyopia

Differential diagnosis in leukocoria

- Unlike PHPV, retinoblastoma is usually not obvious at birth, bilateral more often, almost never associated with microphthalmos or cataract

Treatment
- Lensectomy and removal of membrane to prevent angle closure, vitrectomy, retinal detachment surgery
- Posterior PHPV – differentiate from ROP, toxo, familial exudative vitreoretinopathy

Tunica vasculosa lentis
- Remnants of TVL and hyaloid system common
- Mittendorf's dot – posterior lens capsule nasal + inferior to posterior pole
- Bergmeister's papilla – fibroglial tuft from disc extending into vitreous; normal vessels may grow in forming prepapillary vascular loops (95% arterial); they supply the retina; may bleed, block
- Hyaloid artery may persist in Cloquet's canal

Hereditary hyaloideoretinopathies with optically empty vitreous
- Vitreous liquefaction → optically empty vitreous → thin layer of cortical vitreous behind lens + white membranes on retina
- Perivascular and equatorial lattice
- ERG subnormal

Group 1 – ocular signs only
- Jansen disease – associated with retinal detachment
- Wagner's disease – no associated retinal detachment
- Both autosomal dominant; myopia, strabismus, cataract

Group 2 – with associated systemic abnormalities
- Sickler syndrome, Weill-Marchesani

Familial exudative vitreoretinopathy
- Unlike ROP, full term, normal lungs

Asteroid hyalosis
- Calcium soaps attached to vitreous framework
- Asymptomatic
- May be associated with diabetes, hypercholesterolaemia, hypertension

Synchisis scintillans
- Free floating cholestrol crystals
- May cause symptoms
- Associated with previous injury or inflammation

Posterior vitreous detachment
- Occurs in old age
- Associated with diabetes, inflammation, myopia, trauma, surgery

Pathology
- Loss of hyaluronic acid → collapse of hyaluronic acid-collagen network with release of water → syneresis cavities → posterior rupture of syneresis cavity → posterior vitreous detachment
- Vitreous base cannot detach

Symptoms
- Light flashes, floaters
- Of the flashes and floaters presenting to the clinic – 75% isolated posterior vitreous detachment, 15% retinal detachment, 10% flat tears

Signs
- Posterior vitreous face seen with 90D, also Weiss ring
- Pigment dust = retinal break; occurs in 10–15% of cases
- B-scan
- OCT
- Posterior perifoveal detachment
  - Localised traction over macula

- Static traction + dynamic traction from saccades
- May lead to vitreomacular traction syndrome

Vitreous haemorrhage

- Trauma
  - Bleeding from ciliary body
  - Retinal tear
- Spontaneous
  - Diabetic retinopathy 39–54%
  - BRVO + CRVO 3–10%
  - Vitreous detachment with no tear 7–12%
  - Vitreous detachment with tear 35%
  - Rhegmatogenous retinal detachment 7–10%
  - Any cause of peripheral neovascularisation e.g. pars planitis
  - Vitreous haemorrhage occurs in 70% of retinal breaks

Terson syndrome

- Vitreous haemorrhage with intracranial haemorrhage
- Due to raised central retinal venous pressure
- Due to rupture into vitreous of an intraretinal haemorrhage
- Due to raised intracranial pressure transmitted down optic nerve sheath space → venous stasis via compression of intraorbital veins

Amyloidosis

- Bilateral vitreous opacification – early manifestation of autosomal dominant familial amyloidosis

Vitreous haemeorrhage

Aetiology

- Neovascularisation of the retina + disc
  - Diabetes (38%)
  - Retinal vein occlusions (9%)
  - Sickle Cell disease (2%)
  - Inflammatory diseases + occlusive vasculitis
  - Eale's
  - Ocular ischaemic syndrome
  - ROP
  - Retimins pigmentosa
  - Chronic RRD
- Rupture of a normal retinal vessel
  - PVD + retinal tear (25%)
  - PVD with no tear (8%)
  - Blunt trauma
  - Terson syndrome
  - Hyperviscosity with retinal vein occlusions
  - Anticoagulant therapy
  - Valsalva retinopathy
- Diseased retinal vessels
  - Macroaneurysm
  - Persistant hyaloid artery
  - Retinoblastoma
  - Hamartoma
  - Angioma
  - Hypertensive retinopathy
- Extension through the retina
  - CNV
  - Choroidal melanoma
  - Scleral buckle intrusion
  - Multiple haemorrhagic RPE detachments
- The 5 labelled conditions account for 75–90%

Optic disc tumours

Intraocular origin

Pigmented

- Melanocytoma
  - Locally invasive, non-malignant, from uveal melanocytes
  - More common in blacks
  - Usually at lower temporal disc quadrant
  - May show leakage on fluorescein
- Complications are rare
  - Malignant transformation
  - Tumour necrosis with central retinal vascular obstruction
- Malignant melanoma of choroid

- RPE proliferation and neoplasia

Non-pigmented
- Drusen
- Hamartomas (astrocytoma)
- Retinoblastoma
- Haemangioma

Extraocular origin
- Meningioma
- Optic glioma
- Metastatic tumours

Von Hippel-Lindau disease
- Capillary haemangiomas → retina + disc
- Hereditary or sporadic
- autosomal dominant, incomplete penetrance
- Von Hippel-Lindau = retinal angiomatosis + central nervous system involvement + visceral involvement
- Early lesions small, easily overlooked, seen on angiography
- Later, large, spherical, orange-red tumour
- Multiple tumours in one eye
- 50% bilateral
- Large feeding + draining vessels
- Surrounding exudate + serous detachment ± exudate at macula
- Vitreous haemorrhage, tractional retinal detachment
- Central nervous system tumours in 20% (haemangioblastomas of cerebellum, medulla, pons, spinal cord)
- Visceral lesions – cysts of kidney, pancreas, liver, epididymis, ovary
- Associations: Renal cell caroinoma, meningiomas, phaeochromocytomas
- Leading cause of death → cerebellar haemangioblastoma + renal cell careinoma

Treatment
- Cryo, laser, (PDT)
- Treat early
- Rarely may spontaneously involute

8

Fluorescein and ICG angiography

Fluorescein angiography

- Fluorescence is the property of some molecules to emit light of longer wavelength when stimulated by light of shorter wavelength
- 490 nm peak (blue) for fluorescein

Technique
- Sodium fluorescein 5 ml 10% IVI; (3 ml of 25% if opaque media)
- Minor adverse effects occur in 20%, severe life threatening side effects occur in 0.05%. ; light → blue excitation filter → yellow-green barrier filter → black and white film
- Sodium fluorescein capsules orally 25 mg/kg body weight; take photos at 40 and 60 minutes; there are fewer adverse side effects.

Adverse effects
- Skin + urine discolouration
- Nausea and vomiting, skin itching, flushing, hives, sneezing
- Syncope, bronchospasm, laryngeal oedema, anaphylactic shock

Phases
- Phase 1 – choroidal (pre-arterial)
- Phase 2 – arterial
- Phase 3 – arteriovenous (capillary)
- Phase 4 – early venous
- Phase 5 – late venous
- Phase 6 – late
- Choroidal filling at 12–20 secs
- Retinal circulation at 15–25 secs

Interpretation

Hyperfluorescence
- Window defect
    - RPE atrophy, early hyperfluorescence, increasing in intensity then fading
    - No change in shape or size

- Pooling
  - Subretinal – central serous chorioretinopathy; early hyperfluorescence increasing in size + intensity
  - Sub-RPE – PDE; early hyperfluorescence, increased intensity, not size
- Leakage
  - Abnormal choroidal vessels – CNV; lacy pattern, increased size + intensity
  - Breakdown of inner blood retinal barrier – CMO
  - Abnormal retinal or disc vasculature – neovascularisation
- Staining
  - Prolonged retention of dye; drusen in late phase
- Autofluorescence
  - Optic nerve head drusen, astrocytic hamartoma

Hypofluorescence

- Blockage (masking) retinal fluorescence
  - Vitreous + preretinal lesions e.g. blood
  - Deep retinal lesions – haemorrhage + hard exudates
- Blockage of choroidal fluorescence
  - Subretinal or sub-RPE lesions e.g. blood
  - RPE clumping, hypertrophy
  - Choroidal lesions e.g. naevi
- Filling defects
  - Vascular occlusion e.g. vein/artery occlusions
  - Loss of vascular bed e.g. choroideraemia

Some characteristics

- Window defect → early hyperfluorescence – stays same size
- Sub-RPE leak → later hyperfluorescence, increases in intensity, well demarcated, e.g. occult CNV
- Subsensory leak → late hyperfluorescence, increase in size, fuzzy borders
- CNV → early lacy hyperfluorescence, late leakage; early hot spot

Indocyanine green angiography

- For choroidal circulation study
- Can theoretically fluoresce through pigment and haemorrhage, increasing possibility of detecting abnormalities such as CNV
- 98% protein bound, therefore, does not leak out of choriocapillaris vessels (cf fluorescein 70–85%)
- Excitation peak 805 nm
- Infra-red light is absorbed and emitted by the dye
- Late photographs yield most information because dye remains in neovascular tissue after dye has left the retinal circulation
- Contraindicated in iodine allergy
- Side effects (less common than fluorescein omgrogram): Staining of stool, nausea and vomiting, pruritis, sneezing, syncope, skin eruptions

Normal angiogram

- Early phase (2–60 secs)
  - Disc hypofluorescence
  - Poor perfusion of watershed zone
  - Choroidal artery filling, early choroidal vein filling
  - Visible retinal arteries, not veins
- Early midphase (1–3 mins)
  - Watershed zone filling
  - Choroidal artery fading, veins more prominent
  - Retinal veins and arteries visible
- Late mid phase (3–15mins)
  - Fading choroidal vessels
  - Diffusion of dye from choriocapillaris → diffuse hyperfluorescence
  - Retinal vessels still visible
- Late phase (15–30 mins)
  - Hypofluorescence of choroidal vasculature against a background

8

of hyperfluorescence resulting from staining of extrachoroidal tissue
  - Retinal vessels not visible
  - dye may remain in neovascular tissue

Abnormal fluorescence

- Hyperfluorescence
  - RPE window defect
  - Leakage – retinal or choroidal circulations or disc
  - Abnormal blood vessels
- Hypofluorescence
  - Blockage – pigment, blood, exudates
  - Obstructed circulation
  - Loss of vascular tissue
  - RPE detachment (hyper on fluorescein omgiogram)

Optical coherence tomography

- Imaging modality producing micron resolution cross-sectional images of ocular tissue
- Analogous to B-scan but uses optical waves
- OCT III – 8–10 μm resolution
- Newer experimental models – 2–3 μm
- Brighter colours (red/white) → dense with high reflectivity e.g. RPE
- Darker colours (blue/black) → less dense structures e.g. vitreous, sub renmal fluid
- Uses
  - Differentiating pseudo and macular holes
  - Vitreomacular traction syndrome
  - Monitoring course of central serous chrioretinopathy
  - Evaluating sub renmal fluid
  - Topographical macular thickness map e.g. for monitoring macular oedema
  - Nerve fibre layer around disc in glaucoma

Electrodiagnostics

- Tests are based on a mass response from the entire retina by a flash of light (single or repeating)
- Provides information on the retina and visual pathway
- Electroretinogram (ERG) is the most commonly used test

Electroretinogram

- Is measured using a Ganzfeld dome stimulus, a contact lens electrode and a neutral electrode on the cheek
- Affected by stimulus intensity, pupil size, area of retina stimulated, high myopia, advanced age and newborns

Physiology of ERG waves

- A-wave – negative wave due to photoreceptor hyperpolarisation
- B-wave – positive wave due to Muller and bipolar cells absorbing K released by the photoreceptors
- C-wave – positive wave due to hyperpolarization of RPE cells, due to decreased extracellular potassium between RPE and photoreceptors
- Oscillatory potentials – ? generated by inhibitory feedback circuits
- Early receptor potential(ERP) – biphasic wave, due to changes in spatial orientation of photopigment molecule, as it changes from cis > trans in rod and cone outer segments (cone > rod)

Recordings

- Scotopic ERG – (rod response) dark adapt the eye for 20 mina, then stimulate with a dim blue light; virtually no a-wave, but prominent b-wave
- Photopic ERG – (cone response, contribute 20–25% to total ERG) no dark adaptation, use bright light flicker stimulus at a rate of 25–30 Hz, or red flash stimuli (cone response first followed by rod response)
- Maximal combined response – bright flash in a dark-adapted eye

- Macula/foveal ERG – (foveal cones contribute less than 2% to total ERG) suppress rods and stimulate cones
- Bright flash ERG – used for judging retinal function with opaque media
- Pattern ERG – using checkerboard stimuli, correlates with the integrity of the optic nerve

Applications

General

- Damage to parts of the retina leads to decreased amplitude, but normal wave form
- Diffuse disease leads to decreased amplitude, change in waveform and delayed response
- ERGs are useful for diagnosing and following retinal dystrophies and degenerations, as well as disorders of dark adaptation, colour vision, VA, hysteria and malingering
- Not a direct test for macular function

Specific

- A-wave indicates outer neuroretinal status
- B-wave indicates inner neuroretinal status, but a-wave necessary for b-wave
- Decreased a and b-wave in retinals pigmentosa, CRAO, chorioretinitis, metallosis, retinal detachment and drugs
- Normal a, and decreased b-wave in congenital stationary night blindness, juvenile retinoschisis, optic atrophy, CRAO and retinal ischaemia
- Decreased cone ERG and rod ERG in Rod monochromatism and progressive cone dystrophy
- C-wave is of no clinical use (? RPE)
- Oscillatory potential is reduced in ischaemic states and congenital stationary night blindness
- ERP is of no clinical use

The electro-oculogram

Physiological basis

- 'Standing potential' between positive cornea and negative back of the eye
- Standing potential increases with the light and decreases in the dark
- Reflects activity of RPE + photoreceptors

Measurement and method

- Uses skin electrodes on inner and outer canthi
- Constant light stimuli to a dark-adapted eye
- Patient looks from side to side and voltage between electrodes is recorded
- Recorded as the Arden ratio (light dark ratio) = highest potential in light/lowest in dark. < 1.85 is abnormal; < 1.3 is severely abnormal

Clinical applications

- Dominated by rod system
- Depends on the integrity of the photoreceptor, RPE and inner retinal integrity
- Abnormal in (RPE disorders) Best's disease, chloroquine retinopathy, rubella retinopathy; may be normal in pattern dystrophy
- Increased in albinism and aniridia

Visually-evoked potentials

Physiological basis

- Electrical signal in occipital cortex following light or checkerboard stimulus
- Most of cortex represents macula, therefore, primary test of macular function, especially foveal cones
- Reflects abnormality of entire pathway

Measurement and method

- EEG electrodes on occiput and mastoids
- Single flash or checkerboard stimulation
- Polyphasic graph with 2 positive and 2 negative peaks

- The important features are
  - Latency
  - Contrast threshold
  - Slope

Clinical applications

- Measurement of visual acuity in children and non-verbal patients
- Detection of malingerers
- Optic nerve lesions: Demylinating disease (delayed conductance), compressive lesions (abnormal wave form), unexplained loss of vision

Electrically-evoked potential

- Electrical stimuli to retina perceived as light in cortex
- Method – 0.5 mA signal to retina > EEP measured
- Uses – Retina and visual pathway integrity; and evaluation of eyes with haemorrhage, opaque media, when bright flash ERG is unrecordable

8

Trauma

- Blunt
- Penetrating
- Perforating
- Intraocular foreign body

Traumatic retinal breaks

- Open or closed ocular trauma
- Blunt trauma – caused by coup or contracoup injury → eye deforms → traction on vitreous base
- Contusion injury → large equatorial breaks, dialysis, macular hole → inferotemporal (poor orbit protection here) + superonasal (because of the contracoup injury)
- Dialyses – small or large; usually posterior border of vitreous base, may be anterior border
- Less commonly – horseshoe tears, operculated holes
- Young eyes – rarely develop acute detachments because vitreous not synergetic
- May develop later, when gel liquefies
- Detachments may be shallow and show signs of chronicity (demarcation lines, subretinal deposits, intraretinal cysts)

Vitreous haemorrhage

- Due to damage of the vessels of the iris, ciliary body, retina, choroid, retinal tears
- Do B-scan
- Bed rest with head elevation may give enough posterior view when haemorrhage settles
- Observe with repeat ultrasound

Blunt trauma

- Posterior vitreous detachment – may be associated with vitreous haemorrhage
- Commotio retinae
  - Concussion of the sensory retina
  - Cloudy swelling, mostly temporally
  - Cherry red spot
  - May have subretinal haemorrhage
  - Most resolve without complication in 6 weeks
  - May lead to pigmentary degeneration, macular hole
  - Berlin oedema – commotio of the posterior pole
- Choroidal rupture
  - Direct – anteriorly, at site of impact; parallel to ora serata
  - Indirect – opposite site of impact, white crescent-shaped streak of underlying sclera, often involving macula, concentric to disc
  - Bruch's membrane not very elastic → may tear along with RPE + choriocapillaris
  - May be complicated by CNV
- Retinal breaks – see above
- Retinitis sclopetaria – shock waves generated by high-speed missile → damaging retina
- Scleral rupture
  - Limbus and muscle insertions (thin sclera) especially

  - Boggy chemosis, deep AC, decreased ductions, severe vitreous haemorrhage, usually reduced IOP
- Macular hole – by contusion necrosis or vitreous traction

Penetrating injury

- Extent of damage determined by kinetic energy
- Introduction of micro-organisms often more important than the trauma
- Tractional detachment – secondary to vitreous incarceration in the wound + intragel haemorrhage; fibroblastic proliferation → contraction → tractional retinal detachment

Intraocular foreign bodies

- Mechanical damage
- Infective damage
- Toxicity
- Siderosis
  - Intraocular ferrous foreign body
  - Undergoes dissociation, deposits of iron → retina + lens epithelium
  - Anterior capsular cataract, iris staining reddish-brown, glaucoma, pigmentary retinopathy
  - ERG → progressive attenuation of b-wave
- Chalcosis
  - FB with copper content
  - Endophthalmitis-like picture with progression to phthisis
  - Less retinotoxic than iron, vision may be preserved
- CT scan (not MRI!)
- B-scan
- Prophylactic intravitreal antibiotics

Signs and symptoms of siderosis	
Symptoms	Nyctalopia
	Concentrically constricted visual field
	Decreased vision
Signs	Rust-coloured corneal stromal staining
	Iris heterochromia
	Pupil mydriasis + poor reactivity
	Brown deposits on the anterior lens
	Cataract
	Vitreous opacities
	Peripheral retinal pigmentation – early
	Diffuse retinal pigmentation – late
	Narrowed retinal vessels
	Optic disc discolouration + atrophy
	Secondary OAG from iron in trabecular meshwork

9

The orbit

Anophthalmos 260
Craniosynostoses 260
Cystic lesions of the orbit 261
Dysthyroid eye disease 262
Idiopathic orbital inflammatory disease 265
Lacrimal gland tumours and inflammations 267
Orbital lymphoma 269
Orbital infections 269
Orbitotomy 271
Other orbital tumours 272
Causes of proptosis 274
Orbital radiology 275
Rhabdomyosarcoma 276
Orbital trauma 276
Vascular lesions of the orbit 279

Anophthalmos

- A spectrum of disease with varying degrees of microphthalmos
- True anophthalmos is very rare – complete absence of ocular structures

9

Genetics

- PAX 2 – optic stalk
- PAX 6 – optic vesicle
- Many environmental factors acting on these genes

Management

- Paediatric workup
- Neuroimaging
- TORCH screen
- Chromosomal studies
- Ultrasound
- Electrodiagnostics
- Socket expansion

Socket expanders

- Hydrophilic expansion – dehydrated soft contact lens material
- Balloon expanders
- New generation of hydrophilic expanders
- Dermis fat grafts for use in the first 3 years of life
- Removeable orbital prostheses – progressively enlarging
- Enucleation is usually not necessary

Craniosynostoses

- Premature closure of skull sutures
- Shallow orbit → proptosis and exotropia
- Papilloedema and optic atrophy
- Include
  - Crouzon syndrome
  - Apert syndrome

Crouzon syndrome

- Premature closure of coronal and sagittal sutures
- Autosomal dominant, 25% sporadic mutations
- Shallow orbits due to arrested growth of maxilla and zygoma
- Results in proptosis and hypertelorism
- Associated exotropia
- May be complicated by exposure keratopathy and optic atrophy

Apert syndrome

- Most severe of the craniostenoses

- Premature closure of all sutures
- Autosomal dominant, most are sporadic
- Shallow orbits are less pronounced

Cystic lesions of the orbit

Causes of cystic lesions of the orbit

Cysts of the surface epithelium

- Epithelial cysts
- Dermoid cysts

Teratomatous cysts

Cysts of neural tissue

- Associated with ocular maldevelopment
  - Anophthalmia with cyst
  - Colobomatous cyst
- Associcated with brain tissue
  - Encephalocoele + ectopic brain tissue
  - Orbital optic nerve meningocoele

Secondary cyst from adjacent structures

- Mucocoele
- Dentigerous cyst

Parasitic cyst

Non-cystic lesions with a cystic component

- Adenocystic ca lacrimal gland
- Rhabdomyosarcoma
- Lymphangioma
- Optic nerve glioma

Dacryops

- Ductal cyst of the lacrimal gland
- Round conjunctival cystic lesion in superior lateral fornix
- Treat by aspiration

Dermoid and epidermoid cysts

- Amongst the most common orbital tumours of childhood
- Progressively enlarge
- Anterior ones present early
- Deeper ones may not present until adulthood
- Benign cystic teratoma (choristoma – growth of normal tissue in an abnormal site)
- May be superficial (anterior to orbital septum, usually in superotemporal orbit) or deep (posterior to orbital septum)
- From sequestration of surface epithelium
- Histology → epidermal lining, keratin and cholesterol crystals, sebaceous glands, hair follicles, sweat glands
- May attach to bone or to dura
- Medial lesions should be distinguished from congenital encephalocoeles
- Rupture → granulomatous inflammation

Mucocoele

Aetiology

- Obstructed sinus drainage, due to chronic sinusitis, trauma, fracture, osteoma, polyp
- Important: may lead to mucocoele cystic fibrosis in children

Pathology

- Enlarging cyst lined with respiratory mucosa
- Usually frontal or ethmoidal → proptosis
- Rarely sphenoidal → optic nerve, chiasm, pituitary compression
- May develop pyocoele

Special investigations

- X-ray → cystic mass

Treatment

- Exenteration of involved sinus with establishment of drainage

Encephalocoele

- Herniation of intracranial contents through a congenital defect of the base of the skull
- Orbital encephalocoele may be anterior (fronto ethmoid), or posterior (sphenoid)

9

Dysthyroid eye disease

Definition

- Component of Graves disease – may occur independently (? 2 distinct immune mediated disorders)
- Graves' disease is a triad of hyperthyroidism, infiltrative ophthalmopathy, dermopathy
- Most common cause of proptosis
- 50% of Graves have clinical myopathy
- 95% of Graves have CT scan myopathy
- 5% of Graves have severe clinical myopathy
- 95% of myopathies have thyroid disease

Epidemiology

- Graves' disease alone female : male = 4 : 1
- Graves' disease with dysthyroid eye disease female : male = 1 : 1
- Most common in third and fourth decades

Aetiology

- Almost certainly has an immune basis
- Increased incidence of other immune disease (5% have myasthenia gravis)
- Genetic basis (HLA BG + HLA BW35)
- ? Precipitated by viral infection, ? precipitated by yersina infection
- Immune complexes of thyroglobulin-thyroglobulin antibody bind to extraocular muscles (EOM) membranes
- But ? hormone, ? antibody, ?autoimmune cell mediated mechanism

Pathology

- Type 5 hypersensitivity reaction
- Genetic basis → T-suppressor cell deficiency → B-cells allowed to differentiate → autoantibody production
- Non-specific inflammation of orbital fat, EOM, and optic nerve; mainly by lymphocytes and plasma cells
- Orbital fibroblast is the primary target in the inflammatory attack
- May be distinguished from pseudotumour by mainly perivascular early on + lymphoid follicles less frequent
- Fibroblasts secrete mucopolysaccharides, collagen and glycoprotein → increased orbital volume
- Late fibroblast → collagen replacement of tissues

> **Classification of dysthyroid eye disease**
>
> **Classification 1 – NOSPECS**
> - 0: **N**o signs or symptoms (50% of patients with hyperthyroidism)
> - 1: **O**nly signs, no symptoms (lid retraction, lid lag, stare)
> - 2: **S**oft tissue involvement/**S**ymptoms and signs
> - 3: **P**roptosis
> - 4: **E**OM involvement
> - 5: **C**orneal involvement
> - 6: Optic nerve involvement (**S**ight loss)
>
> **Classification 2 – Grading of active/wet dysthyroid eye disease**
> - Mild – chemosis
> - Moderate – proptosis
> - Marked – diplopia
> - Severe – compressive optic neuropathy

Clinical features
- Upper lid retraction (Dalrymple's sign)
  - ? Due to sympathetic tone, levator infiltration, adhesion of muscle to fixed orbital tissues, inferior rectus restriction
  - Causes of lid retraction
  - Lid lag (Von Graefe's sign) – probably due to adhesions
  - Anisocoria – ? due to increased sympathetic tone
  - Dysthyroid eye disease, irritative sympathetic lesion, dorsal midbrain syndrome, aberrant third nerve regeneration, contralateral ptosis, hypokalemic periodic paralysis, cirrhosis of the liver, systemic steroids
- Proptosis – exophthalmometer reading > 20 or difference >3 mm
- Symptoms – burning, grittiness, tearing, lid swelling, conjunctival injection, chemosis
- EOM involvement – IR 60%, MR 30%, SR 10%
- Injection over EOM insertions, fibrotic contracture of muscle, IOP increase > 4 mmHg on attempted movement, forced duction test positive
- Corneal involvement – unstable tear film occurs in 98%; leads to exposure and drying
- Optic nerve involvement – compression and interference with blood supply; decreased visual acuity, afferent pupil defect, centrocaecal scotoma or inferior arcuate scotoma, decreased colour vision, ± papilloedema and choroidal folds, late optic atrophy
- Pretibial myxoedema is a bad prognostic sign

Differential diagnosis
- Myasthenia gravis
- Pseudotumour
- Lymphoma
- Other orbital tumour

Special investigations
- Thyroid function tests
  - T3/T4 levels
  - T3 suppression
  - TSH stimulation
  - TRH stimulation
- U/S + CT scan → EOM involvement; CT scan muscle volume correlates with the degree of optic neuropathy; if the muscle volume is < 13% of the orbital volume, there is no danger of compressive optic neuropathy; muscle belly is involved in dysthyroid eye disease, cw muscle tendon in myositis
- MRI

9

- Do when there are motility problems
- Do a STIR sequence

Treatment – according to NOSPECS

- Class 0 – no treatment
- Class 1
  - Guanethidine 5% drops (may cause superficial punctate keratopathy)
  - Propanolol 10 mg 6 hourly
- Class 2
  - Tear lubricants, taping of eyelids at bedtime
  - Prednisone 5 mg 6–12 hourly
- Class 3 – temporary tarsorrhaphy
  - weakening of Muller's muscle
  - levator recession
- Class 4
  - Botulinum; within 1 month of EOM involvement, to prevent contractures
  - Prisms for diplopia, prisms for reading (Fresnel)
  - EOM surgery; when stabilised for 6 months – 1 year; recession of involved muscle, ± adjustable sutures
  - IR recession → correction of upper lid retraction
  - Delay adjustment if necessary for 3–4 days
- Class 5 + 6
  - Steroids: 40 mg daily × 2 weeks; stop if no response, tail off if responds
  - Cyclophosphamide if no response, ± cyclosporin A
  - ± Orbit irradiation: If steroids have no effect; if decompression has no effect
  - Orbit decompression: If irradiation has no effect; transantral, transethmoidal, lateral; combined transantral and transethmoidal → 75–80% 'cure rate'

Treatment according to active/wet disease classification

- Mild (chemosis) – lubricants, non-steroidal anti-inflammatories, ± topical anthihistamine, steroid ointment at night
- Moderate (proptosis) – prednisone 15–20 mg daily, ± azathioprine 150 mg daily
- Marked (diplopia) – irradiation 20 Cy, azathioprine 150 mg daily, prednisone 30 mg daily
- Severe (optic nerve compression) – methylprednisone 500 mg IVI 12 hourly × 1–2 days; irradiation 20 Cy, azathioprine 150 mg daily, prednisone 30 mg daily

Prognosis

- Self-limiting, 6 months to 3-year course

Orbitalir radiation/orbital radiotherapy

- Non-specific anti-inflammatory effects on radiosensitive lymphocytes
- Works well but the effect is limited and temporary
- Must be used in conjunction with a long-term anti-inflammatory
- For severe soft tissue signs or optic nerve compression (although proven efficacy in mild + moderate disease as well)
- Response rate ± 60%
- Not useful in inactive disease
- Normal dose: 20 Gy in 10 fractions over 2 weeks
- Low dose 1 Gy over 20 weeks + 10 Gy over 2 weeks may be more effective
- Appears to be a better response with IVI pulsed methylprednisolone, repeated 3 times within 3 weeks of the radiation
- Adverse effects
  - Generally safe
  - Skin irritation + temoral hair loss
  - Conjunctivitis and chemosis
  - Cataract (incidence unknown)
  - Radiation retinopathy (especially in diabetes)
  - Theoretical risk of secondary tumours

Mouritz score

- Inflammatory index for thyroid orbitopathy
- Used to evaluate the patient for soft tissue inflammatory features and to assess the progression of thyroid orbitopathy
- Score > 3 indicates a greater likelihood of active disease
- Best used by assessing changes in the score rather than the absolute value

Mouritz score of thyroid eye disease activity

Soft tissue feature	Rating
Chemosis	0 Absent 1 Mild (to grey line) 2 Moderate (to lid margin) 3 Severe (over lid margin)
Conjunctival injection	0 Absent 1 Present
Lid injection	0 Absent 1 Present
Lid oedema	0 Absent 1 Mild 2 Moderate 3 Severe
Pain at rest (retrobulbar aching)	0 Absent 1 Present
Pain on movement	0 Absent 1 Present
Total possible score	10

Idiopathic orbital inflammatory disease

Definition

- Idiopathic non-specific inflammatory lesion, of variable location and variable histology
- An idiopathic tumorous inflammation made up of pleomorphic inflammatory cellular response and a fibrovascular tissue reaction

Aetiology

- Unknown
- ? Viral, ? secondary to contiguous sinus disease, ? reaction to blood-borne antigen, ? some due to mycoplasma infection
- Systemic evaluation, very rarely, may find SLE, polyarteritis nodosa, dermatomyositis

Classification

- Anterior, posterior, atypical, diffuse, lacrimal, myositic, cavernous sinus (Tolosa-Hunt syndrome)

Clinical features

- Female = male, no racial predilection, most common in middle age
- Adults + children
- Usually unilateral, remitting or chronically progressive – a variable but usually limited course
- Proptosis and pain, fairly rapid in onset

9

- Variable meningeal irritation
- Anterior – chemosis, scleritis, uveitis, exudative retinal detachment, papillitis
- Lacrimal – lacrimal gland swelling (dacryoadenitis)
- Sclerotenonitis
- Trochleitis
- Superior orbital fissure and cavernous sinus
- Posterior – early optic nerve involvement
- Myositis – pain, decreased ocular motility, inferior rectus most commonly involved, diplopia, injection over muscle, haemorrhage – muscle and tendons thickened on CT
- Bilateral pseudotumour in adults suggests a possible vasculitis or a lymphoproliferative disorder
- In children one-third are bilateral and are rarely associated with systemic disorders

Histology

- Two basic types, with spectrum between non-specific chronic inflammatory pseudotumour and reactive lymphocytic hyperplasia
- Non-specific chronic inflammatory pseudotumour
  - Cellular polymorphism (lymphocytes, plasma cells, epithelioid cells, macrophages, giant cells, fibroblasts, eosinophils)
  - Variable histology – lymphoid follicles with germinal centres, variable amount of collagen, plasma cells containing intracytoplasmic Russell bodies and intranuclear Dutcher bodies (precipitated antigen), non-caseating granulomas, 'vasculitis' (inflammatory reaction around blood vessels, a feature of dysthyroid eye disease), myositis, dacryoadenitis, sclerosing lipogranulomas
- Reactive lymphocytic hyperplasia
  - May actually be an early form of lymphoma or may lead to lymphoma
  - Cellular monomorphism, sheets of uniform mature lymphocytes

Special investigations

- X-ray – no bone involvement
- Ultrasound – irregular poor transmission, variable in location and extent
- CT scan – indicates location and extent of pseudotumour; differentiates from lymphoma, where the lesion is more homogeneous
- ESR – minimally elevated
- CSF – elevated protein + mild pleocytosis
- Visual field – variable deficit

9

Management of orbital pseudotumour

■ Biopsy	□ Surgery may exacerbate inflammation, therefore avoid at first
	□ Make the diagnosis on non-invasive U/S and CT scan
	□ Needle biopsy if chronic and recurrent
■ Steroids	□ Oral prednisone 40–60 mg daily for 2 weeks, then decrease; taper over several months
	□ Rapid response is 'pathognomonic' and is seen in 50 % of cases; but some lymphomas also respond to steroids
	□ Intralesional triamcinolone
■ Radiotherapy	□ External beam irradiation (2 500 rads or 25 Gy)

	◻ If steroids contraindicated or if there is an inadequate response to steroids ◻ Response seen in 85% cases
■ Cytotoxics	◻ Chlorambucil, cyclophosphamide, or cyclosporin; if there is inadequate response to steroids and radiotherapy
■ Rifampicin	◻ Empiric treatment if TB a possibility

Lacrimal gland tumours and inflammations

Classification of lacrimal gland enlargement

- 50% inflammatory or lymphomatous
- 50% epithelial tumours
  - 50% lymphoproliferative
  - 50% neoplasms
  - 50% benign mixed
  - 50% malignant

Epithelial tumours

- Benign
  - benign pleomorphic adenoma (benign mixed)
- Malignant
  - Adenocystic carcinoma 60%
  - Malignant pleomorphic carcinoma 20%
  - Mucoepidermoid carcinoma 20%
  - Undifferentiated carcinoma

Clinical presentation

- Mass in upper temporal lid
- Variable tearing and pain, pressure on globe, limitation of movement, proptosis

Benign mixed tumours (pleomorphic adenoma)

- Most common tumour
- Macroscopic
  - Usually smooth, may be nodular
  - Nodule formation is a feature of recurrence
  - May be precipitated by aspiration or needle biopsy
  - Capsule is formed by condensation of surrounding tissues (pseudocapsule)
  - Firm, soft or cystic in consistency
- Microscopic
  - Epithelial derived tissues (ducts, acini, cords, squamous pearls, sheets of cells)
  - Also chondroid, myxofibroma and bone (also originating from epithelium)
  - Micro extensions of tumour into the pseudocapsule cause tumour recurrence unless an adequate margin of normal surrounding tissue is taken

Clinically

- Adults – fourth to fifth decade
- Slow growing, malignant change may occur after years (history > 1 year = benign mixed tumour, not carcinoma)

9

- Progressive, painless downwards + inwards displacement of the globe with axial proptosis
- CT scan: Well-circumscribed with a slightly nodular configuration

Adenocyctic carcinoma

- Highly malignant
- Macroscopic – no capsule, infiltrative
- Microscopic – histology variable; primarily epithelial with sheets of cells, ± invades nerves, blood vessels, bone; later lids and brain

Clinically

- Rapid growth, painful due to perineural invasion + bone destruction
- Rapid course < 1 year locally invasive, lymph node metastases uncommon
- Invades nerves, therefore painful
- Perineural extension often occurs – intracranial or systemic metastases usually occur within 1 decade of presentation

Special investigation

- X-ray – hyperostosis = bone invasion, erosion = bone invasion, expansion = compression
- CT scan
  - Tumours → isolated globular mass, displacing + indenting the globe
  - Inflammation + lymphoproliferative → diffuse enlargement, contours around the globe

Management

- Aspiration + needle biopsies are contraindicated
- Treatment is entirely surgical; complete extirpation is necessary for cure
- Radiotherapy may be used only pre-op to prevent dissemination or for inoperable or recurrent tumours; some tumours are radioresponsive, none are radiocurable
- Surgical exposure of tumour; if encapsulated, complete excision + orbitotomy; if invasive, excision biopsy → exenteration

Prognosis

- Worse prognosis than salivary gland tumours
- Mortality is from local recurrence and intracranial spread
- Benign mixed
  - 30% recurrence after 30 years
  - 0.5% mortality from recurrence and malignant change
- Adenocystic carcinoma – 70% 15 year mortality

Lacrimal gland inflammations

Infections/dacryoadenitis

- Viral – mumps, cytomegalo inclusion, coxsackie A, echo, zoster, infectious mononucleosis
- Bacterial (with pre-auricular adenopathy) – staph, strep, gonococcus, trachoma, tuberculosis, leprosy, syphilis
- Fungal – blastomycosis, histoplasmosis, actinomycosis, nocardiosis

Non-infectious chronic inflammation

- Radiation
- Ectopic tissue → build up of secretions and eruption → chronic inflammatory response
- Sarcoidosis – lacrimal gland involved in 7%
- Sjögren's syndrome → keratoconjunctivitis sicca due to also accessory lacrimal gland involvement
- Mikulicz's disease – infiltration of lacrimal gland by lymphocytes, no associated systemic disease, asymptomatic, often unilateral, common in middle-aged females

Lacrimal gland lymphoma

- Pseudotumour
- Lymphoma

Sialadenosis of the lacrimal gland

- Malnutrition
- Diabetes
- Alcoholism

Orbital lymphoma

Incidence

- Primary orbital lymphoma is very rare; ? may arise from pseudotumour
- Systemic lymphoma
  - Orbit involvement in 1% of cases (classified as extranodal)
  - Conjunctival involvement in 2% of cases (classified as nodal)
- Usually non-Hodgkin's; Hodgkin's documented but rare
- Never involves the globe
- Often bilateral if it occurs in the orbit

Histology: Rappaport classification

- Hodgkins (T-cells)
  - Lymphocytic predominant
  - Mixed
  - Nodular sclerosing
  - Lymphocytic depleted
- Non-Hodgkin's (B-cells)
  - Lymphocytic lymphoma, well differentiated
  - Lymphocytic lymphoma, poorly differentiated (most common orbital lymphoma)
  - Mixed lymphoma
  - Histiocytic lymphoma
  - Undifferentiated lymphoma

Treatment

- Radiotherapy
- Some evidence to suggest that treatment of low-grade lymphomas with chemotherapy may contribute to the development of a more aggressive tumour

Other haemopoetic tumours of the orbit

- Burkitt's lymphoma – starts in maxilla, may spread to orbit
- Multiple myeloma
- Histiocytosis → exophthalmos, diabetes insipidus, bone lesions
- Juvenile xanthogranoloma → iris, skin, + orbit tumours
- Acute leukaemia – involves eye in 75% of cases
- Chloroma – deposits of blast cells in myeloblastic leukaemia; green due to myeloperoxidase
- Lethal midline granuloma – encompasses lymphoma, atypical lymphoma, Wegener's granulomatosis, syphilis and fungal infection

Orbital infections

Bacterial orbital cellulitis and orbital abscess

Bacteriology

- Staph aureus, Staph epidermidis, Streptococcus, Escherichia coli
- Haemophilus influenzae in children under 3 years

Pathogenesis

- Gain access by three routes
  - Implantation with foreign bodies
  - Systemic circulation in a bacteraemia
  - Direct spread from adjacent structures (sinuses, teeth, lacrimal sac, lids)
- 80% result from paranasal sinus infection
- Ethmoid sinus is most commonly affected in the first decade, later frontal sinus
- Spread via lamina papyracea or blood vessels

Classification

- Preseptal cellulitis
- Orbital cellulitis
- Subperiosteal cellulitis/abscess
- Orbital cellulitis
- Cavernous sinus thrombosis

9

Clinical features

- Of acute inflammation-tumour, rubor, colour, dolor, functio laesa

Diagnosis

- X-ray → air fluid level in sinus + air in orbit
- Ultrasound → demonstration of anterior orbit abscess
- CT scan → demonstration of intraorbital abscess, sinusitis, intracranial involvement

Treatment

- Broad spectrum IVI antibiotics (penicillin, chloramphenicol, metronidazole)
- Nasal decongestant
- Incision and drainage if indicated
- Heparin and steroids if there is a cavernous sinus thrombosis

Complications

- Osteomyelitis, meningitis, brain abscess, blindness
- In pre-antibiotic era – 25% blind + 25% mortality

Pointers for diagnosing cavernous sinus thrombosis

- III, IV, V, VI palsies
- May be bilateral
- Systemically sicker
- CSF evidence of meningitis
- Papilloedema
- Paresis in other eye
- Evidence of hypopituitarism

Fungal infections of the orbit

Mucormycosis

- In diabetic and immunosuppressed patients
- Spread from paranasal sinuses
- Invades blood vessels
- Treat with amphotericin + surgical excision
- Poor prognosis

Aspergillosis

- In healthy persons
- Spread from the sinuses
- Chronic, low grade, slow

Other

- Penicillium, histoplasma, blastomycosis, sporotrichosis

Parasitic infections of the orbit

Hydatid cyst

- Echinococcus (sheep tape worm)
- 1% of cysts occur in the orbit
- Rupture of cyst can cause progressive inflammation and a severe immune response
- Slow growing, x-ray shows calcification, eosinophilia in 25%

Cysticercosis

- Taenia solium – pork tape worm
- May occur in the eye or in the orbit

Other

- Microfilaria, ascaris, shistosoma, amoebiasis

Orbitotomy

Orbitotomy approaches	
■ Transeptal	□ Through skin crease + septum; above, below, medial, lateral □ To get to an anterior orbital lesion
■ Transconjunctival	□ Above, below, medial, lateral □ To get to an anterior orbital lesion □ Can get to a more posterior lesion by massaging the eye and taking off the medial rectus
■ Extraperiosteal	□ To get further posteriorly, without damaging intraorbital structures □ Skin incision 5 mm outside orbital margin, down to and through periosteum, strip periosteum back from the bone □ Useful to drain ethmoid sinus
■ Lateral orbitotomy	□ Curved s-shaped incision down to zygoma, drill holes for wires, cut through with a Stryker saw, flap the bone back, +/− remove lateral rectus □ To get to a posterior lesion
■ Transfrontal (neurosurgical)	
■ Transantral (maxillary sinus – Caldwell-Luc)	

Anterior orbitotomy

- Superior approach
  - Most lesions are in the anterior and superior orbit
  - Transcutaneous – upper lid crease; coronal scalp flap – avoids visible facial scars
  - Transconjunctival
  - Vertical eyelid splitting – at the junction of the medial and central thirds
- Inferior approach
  - Visible or palpable masses inferiorly; deep, inferior extraconal masses
  - Transcutaneous – infraciliary blepharoplasty incision; dissection below orbicularis to expose the orbital septum + orbital rim; don't cut skin perpendicular to normal horizontal skin lines → disruption of lymphatics
  - Transconjunctival – has largely replaced transcutaneous for tumours + fractures; may combine with a lateral canthotomy for exposure
- Medial approach
  - Transcutaneous – fronto-ethmoid (Lynch) medial orbitotomy
  - Transconjunctival – detach medial rectus to expose central surgical space – especially access to anterior optic nerve
  - Transcaruncular – better cosmetically than Lynch; repair of medial wall fractures, medial orbital decompression, abscess drainage

Lateral orbitotomy

- Tumours within muscle cone; in lacrimal gland fossa; behind equator of globe
- Several skin incisions possible
  - S-shaped incision extending from eyebrow along zygomatic arch
  - Lateral canthotomy + skin incision 3–4 cm (Berke)

9

- Expose the orbital rim + anterior portion of the zygomatic arch
- Bone saw to remove the bony rim, exposing periorbita
- Retraction of LR
- Drain often placed before closure
- Post-op steroids for swelling

Orbital decompression

- Thyroid eye disease primary indication → reduce optic nerve pressure; decrease expophthalmos
- Removal of the medial wall and much of the floor → expansion into ethmoid + maxillary sinuses
- Approaches
  - Through maxillary sinuses (Caldwell-Luc)
  - Transcutaneous anterior orbitotomy
  - Transconjunctival with lateral cantholysis
  - Transnasal endoscopic to medial wall
- Roof approach not advisable

Complications of orbital surgery

- Decrease/loss of vision – excessive traction on ON, contusion, haemorrhage
- Orbital haemorrhage
- Downward displacement of the globe
- Motility disorders in one-third
- EOM damage
- Ptosis
- Neuroparalytic keratopathy
- Pupillary changes
- Vitreous haemorrhage
- Detached retina
- Hypoaesthesia of the forehead
- Keratitis sicca
- CSF leak
- Infection

Other orbital tumours

Optic nerve glioma

Incidence

- Uncommon
- Mostly children, first decade
- 25–50% will have neurofibromatosis

Clinical

- Gradual, painless, unilateral axial proptosis, ? actually a benign hamartoma
- Loss of vision, APD – chronic optic nerve dysfunction
- Optic atrophy, papilloedema, strabismus
- Rarely optociliary shunt vessels
- Hypothalamic + pituitary hypofunction, raised intracranial pressure
- (May resemble optic neuritis in adults → rapid blindness + death

Diagnosis

- CT, MRI – fusiform enlargement of the optic nerve

Pathology

- May infiltrate optic nerve or be confined to the subarachnoid space

Histology

- A juvenile pilocytic astrocytoma
- Paucity of atypia, mitoses or tumour necrosis – appears benign

Treatment

- Controversial – individualise treatment
- Observation – slow growing, good vision, confined to orbit
- Surgery – rapidly growing tumours or extending beyond orbit, cosmetically unacceptable, etc., intracranial approach
- Radiation – tumour cannot be resected + symptoms progress
- Chemotherapy – actinomycin D + vincristine

Predictors of clinical course

- Benign course: Mild proptosis, disc pallor, neurofibromatosis
- Aggressive course: Moderate to severe proptosis, disc swelling, no neurofibromatosis

Meningiomas

- Invasive tumour arising from arachnoid villi
- Originate intracranially with secondary orbital invasion
- Sphenoid wing meningiomas → temporal fossa mass + proptosis
- Meningiomas arising near the sella + optic nerves → visual field defects + papilloedema
- CT: Localised bone thickening (hyperostosis) + tumours calcifications
- Intracranial spread + death within a few months inevitable
- No role for radiation
- Use of hormonal treatment

Optic nerve sheath meningioma

- < 1% of meningiomas, 3–4% of orbital tumours
- Age: 30–50, female : male = 3 : 1
- Arise from the arachnoid of the optic nerve sheath

Histology

- Presence of whorls + psammoma bodies
- Affect vision early – present with unilateral or bilateral visual loss
- Classic triad: Optociliary shunts, disc pallor + visual loss
- Also: Lid oedema, chemosis, choroidal folds, motility disorder
- CT
  - Tumour has a radiolucent centre (glioma → dense centre)
  - Fusiform enlargement of the optic nerve
  - Circumferential calcification that looks like railroad tracks
- In children → aggressive, potentially lethal
- Adults → aggressive
- Only rarely extend intracranially in contrast to meningiomas which begin intracranially and are very aggressive

Clinical

- Normal disc or oedema + atrophy
- ± Proptosis, ophthalmoplegia, chemosis, venous stasis retinopathy

Treatment

- Surgical manipulation of optic nerve sheath → blindness
- Therefore, surgical resection only if intracranial spread threatened (transcranial orbitotomy)
- Radiation

Schwannoma (neurilemmoma)

- Proliferations of Schwann cells that are encapsulated in perineurium
- Characteristic biphasic pattern of solid areas with nuclear palisading (Antoni A pattern) + myxoid areas (Antoni B pattern)
- May undergo malignant transformation
- Well-encapsulated, easily excised

Neurofibroma

- Composed of proliferating Schwann cells within their nerve sheaths
- Axons, endoneural fibroblasts + mucin also seen
- Plexiform neurofibromas – infiltrative tumours usually occurring in neurofibromatosis type 1 → well-vascularised + can seldom be removed surgically

Orbital neuroblastoma

- Abrupt ecchyymotic proptosis, may be bilateral
- May lead to the mistaken impression of injury
- Commonly causes bone destruction of the lateral orbital wall
- These metastases usually occur late in the primary disease
- Congenital neuroblastoma of the cervical ganglia → Horner's syndrome with heretochromia

Leukaemia

- May produce unilateral or bilateral proptosis
- Most common form involving the orbit is lymphoblastic leukaemia
- Granulocytic sarcoma (chloroma)
- Typically presents several months before bone marrow or blood signs

Adult metastatic tumours

- Any internal organ carcinoma + cutaneous malignant melanoma
- Mostly breast + lung
- In 75% there is a known primary; in 25% the orbital metostases is the presenting sign
- Treatment usually palliative radiation
- Some warrant excision e.g. renal cell carcinoma

Orbital invasion by sinus tumours

Causes of proptosis

Common causes of paediatric proptosis

- Congenital
  - Craniostenosis
  - Dermoid and epidermoid
- Traumatic – haemorrhage
- Inflammatory – orbital cellulitis (usually secondary to ethmoiditis)
- Neoplastic – benign
  - Capillary haemangioma
  - Lymphangioma
- Neoplastic – malignant
  - Rhabdomyosarcoma
  - Optic nerve glioma
  - Secondary/metastatic – neuroblastoma (zygomatic bone); chloroma/leukaemia
- Metabolic – dysthyroid eye disease

Less common causes of paediatric proptosis

- Meningocoele
- Encephalocoele
- Cavernous sinus thrombosis
- Histiocytosis
- Mesenchymal tumours
- Teratoma
- Neurofibroma
- Ewing's sarcoma
- Retinoblastoma

Common causes of adult proptosis

- Congenital
- Traumatic
  - Haematoma
  - Carotid cavernous fistula
- Inflammatory
  - Orbital cellulitis
  - Mucocoele
- Neoplastic
  - Benign – cavernous haemangioma; pseudotumour; benign lacrimal gland tumour
  - Malignant – lymphoma; malignant lacrimal gland tumours; meningioma
  - Metastases – carcinoma bronchus; carcinoma breast; carcinoma kidney
  - Secondaries – nasopharyngeal carcinoma; malignant melanoma of choroid
- Metabolic – dysthyroid eye disease

Less common causes of adult proptosis

- Benign neoplasms
  - Benign peripheral nerve tumours (neurofibroma, schwannoma)
  - Benign mesenchymal tumours
  - Glioma optic nerve
- Malignant neoplasms
  - Malignant peripheral nerve tumours
  - Malignant mesenchymal tumours
- Post-irradiation osteosarcoma
- Squamous cell carcinoma conjunctiva and lids
- Basal cell carcinoma lids
- Sebaceous cell carcinoma lids

- Carcinoma lacrimal sac
- Melanoma conjunctiva
- Carcinoma sinus
- Sinus sarcoma
- Meningioma

Histiocytosis

- Also known as Langerhans cell histiocystosis
- A collection of disorders of proliferation of dendritic histiocytes (macrophages)
- Represent abnormal immune regulation
- Range of benign, self-limiting to chronic, disseminating and death
- Most frequent orbital presentation → lytic defect of the orbital roof with progressive proptosis
- ± Overlying soft tissue inflammation
- Young children need ongoing follow up for multiorgan involvement; less likely to develop in children > 2 years

Prognosis

- < Two years – 50% survival; > 2 years – 87% survival

Management

- Confirmatory biopsy
- Debulking
- Intrastromal steroid
- Low dose radiation
- Spontaneous remission may occur

Orbit radiology

X-ray

- Waters position
  - Standard antero-posterior, head extended with chin on table
  - Shows paranasal sinuses as well
- Caldwell views
  - antero-posterior, forehead and nose on table
  - Dense middle ear bone is below orbital floor, therefore, allows full view of orbits
- Base projection
- Optic canal view (Rhese position)
- Lateral view

CT and MRI

- Shows globe, extraocular muscles, optic nerve

Ultrasound

- A, B, M modes

Normal

- Reflections from eye and retrobulbar
- Eye – anterior and posterior corneal surfaces, anterior and posterior lens surfaces, retina, choroid, sclera
- Retrobulbar – anterior orbital fat and posterior muscle–bone region; nerve and muscles blank

Ocular pathology

- Corneal thickness, anterior chamber depth, lens position, vitreous haemorrhage, retinal detachment, proliferative retinopathy, IOFB localisation, choroidal melanoma, choroidal haemangioma, choroidal metastases, retinoblastoma

Orbital pathology

- Tumours – rounded – poor transmission (solid)
  - Meningioma
  - Glioma
  - Neurofibroma
- Tumours – rounded – good transmission (cystic)
  - Mucocoele
  - Dermoid
  - Cavernous haemangioma
- Tumours – irregular – good transmission (angiomatous)
  - Haemangioma
  - Lymphangioma
- Tumours – irregular – poor transmission (infiltrative)
  - Lymphoma
  - Pseudotumour
  - Metastases

Inflammations

- Cellulitis – wider spaced echoes in orbital fat
- Dysthyroid eye disease – enlarged extraocular muscles
- Optic neuritis – doubling of optic nerve outline pseudotumour – variable appearance

Rhabdomyosarcoma

Epidemiology

- Most common primary malignant orbital tumour of childhood
- Male > female
- Experimental evidence for a viral aetiology

Histology

- Arises from undifferentiated pluripotential mesenchymal elements
- Three types – embryonal (most usual orbital type), pleomorphic, alveolar

Clinical features

- Usually presents in first decade
- Highly malignant
- Rapidly evolving proptosis, may mimic orbital cellulitis
- Retrobulbar is the most common site, then superotemoporal
- Metastases → cervical lymph nodes, lungs and bone
- Direct spread → brain

Histology

- Four categories: Embryonal, alveolar, pleomorphic, botryoid
- Embryonal
  - Most common
  - Arises from soft tissues, not muscle
  - Predilection for superotemporal orbit
  - Loose fascicles of undifferentiated spindle cells
- Alveolar
  - Predilection for the inferior orbit
  - Regular compartments of fibrovascular strands
  - Most malignant form
- Pleomorphic
  - Most differentiated, strap-like or rounded cells with cross-striations
  - Best prognosis + rarest
- Botryoid
  - Rare variant of embryonal
  - Grape-like form
  - Only found in the orbit as a secondary invader from paranasal sinuses or conjunctiva

Management

- Radiotherapy
- Adjuvant chemotherapy
- Exenteration, if recurrent, tumour unresponsive to treatment
- Metastatic screen – CXR, bone marrow, CSF

Prognosis

- 90% survival if confined to the orbit
- 65% survival if extended beyond the orbit

9

Orbital trauma

Orbital fractures

Classification of orbital fractures	
■ External (involving rim)	□ Inferolateral □ Inferomedial □ Superior
■ Blowout	□ Floor □ Medial wall

- Orbital apex + optic canal
- Internal
  - Involves just the internal orbital skeleton
- Rim
  - Involves just the rim
- Complex
  - Involves the orbit + other facial bones
- Open or closed

Midfacial fractures

- Involve the maxilla; often complex + asymmetric; extend posteriorly through the pterygoid plates
- Treatment: Dental stabilisation + open reduction
- Le Fort I: Low transverse maxilla – no orbital involvement
- Le Fort II: Pyramidal configuration, involving nasal, lacrimal + maxillary bones, including floor of orbit
- Le Fort III: Entire facial skeleton detached from skull. Orbital floor, medial + lateral orbital walls

Zygomatic fractures

- Usually involves the orbital floor, but may not involve the orbit at all
- Can cause a downward displacement of the lateral canthus
- Treatment: May not be required, or open reduction + internal fixation

Orbital apex fractures

- Usually occur in conjunction with fractures of the rest of the skull
- May involve optic canal, superior orbital fissure
- Damage to optic nerve through ischaemia, bone compression, oedema
- Treatment
  - Steroids
  - Medial wall decompression within 5 days

Orbital roof fractures

- Uncommon
- Blunt trauma or missiles
- Brain + frontal sinuses may be involved

Complications

- CSF rhinorrhoea, pneumocephalus, intracranial injuries, ptosis, EOM imbalance
- Manage with neurosurgeon

Medial orbital wall fractures

- Often have a traumatic telecanthus → transnasal wiring
- Surgery seldom necessary unless the MR is entrapped

Blowout fractures

Mechanisms

- Blunt injury → increased intraorbital pressure (hydraulic theory)
- Trauma to inferior orbital rim → temporary distortion, transmitted to orbital floor (buckling force theory)

Anatomy

- Floor
  - Thinnest posteriorly, weakened by groove
  - Fracture → IR + IO entrapment; III inferior division injury (IO branch most vulnerable)
- Medial wall
  - Thinnest over ethmoid plate (lamina papyracea)
  - Fracture → MR entrapment rarely; disruption of medial canthal tendon; lacrimal sac and duct injury

Clinical presentation

- Diplopia and limitation of movements
  - Due to muscle injury, muscle entrapment, or nerve injury
  - IR and IO limitation results from entrapment or damage

9

- SR limitation results from IR entrapment
- FDT differentiates palsy and entrapment

■ Enophthalmos
- Due to prolapse of fat and tissues, fat necrosis and muscle fibrosis

■ Infraorbital nerve sensory disturbance
- If absent, the fracture may be medial or lateral to groove
- Zygomatic nerve sensory disturbance may occur in lateral fractures

■ Unilateral epistaxis
■ Surgical emphysema, more usually with medial wall fractures
■ Loss of vision, commotio retinae

Special investigations

■ Hess charts, single binocular field
■ X-ray orbits
- Straight – prolapse of orbital contents
- Ultrasound – into maxillary sinus
- Tomography – fragmentation of orbital floor, opacity of sinus, orbital emphysema

■ Forced duction test – IR tendon is grasped and moved
■ CT scan – may be helpful to assess
- Size of fracture = degree of orbital herniation
- Depth of surgical exploration

Management

■ Prophylactic antibiotics only for open fractures, chronic sinusitis, the immunosuppressed
■ Avoid nose blowing → orbital emphysaema
■ Prednisolone used by some
■ Trend towards earlier surgery (within 7–10 days)
■ Intermediate repair probably favourable → 10 days
■ In cases of obvious + clinically significant entrapment → surgery within 48 hours

Very early treatment (within 1–2 hours)

■ Contraindicated, as swelling and haemorrhage can cause limitation and 50% of small fractures recover spontaneously

Early treatment (within 2 weeks)

■ Indications are – enophthalmos > 3 mm, diplopia, obvious fracture with herniation into antrum, incarceration with positive forced duction test
■ Medial wall fracture rarely requires repair
■ Optimum time is 10–14 days, before union occurs
■ May be via Caldwell-Luc approach (canine maxillary) or lower lid approach
■ Tissues freed and integrity of floor restored with silicone graft/silastic plate
■ May be complicated by optic nerve injury, either directly by graft or indirectly by fat traction

Late treatment (after 3–6 months)

■ Contraindicated due to increased complications and poorer results
■ If present late with restricted vertical movements, do the following:
- Orthophoria in the primary position but diplopia in elevation → either nil or recess contralateral SR
- Orthophoria in the primary position but diplopia in depression → contralateral IR Fadens or contralateral SR + IR recession
- Hypophoria in the primary position → ipsilateral IR recession on an adjustable suture, to align in the primary position; wait 6 months, then transpose ipsilateral MR and LR
- Hypertropia in the primary position → ipsilateral SR recession, ipsilateral IR resection, ? contralateral IR recession or transposition down of MR and LR (< 10 D hypertropia, to IR insertion; > 10 D hypertropia, to 3 mm posterior to IR insertion)

9

- The aim of treatment is to achieve binocular single vision in the primary position and in downgaze
- If present late with a medial wall fracture, do the following:
  - Forced duction test positive – ? free up subperiosteal tissue, recess MR, wait 6 months, transpose SR and IR to MR insertion
  - Forced duction test negative – transpose SR and IR to MR insertion; or treat LR with botulinum

Orbital haemorrhage

Aetiology

- Trauma, iatrogenic, associated with neoplasms + vascular malformations, spontaneous

Sites

- Retrobulbar (intraconal), extraconal, subperiosteal, subtenons, subdural (optic nerve sheath)
- Retrobulbar – most common
  - Post-blunt or penetrating trauma
  - Post-retrobulbar anaesthetic

Orbital compartment syndrome

- Pathological compression of orbital structures → globe + optic nerve ischaemia
- Ophthalmic emergency
- Emergency canthotomy + cantholysis – can be left to heal spontaneously or a secondary canthoplasty can be performed after 2–5 days when swelling down

Traumatic optic neuropathy

- Posterior indirect – most common
  - Due to a frontal or midfacial blow (e.g. car accident)
  - Decreased VA, APD, optic canal fracture on CT
  - Treatment controversial: Observe, steroids, optic canal decompression
- Direct
  - Penetration – nerve transection, contusion, compression
  - Remove foreign body in theatre, canthotomy/cantholysis if retrobulbar haemorrhage present, drain subperiosteal blood, optic nerve sheath fenestration for sheath haematoma or oedema
- Anterior indirect
  - Injury at level of lamina cribrosa
  - Sudden rotation or displacement of globe (e.g. by a finger)
  - Vitreous haemorrhage, nerve head avulsion, optic nerve swelling, CRVO
- Chiasmal – severe closed head injuries

Vascular lesions of the orbit

Capillary haemangioma

Clinical features

- High flow hamartoma
- Common tumour of neonates and infants
- Strawberry naevus of skin, may affect lids or orbit
- Grows after birth, involutes after 6 months to 2 years of age, involution complete by 4–7 years of age
- 40% have resolved by age of 4 years, 70% by age of 7 years
- +/– Associated thrombocytopenia (Kassabach-Merritt syndrome) and high output cardiac failure
- No associated ocular malformations
- Ulceration, secondary infection, ptosis → amblyopia may occur

Treatment

- Avoid intervention as long as possible
- Indications for treating – anisometropia, strabismus, amblyopia
- Systemic steroids (rebound growth when discontinued), injection of steroid, injection of sclerosing agent

9

(scarring is a problem), cryotherapy, radiotherapy (cataract, bone growth depression, future malignancy), surgical excision, pulsed dye laser treatment (controversial – may only treat superficial vessels)
- Repository steroid injection is the treatment of choice; ? acts by producing local vasoconstriction with thrombosis, hypoxia and enhanced involution; may be complicated by fat atrophy, lid necrosis, adrenal suppression
- Treat amblyopia

Cavernous haemangioma

Clinical features

- Low flow system
- Most common benign primary orbital tumour
- Tumour of adolescents and young adults; female > male (middle-aged females most common)
- Slowly progressive proptosis, late loss of vision
- Increased growth during pregnancy
- May be intra or extraconal
- Retinal striae, hyperopia, optic nerve compression, glaucoma, strabismus

Diagnosis

- CT, US

Histology

- Encapsulated, large cavernous spaces containing red blood cells, walls contain smooth muscle

Treatment

- Surgical excision if ocular function compromised → usually lateral orbitotomy
- Steroid injection – 60 mg methyl prednisone into lesion + 4 mg dexamethasone sodium phosphate around lesion; repeat 3 times at 6 week intervals

Lymphangioma

- Uncommon

Pathology

- Congenital abnormality of orbital veins
- Occur most commonly in medial and upper half of orbit
- Large, serum-filled spaces lined by endothelium
- No smooth muscle or pericytes in the walls
- Scattered follicles of lymphoid tissue in the interstitium
- Can be found in the conjunctiva, eyelids, orbit, oropharynx, sinuses

Clinical features

- Onset in childhood or early adulthood
- Slowly progressive proptosis; may be intermittent due to hyperplasia of associated lymphoid tissue with upper respiratory tract infection
- Increase in size with valsalva
- Haemorrhage → chocolate cyst
- Variable + unpredictable natural history; some are localised while others diffusely enlarge

Treatment

- Surgical excision not advised (bleeding can become uncontrolled necessitating exenteration)
- Drain choclate cyst ± under CT guidance

Venous malformations – varices

- Intermittent exophthalmos with increased venous pressure
- ? Left orbit more commonly affected than right orbit
- Secondary glaucoma may occur
- Contrast-enhanced CT or venography ± phleboliths
- Treatment: Usually conservative; surgery if varix threatening vision due to opric nerve or globe damage

Arteriovenous malformations – carotid cavernous fistula

- Intraorbital rare, intracranial more common

- Carotid cavernous fistula may be spontaneous (rupture of aneurysm or atherosclerotic artery) (25%), or secondary to trauma (75%) (high vs low flow)
- Proptosis, engorged conjunctival veins, pulsation, bruit, retinal venous engorgement, stasis retinopathy, glaucoma from increased episcleral venous pressure, rubeosis iridis

Treatment

- By surgical excision of arteriovenous malformations
- Selective embolisation of carotid cavernous fistulae

Orbital vasculitis

- Wegener's granulomatosis
    - Involves orbit in 25% of cases
    - Full-blown disease = sinus mucosa involvement with bone erosion, tracheal bronchial necrotic lesions cavitatory lung lesions and glomerulonephritis
    - Usually from contiguous spread from paranasal sinuses or nasopharynx
    - May be bilateral
    - Classic triad of vasculitis, granulomatous inflammation + tissue necrosis
    - Antineutrophilic cytoplasmic antibody (ANCA) is the serologic test
    - Presents in fifth decade with upper and lower respiratory tract disease and nephritis

Idiopathic midline destructive disease

- Relentless, progressive destructive lesions of the nose, paranasal sinuses, pharynx + palate
- Try to differentiate Wegener's or localised granulomatous vasculitis e.g. syphilis
- Treatment: High dose irradiation, prednisone, cyclophosphamide

Thrombophlebitis

- Idiopathic or due to peri-orbital infection + cavernous sinus thrombosis
- Pain, conjunctival injection + varicosities of the eyelids

10

Strabismus

Prevalence classification	282	Syndromes	296
Versions and vergences	283	Miscellaneous strabismus	298
Congenital esotropia	285	Amblyopia	298
Accomodative esotropia	287	Monofixation syndrome	300
Other esotropias	288	Motor adaptations (abnormal postures)	301
Exotropia	290	Sensory adaptations	301
Vertical deviations	292	Surgery	303
Obliques	293	Surgical complications	305
Paralytic and restrictive strabismus	295	Botulinum toxin (Botox)	306

Prevalence classification

Prevalence of strabismus

- Only 2% of people have totally balanced eyes; majority have phorias
- Prevalence of strabismus
  - In preschool children – 5%
  - In school children – 4%
- Prevalence of amblyopia in school children is 2%
- 50% of squints occur before 1 year, 80% before 4 years
- Prevalence of strabismus in children with cerebral palsy is 44%

Classification of strabismus

True strabismus

■ Comitant: 99% horizontal	□ 80% eso – 50% infantile; – 50% accommodative □ 20% exo – 90% intermittent; 10% constant
■ Comitant: 1% vertical	
■ Incomitant	□ III, IV, VI nerve palsy □ Dysthyroid eye disease □ Myasthenia gravis □ Post-trauma □ Fibrosis syndromes □ Duane's syndrome □ Möbius syndrome

Pseudostrabismus	
Pseudo eso	Epicanthic folds
Pseudo exo	Hypertelorism
Pseudo hyper	Facial asymmetry
Angle kappa	Angle between visual axis and pupillary axis i.e. patient appears to have a strabismus because the pupils are not aligned, although the visual axes actually are Measure on perimeter; fixate target, move light until corneal reflex centred, measure difference Positive up to 5 degrees Positive simulates exo + masks eso; negative simulates eso + masks exo

Preschool screening for amblyopia and strabismus

- Gross observation – 7 degrees deviation is the minimum detectable
- VAs to detect amblyopia and refractive error
- Simultaneous corneal and fundus reflex photography – fundus reflex brighter off macula than on macula
- Cover test and 4D base out prism test
- Asymmetric optokinetic nystagmus – normal response to stripes moving nasally but not to stripes moving temporally in prebinocular infants and older children not binocular
- Stereopsis – best method using random dot stereogram (no monocular clues)

Versions and vergences

Classification of versions and vergences	
Convergence	Voluntary Reflex – accommodative; fusional; tonic
Divergence	Fusional
Vertical fusional	

Accommodative convergence

Definition

- Part of optokinetic near response, involving accommodation, miosis, convergence

Stimulation

- Blurred retinal images, bitemporal retinal disparity, awareness of near, voluntary convergence

AC/A ratio (accomodative convergence to accommodation ratio)

Measurement

- Distance-near measurement
  - Measure deviation at 6 m and measure pupillary distance
  - $AC/A = PD + \frac{\text{Deviation difference}}{\text{Near fixation distance}}$

- Lens gradient method
  - Measure the deviation at either 6 m or 0.33 m with + 3.00 lenses and –3.00 lenses
  - AC/A = $\frac{\text{Deviation with } +3 - \text{Deviation with } -3}{6}$
- Normal values – 4–6 D
- High AC/A → patient will overconverge at near
- Low AC/A → lack of convergence or relative divergence
- Pliable in children
- Increased with myopia and exodeviation, to compensate
- Miotics → increased acetylcholine transfer across myoneural junction → increased ciliary body contraction → decreased AC/A
- Cycloplegics → increased AC/A
- AC/A may be high or low, primary or secondary (to offset the deviation)

High AC/A

- Associated with
  - Convergence excess (primarily defective)
  - Divergence excess (compensatory)
- Improves after 7 years of age
- Treat with miotics and surgery
- Clinical indicator of high AC/A ratio is a convergent deviation for near 15D greater than the deviation for distance

Low AC/A

- Associated with
  - Convergence insufficiency (primarily defective)
  - Divergence insufficiency (compensatory)
- Never improves
- Treat with cycloplegics

Clinical applications of AC/A ratio

- High AC/A ratio in minimal hypermetropia → esotropia for near; treat with bifocals
- Surgical correction of exodeviation with primarily high AC/A ratio → esodeviation at near
- Low AC/A ratio may cause exotropia for near

Convergence insufficiency

- Near point of convergence > 8 cm

Treatment

- Convergence exercises
- Base in prisms (1.5–2 D per eye)

Fusional vergence

- Reflex to overcome retinal image disparity
- Horizontal, vertical or torsional
- Measure with prisms
- Horizontal convergence
  - To correct bitemporal disparity
  - Amplitude at 6m is 15D for fusion break and 12D for fusion restoration
  - Amplitude at 0.33m is 20-25 for fusion break and 18-22 for fusion restoration
- Horizontal divergence
  - To correct binasal disparity
  - Amplitude at 6m is 8/6D
  - Amplitude at 0.33m is 12/9D
- Vertical – normal amplitude 3–6D
- Torsional
  - Normal amplitude – incyclovergence 6–10 degrees
  - Normal amplitude – excyclovergence 8–12 degrees

Normal fusion vergence amplitudes

	For 6m	For near
Convergence	20–25D	30–35D
Divergence	6–8D	8–10D
Vertical vergence	2–3D	2–3D

Tonic vergence

- Convergent and divergent
- Normally balance; disturbance → horizontal tropias

Congenital esotropia

Prevalence

- 50% of esotropias, 40% of all comitant squints
- Equal gender incidence; may be familial

Pathogenesis

- Multifactorial
- May be autosomal dominant, autosomal recessive, often no family history
- Delay in III nerve myelination causes a MR paresis
- The cause of infantile esotropia remains unknown

Aetiology

- Appears to be comprised of two groups of patients – no fusion potential and early deviation, and normal sensory components with later onset of deviation
- No fusion potential and early deviation
  - These demonstrate asymmetry of optokinetic nystagmus, dissociated vertical deviation, and latent nystagmus
  - No potential to develop monofixation syndrome
- Normal sensory components
  - Motor factors cause late onset deviation + secondary interference in normal binocular development
  - Due to failure of maturation and development of binocular connections of motor processing neurones

Clinical features

- Onset – 0–6 months of age
- 50% amblyopia
- Size of deviation – large (40–80D), equal for near and far, stable angle
- Refractive errors
  - Cycloplegic refractions are similar to those of normal children at this age
  - 80% low hypermetropia (< 3D), 16% high hypermetropia, 4% myopia
  - 55% later develop significant hypermetropia
- Associated findings
  - Dissociated vertical deviation – may be associated in 75% of cases
  - Inferior oblique overaction – may be associated in 70% of cases
  - Latent nystagmus – may be associated in 50% of cases
- Patients with late onset, acquired esotropia may have intermittent esotropia with large fusional divergence amplitudes and have a much better prognosis for binocular fusion
- Associations – Down's syndrome, albinism, cerebral palsy
- Face turn – may occur with cross-fixation

Differential diagnosis

- Pseudoesotropia (–ve angle kappa, epicanthic folds)
- Duane's retraction syndrome types 1 and 3
- Möbius syndrome
- Nystagmus blockage syndrome (fixate in adduction)
- Congenital VI nerve palsy
- Early onset accommodative esotropia
- Sensory esotropia
- Esotropia in the neurologically impaired
- Congenital fibrosis syndrome
- Infantile myasthenia gravis

Treatment

Aims of treatment

- Patients with congenital esotropia never become bifixators i.e. they do not develop stereoscopic acuity of 40 secs of arc

10

- But alignment to < 10D before 2 years of age may result in peripheral fusion and central suppression i.e. monofixation syndrome with some binocularity + fusion
- To achieve monofixation, the eyes must be aligned within 8–10 D before 2 years of age
- This occurs in 20% of patients
- It will prevent consecutive exotropia occurring later

Non-surgical treatment

- Treat amblyopia before surgery
- Treat refractive error; prescribe full cycloplegic refraction if refraction > 2.00 D; reassess angle after 2 months, operate if eso persists
- Full-time alternate occlusion; this may delay or preserve potential binocularity

Surgical treatment

- Operate between 6 months and 2 years of age
- Excellent fusion possible if surgery done before 6 months of age
- After 6 months of age, stable angle, freely alternating, no accommodative element
- Correct deviation to < 10 D; 1 operation (bilateral medial rectus recessions) in 70%, > 1 operation (bilateral lateral rectus resections) in 30% (after 6 weeks)
- If eyes are aligned before 2 years of age, 75% will develop peripheral fusion and gross stereopsis (monofixation syndrome)
- If eyes are aligned after 2 years of age, 15% will develop peripheral fusion and gross stereopsis
- If there is minimal brain dysfunction or other neurologic disturbance, postpone surgery to 3 years of age, then undercorrect by 15D
- If present late, undercorrect by 15D to prevent late development of divergence

Post-surgery treatment

- Over and undercorrection
    - Alignment is unstable for up to 10 years
    - Consecutive exo > 15D after 6 weeks requires recorrection (medial rectus advancement if underacting, or lateral rectus recessions)
    - Consecutive exo > 10D after 6 weeks may respond to correction of hypermetropia > +1.50D
    - Residual eso > 15D after 6 weeks requires further correction
- Accommodative esotropia – 50% of patients develop accommodative eso
- Dissociated vertical deviation – treat for cosmesis by SR recession, ± IR resection or IO advancements
- Inferior oblique over action – weakening surgery indicated for cosmesis
- Amblyopia
    - 20% develop amblyopia post-op
    - Therefore, follow up carefully and treat

Delayed surgery in low income communities

- 50% of patients undergoing early surgery require ongoing treatment for amblyopia or develop amblyopia if unsupervised
- If not surgically aligned, risk of amblyopia is only 25% (increased risk with dissociated vertical deviation or latent nystagmus, decreased risk without)
- Therefore, defer surgery until 6 years old

Classification of surgical results

- Optimal – orthotropia or asymptomatic heterophoria; 25%
- Desirable – microtropia; 25%
- Cosmetically acceptable – small angle (< 15D) cosmetically acceptable residual esotropia or consecutive exotropia; 40%
- Cosmetically unacceptable – large angle (> 15D) residual esotropia or consecutive exotropia requiring additional surgery; 10%

Accomodative esotropia

Incidence

- 50% of esotropia, 40% of all comitant squints

Aetiology

- May be hereditary

Classification of accommodative esotropia	
■ Refractive (hypermetropia)	□ Fully accommodative □ Partially accommodative
■ Non-refractive (high AC/A ratio)	□ With convergence excess □ With accommodation weakness (hypoaccomodative)
■ Mixed accomodative	

Features of accommodative esotropia

Accommodative esophoria

- The squint is within fusional divergence amplitude therefore not manifest
- Usually asymptomatic; asthenopia may occur with prolonged near work
- Breakdown → alternating blurring and diplopia
- If due to hypermetropia, symptoms occur at near
- If due to high AC/A, symptoms occur at near and far

Accommodative esotropia

- Onset 6 months – 7 years of age, average $2\frac{1}{2}$ years of age
- Intermittent → constant
- Initial diplopia, later sensorial adaptation, amblyopia may develop
- May be superimposed on infantile esotropia
- Secondary medial rectus hypertrophy or contracture may result in superimposed non-accommodative esotropia in 50% cases

Refractive accommodative esotropia

- Distance–near deviation differs by < 10D
- Usual refractive error +4.00D to +7.00D, average +4.75D
- Average size of deviation 25–30D

Non-refractive accommodative esotropia (high AC/A ratio)

- Straight for distance, esotropia for near
- Usual refractive error +2D to +3D, average +2.25D
- Due to high AC/A ratio
- Two types
  - Convergence excess – accommodation is normal, convergence is exaggerated
  - Hypoaccommodation – accommodation is weak necessitating a strong convergence and extra accommodative effort for near

Mixed accommodative

- Refractive + high AC/A components

Examination

- Cycloplegic refraction
  - g. atropine 1% twice × 3 days; subtract 1.5 D for resting tone
  - Or g. cyclopentolate 1% 2 drops 5 mins apart – then wait 30–45 mins; subtract 0.75D for resting tone
- AC/A ratio measurement
  - Alert to high AC/A ratio if near deviation is 15D more than distance deviation
  - Measure by lens gradient method
- Sensory tests
  - Tests of suppression and anomalous retinal correspondence

Treatment of accommodative esotropia

Age < 4–6 years

- Spectacles
  - Full cycloplegic correction (deduct working distance only); if refraction is ≥ + 1.50 to 2.00D or if there is any anisometropia
  - Add + 2.50 D for near if – > 6 D hypermetropia; or if due to high AC/A ratio
  - Prescribe executive bifocals, place reading segment 1 mm below the visual axis
  - Prescribe plastic lenses; use velcro tape on ear-pieces if necessary
- Miotics (pilocarpine)
  - Temporary, for patients who cannot wear glasses
  - 0.125% drops daily, decrease to once weekly; → miosis; but may precipitate retinal detachment, iris cysts (preventable with phenylephrine 2.5%)
  - Stop 3 weeks before surgery to prevent post-op apnoea; works by inducing peripheral accommodation → less accommodation effort needed for near → less accommodative convergence needed (helpful for a high AC/A ratio)
- Surgery – for any residual deviation after spectacles worn for 1 month (accommodative esotropia superimposed on infantile esotropia, secondary medial rectus changes)

Age 6–8 years

- Prescribe least plus to keep eyes straight; should have an esophoria

Age > 8 years

- Decrease the plus; ultimately withdraw glasses if possible
- Patients do not usually outgrow hypermetropia
- Prescribe a mild reading add for asthenopic symptoms due to a slight esophoria
- Prognosis for binocular vision is better than infantile esotropia because the eyes are often straight during the critical period of visual development

Other esotropias

Esotropia associated with impaired sight

- Due to disturbance of tonic vergence mechanism
- Apparent after 6 months of age
- Angle is less than that in congenital esotropia
- Important to identify the cause (fundoscopy)
- Surgery is cosmetic; undercorrect by 15D, limit surgery to the involved eye (recess-resect)
- Visual loss before 2 years of age → esotropia
- Visual loss after 2 years of age → exotropia

Divergence paralysis

- Abrupt onset of acquired comitant esodeviation, maximal for distance, decreased to orthophoria for near
- Onset is at any age
- Associated with head injury, raised intracranial pressure, encephalitis, intracranial tumour

Treatment

- Occlusion or prisms × 6 months; surgery (bilateral medial rectus recessions) after 6 months of age

Convergence spasm

- Simulates esotropia at near
- Usually hysterical in origin
- May be a feature of dorsal midbrain syndrome
- Spasm of accommodation + convergence

- Induced myopia, miosis, esotropia, diplopia
- Cycloplegic refraction → true refractive error

Treatment
- Refractive correction, cycloplegia, psychotherapy

Consecutive esotropia

- Following surgery for an exo deviation
- Spontaneous improvement may occur

Stress induced esotropia

- Breakdown of previously efficient fusional divergence mechanism
- Treat with surgery once angle is stable

Non-accomodative convergence excess

- Rare
- Large angle eso at near
- AC/A normal or low
- Onset 1–3 years of age

Treatment
- Bilateral medial rectus recessions and bilateral Faden procedure (posterior fixation suture 12 mm behind muscle insertion)

Nystagmus blockage syndrome

Pathogenesis
- Convergence dampens nystagmus, therefore eyes are converged to decrease nystagmus
- Not the only cause of the esotropia
- Seen in 10% of esotropic infants

Features
- Variable angle esotropia in a young child with congenital nystagmus
- Pseudoparesis of lateral rectus muscles
- Best visual acuity at near, fixation with adducting eye

Treatment
- Controversial
- Treat if there is face turn abnormal head posture
- Bilateral medial rectus recession, lateral rectus resection, Faden procedure on medial rectus, base out prism
- Results of surgery are unpredictable

Spasm of the near reflex/ convergence spasm

Causes
- Anxiety/hysteria, seizure, head injury, Parinaud's syndrome, craniocervical junction lesion

Features
- Spasm of accommodation, convergence, induced myopia, miosis, esotropia, diplopia

Treatment
- Cycloplegic refraction → true refraction; give correction
- Cycloplegic–mydriatic drops
- Psychotherapy

Cyclic esotropia

Aetiology
- Possible effect in superior colliculi or oculomotor nuclei
- Associated with EEG changes and behaviour pattern changes

Features
- Onset 3–4 years of age
- 48 hour cycle normally, sometimes longer
- Straight on some days, large angle esotropia (35–40D) on others
- Lasts months to years, → constant esotropia

Treatment
- Full correction of maximum esotropia

Acute acquired comitant esotropia

Clinical features
- Dramatic onset large angle esotropia with diplopia and minimal refractive error
- May be intermittent initially, constant later

Classification of acute acquired comitant esotropia	
■ Type 1	□ Follows occlusion of 1 eye or loss of vision in 1 eye secondary to injury or disease □ The result of interruption of a previously well-functioning fusion mechanism, causing a latent deviation to become manifest
■ Type 2	□ No precipitating cause
■ Type 3	□ Actually divergence insufficiency; esotropia at distance, orthophoria for near

Treatment
- Base out prisms to maintain binocular function until angle of deviation stabilises
- Then surgery

Exotropia

Comitant exodeviations

- Usually intermittent with high-grade stereopsis, amblyopia rare
- This may be because fusional convergence amplitudes are strong, making exodeviations well controlled

Incidence
- 20% of comitant squints
  - 90% intermittent
  - 10% constant

Aetiology
- Disturbance of horizontal tonic vergence ie excess divergence or deficient convergence
- Secondary changes in muscles (lateral rectus hypertrophy)

Classification
- Exophoria
- Intermittent exotropia
- Constant exotropia
- Secondary comitant exotropia

Differential diagnosis
- Positive angle kappa
- Exo Duane's
- Partial III nerve palsy

Exophoria

Features
- Latent deviation with good fusional vergence amplitude, normal stereoacuity, no amblyopia
- < 10D asymptomatic
- > 10D symptomatic – asthenopia, alternating diplopia and blurring
- Most have low AC/A (symptoms for near); some have high AC/A or normal AC/A

Treatment
- Asymptomatic – nil
- Symptomatic
  - Orthoptic fusional convergence training
  - Accommodative convergence training with –2 to –3D correction
  - Base in prisms (half measured deviation) in old patients

Intermittent exotropia

Features
- Onset 1–6 years
- Usually gradually deteriorate (75% progress); may → exophoria or constant exotropia
- Precipitated by fatigue, illness, bright sun (disrupts fusion possibly causing diplopia – children close one eye in bright light)
- Normal fusional vergence amplitude, good stereopsis, no amblyopia
- < 10 years – suppression and ARC when divergent (scotoma large

10

and temporal); normal retinal correspondence and stereopsis when straight
- > 10 years – diplopia when divergent
- Most have high AC/A (i.e. worse for distance)
- Lateral incomitance if present indicates tight medial rectus; therefore reduce surgery amount
- May be associated inferior oblique over-action or superior oblique overaction with A or V + vertical deviation; differentiate from a tight lateral rectus
- Make sure to measure the full exotropia – do the monocular patch test to break down fusion

Treatment
- Correct refractive error; over minus by 2D
- Surgery indicated if
  - Exotropia persists with correction
  - Convergence is lost
  - Deviation is > 15 D (defer if <)
  - Prism fusional range < 20 D
  - Exotropia worsens
  - Exotropia for more than 50% of time
  - Diplopia troublesome
- Do sooner rather than later; if becomes constant, will lose fusion, therefore, do before this happens
- Best done at 4–5 years of age; poor post-op co-operation if earlier, persistent anomalous retinal correspondence and suppression with recurrence of deviation if later
- Do recess-resect in one eye, or bilateral lateral rectus recessions; also correct A or V
- Aim for overcorrection of 5–10D; will diverge and fuse; warn patient of hemiretinal trigger with diplopia following over correction
- Blind spot syndrome
  - Consecutive eso after 6 weeks – will seek blind spot for suppression → increasing eso (to 25–30 D)
  - Treat this with full plus-correction, miotics, prisms, occlusion; recorrect after 6 months
  - Undercorrection > 15D – re-operate
  - Undercorrection < 15D – Fresnel base in prisms
- Basic intermittent exotropia
  - Distance and near deviation within 10 dioptres
  - Operate for the largest deviation
- Pseudodivergence excess
  - The distance deviation seems > 10D than the near, but prolonged monocular occlusion (30 minute patch test) increases the near to within 10D of far
- Divergence excess
  - Exotropia > 10D greater in distance or near
  - Caused by a high AC/A ratio or increased proximal convergence

Constant exotropia

Features
- May be congenital exotropia, blind eye, or degenerated intermittent exotropia
- AC/A usually normal or low; usually present at birth
- Amblyopia or alternate fixation may occur, with suppression + anomalous retinal correspondence

Treatment
- Occlusion treatment of amblyopia
- Surgical correction before 18 months of age

Secondary comitant exotropia

- Consecutive exotropia – following esotropia correction; will have diplopia
- Sensory exotropia – in adults and infants, cw esotropia in children
- Wall-eyed bilateral internuclear ophthalmoplegia (WEBINO) syndrome – longstanding bilateral internuclear ophthalmoplegia
- Convergence paralysis
  - Feature of Parinaud's syndrome

  - Also seen in encephalitis, multiple sclerosis, cerebral concussion and other lesions
- Exotropia secondary to ectopic foveas – retinopathy of prematurity, autosomal dominant proliferative vitreoretinopathy

Congenital exotropia

- Very rare
- Usually associated with systemic problems like albinism, craniofacial abnormalities, cerebral palsy
- Treatment: Bilateral LR recessions

Convergence insufficiency

- Inability to converge resulting in an exodeviation for near
- Asthenopia, reading fatigue, diplopia for near
- Exophoria at near breaks down into an exotropia

Treatment

- Near point exercises (pencil push-ups)
- Base out prism convergence exercises

Vertical deviations

Small primary vertical deviations

- < 4D common
- Usually overcome by fusional vergence
- Elicited with Maddox rod
- Treat with prisms if necessary

Large primary vertical deviations

- Rare
- Often due to orbit asymmetry (shallow orbit → hypertropia)
- Treat with prisms or surgery

Skew deviations

- Sudden onset large variable vertical deviations (disconjugate vertical gaze palsy)
- Associated with cerebellar, brainstem and labyrinthine lesions (tumour, vascular, demyelinating)
- May disappear once aetiological factor is removed

Inferior oblique overaction

- Primary or secondary; weak contralateral superior rectus (Hering's law), or ipsilateral superior oblique (Sherrington's law)
- Primary may occur in isolation or with a horizontal deviation
- Over elevation in adduction, ± V pattern

Superior oblique overaction

- Primary or secondary; secondary rare, due to weak contralateral inferior rectus or ipsilateral inferior oblique
- Overdepression in adduction, ± A pattern

A, V and X patterns

Aetiologies

- A – SOOA, ± IOUA ± LRUA
- SOs act as abductors in downgaze
- V – IOOA, ± SOUA ± MROA
- IOs act as abductors in upgaze
- X – SOOA + IOOA

Diagnosis

- Prism cover test in primary position, 30 degrees up, 30 degrees down; 10–15 D difference is diagnostic

Surgery

- Weaken overacting obliques
- Vertically transpose horizontal recti if obliques are not overacting

Obliques

- Weakening procedures
  - IO weakening; recession; antero positioning; disinsertion; IO weakening → 20 D correction in upgaze and in the primary position

- SO weakening
  - Posterior two-thirds tenotomy; → 20 D correction in downgaze
  - Z plasty
  - Total tenotomy; → 50 D correction in downgaze
- Strengthening procedures

Horizontal recti

- MR more effective in downgaze
- LR more effective in upgaze
- → 10 D correction in primary position
- Recessions + resections
  - Eso V – MR recessions
  - Eso A – LR resections
  - Exo V – LR recessions
  - Exo A – MR resections
- Transpositions
  - If there is an A or V pattern without superior or inferior oblique over action
  - Insertion moved in direction in which one wishes to reduce the action of the muscle
  - MR moved towards apex, LR moved towards base
  - i.e In an A pattern: MR up, LR down In a V pattern: MR down, LR up
  - Transpose 0.5–1 muscle width

Vertical recti

- Weakening or strengthening
- Horizontal transpositions

Dissociated vertical deviation (DVD)

Aetiology

- Congenital dysfunction of supranuclear downgaze signal

Features

- Onset most common during second year of life, may occur up to 5 years of age
- Usually bilateral, may be asymmetrical
- Upward turn and extorsion of covered eye on alternate cover test
- No hypertropic shift of fellow eye when DVD eye is covered
- May be present as a phoria or a tropia; tropia is more often manifest at distance fixation
- May be intermittent (fatigue or daydreaming) or constant
- Bielschowsky phenomenon; deviating eye moves down when illumination in the fixing eye is increased or decreased; this is also seen in latent nystagmus
- Absence of stereopsis, due to chiasmal cross-over of temporal fibres; DVD + no fusion potential
- Associations – infantile esotropia, orthophoria, exodeviations, inferior oblique overaction, superior oblique over acction, latent nystagmus
- 80–90% of congenital squints have DVD
- If it occurs with inferior oblique over action or superior oblique over action, it is incomitant i.e. different size in different horizontal gaze fields

Treatment

- Cosmetic surgery if present as a tropia
- SR recessions or IR resections or SR recessions ± Faden procedures
- ID anterior transposition if associated with IODA
- SR recessions should be large (7–9mm)

Dissociated strabismus syndrome

- Dissociated vertical deviation (DVD)
- Dissociated horizontal deviation (DHD)
- Dissociated torsional syndrome (DTD)
- Latent nystagmus
- One or more component may predominate

Obliques

Inferior oblique overaction

Aetiology

- Primary or secondary
- Primary – idiopathic

- Secondary
  - To contralateral SR weakness (yoke muscles – Hering's law)
  - To ipsilateral SO weakness (antagonist; Sherrington's law)

Head tilt test
- To differentiate primary + secondary
- Positive tilt test → vertical deviation changes by > 5D → paresis

Features
- Vertically incomitant deviation
- Upshoot of eye in horizontal adduction and/or over elevation of eye in adduction
- How to differentiate it from a DVD which will also do this: Occlude the eye and then check the deviation for abduction + adduction; if it is the same → DVD
- Graded 1–4, according to 1–4 mm upshoot on adduction
- Primary onset 2–3 years of age, usually bilateral
- May occur alone, or with esotropia or exotropia (eso > exo)
- Vertical deviation is rarely present (cw secondary form)
- May result in V pattern
- Large V patterns of ≥ 20D are indicative of 2 + IOOA or more

Treatment
- Generally needed for 2+ or more
- IO weakening; recurrence is common
- Myectomy, recession (for small) or anteriorisation (for large + only for bilateral surgery – makes the muscle act as a depressor)

Superior oblique overaction

Aetiology
- Primary or secondary
- Primary – idiopathic
  - Due to hypercontraction
  - Due to sagitalisation of superior obliques, probably as a result of an anomaly of orbital development → torsional effect weakened → overcontraction to prevent torsional diplopia
- Secondary
  - To contralateral IR weakness (yoke; Hering's law)
  - To ipsilateral IO weakness (antagonist; Sherrington's law)

Features
- Vertically incomitant deviation
- Downshoot of eye in horizontal adduction and/or over depression of eye in adduction
- Limited elevation in abduction
- Primary usually bilateral
- May occur alone, or with exotropia or esotropia (exo > eso)
- Vertical deviation is rarely present (cw secondary form)
- May result in A pattern

Differential
- Brown's (no SOOA, positive forced ductions)
- IO paresis (positive head tilt test)

Treatment
- SO weakening
- Tenotomy – cutting the tendon in two
- Wright silicone tendon expander
- V + A patterns can be treated by transposition of the horizontals

Superior oblique palsy

- Most common cause of an isolated vertical deviation
- Ipsilateral hypertropia, worse on ipsilateral head tilt + contralateral side gaze
- Ipsilateral SOUA + IOOA
- Can be bilateral
  - Bilateral SOUA + IOOA
  - Right hypertropia in left gaze + left hypertropia in right gaze

Aetiology
- Traumatic – severe head trauma; almost always bilateral

- Congenital – cause unknown
- Vascular disease
- Neoplasms
- Zoster

Congenital superior oblique palsy

- Usually unilateral or asymmetrical bilateral
- Large hypertropia in primary position with IOOA
- Paresis present from birth but often only manifests in late childhood or early adulthood
- This is because these patients develop large vertical fusional amplitudes
- Also have a compensatory head tilt opposite to the side of the palsy
- Good stereopsis
- Show the deviation intermittently when fatigued
- Good suppression therefore no diplopia

Treatment

- Pattern of strabismus critical
- Identify where the deviation is the greatest
- May just need an ipsilateral IO weakening – small deviation < 10D
- Or a bilateral IR recession – > 10D
- Bilateral SO tucks + bilateral MR recessions – for bilateral SO palsies
- Harada-Ito – for extorsional diplopia (selective tightening of the anterior 25% of the SO tendon fibres – disinsert fibres + reinsert at superior border of LR)

Paralytic and restrictive strabismus

- Paresis
  - Cranial nerve palsy, congenital agenesis, traumatic rupture, slipped muscle post-surgery
- Restriction
  - Thyroid, congenital fibrosis syndrome, Brown's syndrome, periocular scarring, orbital fracture with fat or muscle entrapment
- Diagnostic tests to differentiate
  - Forced duction test
  - Forced generation test
  - Saccadic velocity measurements – normal muscle is required to generate a saccadic movement; paretic muscle → slow eye movement that does not generate a saccade; restriction → saccade that abruptly stops
  - Differential IOP changes
  - Lid fissure changes in side gaze

Palsies

III palsy

- Observe for at least 6 months
- Secondary contracture of the antagonist muscle may occur; prevent with botulinum

Treatment

- No good procedure
- Large ipsilateral LR recession + MR resection + SO tenotomy
- Brow sling for ptosis

VI palsy

- Observe for at least 6 months
- Secondary contracture of the antagonist muscle may occur; prevent with botulinum
- Treatment
  - Depends on degree of LR function
  - If < 50% function: Ipsilateral MR recession + vertical muscle transposition
  - Knapp procedure – full tendon transfer of SR + IR laterally
  - Hummelsheim + Jensen's operations – split tendon transfers – effect less, but less anterior segment ischaemia
  - If > 50% then recess MR + resect LR

Slipped and lost muscle

- Try to find, otherwise transposition

Congenital absence of an extraocular muscle

- IR most common
- Transposition

Restrictions

Fat adherence syndrome

- Fat adherence to sclera post-trauma e.g. orbital or retinal surgery
- Very difficult to treat
- Do not penetrate the posterior tenons during surgery

Graves' ophthalmopathy

- Strabismus in the cicatricial phase
- Surgery should be limited to recession procedures to release tight muscles

Orbital floor fracture

- Restriction of elevation and postitive forced ductions
- Limited depression → IR gets tethered to the globe by scarring

Double elevator palsy

- Limited elevation in one eye in all gaze positions
- A misnomer because in 70% the cause is restriction secondary to a tight IR
- Hypotropia with chin elevation + ptosis

Syndromes

Duane's retraction syndrome

Aetiology

- Paradoxic innervation of horizontal recti
- LR co-contracts on adduction → retraction + limitation of adduction and convergence

Classification (Huber's)

- Eso – retraction on adduction
- Exo – retraction on abduction
- Vertical – retraction on downgaze; ? due to fibrous band between SO and SR
- Type 1 – abduction limited
- Type 2 – adduction limited
- Type 3 – abduction and adduction limited

Features of eso Duane's

- Retraction on adduction; limitation of adduction and convergence
- Absent abduction
- ± Up or down shoot on adduction; due to bridle effect of co-contraction of MR and LR
- ± contracture of MR with positive forced duction test, esotropia, and abnormal head posture
- Usually orthophoric in primary position during infancy and early childhood, become eso subsequently
- May be autosomal dominant or sporadic
- Female : male = 2 : 1, left > right
- Bilateral in 20% of cases
- Systemic associations occur in 30–50% of cases
- Include labyrinthine deafness, Goldenhar's syndrome
- Ocular associations include anisocoria, microcornea, coloboma, nystagmus, anisometropia

Differential diagnosis

- VI palsy
- Myasthenia gravis
- Möbius syndrome
- Dysthyroid eye disease

Special investigations

- Forced duction test

Treatment

- Only if
  - Abnormal head posture present (> 30 degree turn)

- Narrowed palpable fissure cosmetically unacceptable
- Strabismus in primary position
- Bilateral medial rectus recessions
- Avoid > 6 mm recession
- ± Ipsilateral lateral rectus recession at same time, to avoid 'splits' and to overcome upshoot and downshoot

Brown's superior oblique tendon sheath syndrome

Pathology

- Congenital – shortened or thickened SO tendon
- Acquired – secondary thickening of SO tendon sheath (regional inflammation, rheumatoid arthritis); therefore, unable to slide through trochlea

Features

- Inability to elevate adducted eye above the horizontal plane
- May be widening of palpebral fissure on attempted elevation, hypotropia with chin up AHP, palpable snap at trochlea on elevation in adduction (click syndrome, evident during recovery)
- Forced duction test is positive

Differential diagnosis

- Inferior oblique palsy – also has superior oblique over action, A pattern, negative forced duction test
- Monocular elevation deficit – unable to elevate 1 eye in any position

Treatment

- Only for abnormal head posture
- SO tenotomy or tenectomy
- SO loop recession
- Forced duction test, if positive → cut Lockwood's ligament
- Forced duction test, if positive → IR recession
- Forced duction test, if positive → IO recession
- Local steroids if required

Prognosis

- Most congenital cases recover spontaneously; therefore, avoid surgery if possible

Möbius syndrome

Aetiology

- Aplasia of nuclei of VI, VII, IX and XII
- May be autosomal recessive or sporadic
- May be associated with autism
- May be associated with use of misoprostol (prostaglandin abortive)

Features

- VI palsy → absence of horizontal versions; often esotropia; may maintain fixation of laterally moving target by voluntarily converging
- VII palsy → smooth expressionless face
- IX + XII palsy → atrophic tongue and delayed speech development, paresis of soft palate, feeding difficulties
- Associations – mental retardation, deafness, musculoskeletal abnormalities (hypoplasia of pectoral muscles, syndactyly, club feet)

Treatment

- Esotropia if present

Fibrosis syndromes

Pathology

- Extraocular muscle(s) replaced by fibrous tissue → globe retraction and loss of movement, positive forced duction test
- Congenital or acquired, unilateral or bilateral, may affect all muscles or 1 muscle

Congenital generalised fibrosis

- Autosomal dominant, levators also involved
- IR maximally involved → eyes drawn down
- Treatment – levator sling for ptosis + IR recessions

Congenital fibrosis of the inferior rectus

- A variant

Vertical retraction syndrome

- Fibrosis of SR

Strabismus fixus

- Fixed in adduction or abduction, due to fibrosis of MR or LR

Miscellaneous strabismus

Chronic progressive external ophthalmoplegia

Aetiology

- Autosomal dominant or sporadic

Pathology

- Bilateral myopathy of extraocular muscles

Features

- Starts in second decade, slowly progressive
- Ptosis → MR involvement with exo → elevation weakness with chin up abnormal head posture → ultimately eyes fixed in primary position

Associations

- Sternomastoid, trapezius and deltoid weakness
- Oculofacial dystrophy
- Pharyngeal muscle dystrophy
- Retinal dystrophy (Kearns-Sayre-Daroff syndrome)
- Neurodegenerative disorders (cerebellar and corticospinal)

Differential diagnosis

- Progressive supranuclear palsy
- Parkinson's disease
- Myotonic dystrophy – chronic progressive external ophthalmoplegia, ptosis, lack of smooth pursuit, orbicularis weakness, cataracts, RPE changes, testicular atrophy, frontal balding

Treatment

- Spectacle crutches for ptosis

Double elevator palsy (IO + SR)

Causes

- Dysthyroid eye disease
- Myasthenia gravis
- Blowout fracture orbital floor
- Vascular insufficiency of relevant part of III nucleus
- Congenital

Treatment

- Transposition of LR and MR insertions (Knapp procedure); not for restrictive double elevator palsy

Double depressor palsy (IR + SO)

- Rare
- Usually congenital, due to IR weakness with spread of comitance
- Treat by inverse Knapp procedure

Marcus Gunn jaw winking phenomenon

- Due to anomalous connection between nuclei of
  - External pterygoid muscle and levator (open mouth and move jaw to opposite side)
  - Internal pterygoid muscle and levator (teeth clenched)
- Left > right, less conspicuous with age
- Ptosis with lid retraction on chewing

Amblyopia

Definition

- Unilateral or bilateral impaired foveal vision in the absence of organic disease, due to non-use of the fixation reflex

Visual development

- Critical period of visual development → first 3–4 months of age

10

- Fixation + smooth pursuit → by 2–3 months of age
- 70% of neonates have a variable exodeviation
- 30% are straight
- < 0.5% have a variable esodeviation
- By 2 months of age most are aligned, but a small exodeviation may persist up to 6 months of age
- Binocularity is established by 2–3 months of age
- Stereopsis is established by 3–6 months of age

Classification
- Strabismic
- Anisometropic
- Stimulus deprivation (e.g. cataract, corneal opacity, occlusion)
- Ametropic
- Meridional

Strabismic amblyopia
- Monocular suppression occurs as an active cortical inhibition; to eliminate diplopia
- Eventually persists, even on occlusion of fixing eye
- Eliminates form perception, not perception of light and colour

Anisometropic amblyopia
- Foveal images of different sizes (> 8%) preclude fusion
- Fovea of the more ametropic eye is deprived of form vision, and suppression of the more blurred image occurs
- > 2D anisometropia in hypermetropia → amblyopiogenic
- > 4D anisometropia in myopia → amblyopiogenic

Visual deprivation amblyopia
- May be unilateral or bilateral
- Media opacity → no clear image on fovea, active suppression occurs
- Prolonged occlusion may similarly result in amblyopia
- Experimental evidence for atrophy of relevant laminae in lateral geniculate nucleus and columns in visual cortex

Ametropic amblyopia
- Bilateral, due to high refractive error

Meridional amblyopia
- Uncorrected astigmatism

Diagnosis
- Visual acuity
  - Preferential looking, Snellen chart
  - Decreased photopic acuity, scotopic acuity about the same
  - Crowding phenomenon; due to contour interaction, origin ? retinal or cortical
- Neutral density filter
  - To distinguish functional and organic amblyopia; decreased visual acuity if organic, no change if functional
- Fixation behaviour
  - Central fixation → eccentric viewing → eccentric fixation
  - Test with – visuoscope motor test and visuoscope sensory test
  - Alternate cover test; grade binocular fixation pattern grade 0 (freely alternating) → grade 4 (no fixation)
- Up to 33% have subtle afferent pupil defect; ? due to defect at ganglion cell level

Treatment
- Occlusion
- Penalisation

Occlusion
- Full time – rarely used now
  - Three months or until no further improvement
  - Use opticlude or occlusor, with skin prep dressing
  - Review after (months of age) days or (years of age) weeks

10

- Part time
  - Mild – 1 hour per day
  - Mod – 2 hours per day
  - Severe – 4 to 6 hours per day

Penalisation

- As an alternative to patching; better tolerated in school children
- Atropine
  - Penalises for near
  - 1 drop 1% daily
  - Use ultraviolet filter sunglasses
- Plus lens
  - Penalises for far
  - Use +1.25D to +1.50D
  - Suitable if visual acuity > 6/12
- Other methods
  - Diffuser lens, opaque contact lens

Follow-up

- Maintenance treatment may be necessary up to age 7, as visual acuity may slip back
- Visual acuity slips back about 1 line in about 50% over the next 6 years; a low initial visual acuity + strabismic amblyopia are risk factors for deterioration

Treatment problems

- Skin injury
- Prevention of removal of patch (water wings, splint)
- Occlusion amblyopia

Prognosis

- Compliance on treatment is most important factor in predicting outcome
- Age of child, type of amblyopia, and degree of amblyopia are less important
- If children are screened at 4 years of age and amblyopia is treated then, most are cured within 3 months
- Strabismic amblyopia is treatable up to age of 7 years
- Anisometropic amblyopia is treatable up to age of 12 years or longer

Surgical correction of squint in untreated amblyopia

- Correction of esotropia → functional improvement in field, as temporal monocular crescents are not involved in amblyopia suppression
- Correction of exotropia → reduction in binocular field

Monofixation syndrome

Definition

- Manifest eso/exodeviation of 0–5 degrees, with absent foveal fusion and unilateral foveal scotoma
- A phoria co-existing with a small tropia
- Peripheral fusion (gross stereopsis), central fixation of the preferred eye and central suppression of the fellow eye

Incidence

- 1.5% of the general population

Aetiology

- Primary
  - Inherent inability to fuse similar images on the maculae
- Secondary
  - Anisometropia
  - Unilateral macular lesion (toxoplasmosis)
  - Strabismus; eso > exo, often seen in treated deviations

Examination

- The simultaneous prism cover test
- A prism is added to the cover/uncover test
- To measure the size of a small tropia in patients with a co-existing phoria (i.e. monofixation syndrome)
- Cover the fixing eye and place a prism over the deviating eye simultaneously
- When the appropriate prism is used, no shift will occur in the deviating eye
- The prism that neutralises the tropia shift is the size of the tropia

Features

- Small angle deviation 0–5 degrees; usually eso
- Monocular foveal scotoma, 3–5 degrees in diameter, not due to suppression or organic foveal lesion, may be detected with Bagolini striated glasses or 4D base out prism test
- Normal peripheral fusion, gross stereopsis (down to 60 secs), normal vergence amplitudes
- Alternate cover test measurement (latent deviation) may be greater than simultaneous prism cover test
- Amblyopia may be present

Treatment

- Motor – usually unnecessary, surgery may be indicated
- Sensory
  - Correct anisometropia
  - Occlusion for amblyopia
  - No treatment for macular scotoma

Motor adaptations (abnormal head postures)

Headturn

- VI palsy
- Duane's syndrome
- IO palsy/SR contracture
- Nystagmus null point
- Medial wall fracture

Chin tip

- A or V
- Dysthyroid eye disease
- Orbital floor fracture
- IR fibrosis
- Vertical rectus palsy
- Brown's syndrome
- SO palsy
- Ptosis
- Accommodative esotropia with high AC/A (no fixation through bifocal seg)
- III palsy

Heat tilt

- SO palsy
- Posterior fossa tumour
- Torticollis

Sensory adaptations

Types

- Occur if strabismus occurs under 9 years of age
- To eliminate diplopia and visual confusion (diplopia = simultaneous appreciation of 2 images of 1 object; confusion = simultaneous appreciation of 2 superimposed but dissimilar images caused by stimulation of corresponding points by images of different objects)
- Manifest only during binocular viewing, not during monocular viewing

Suppression

- Positive cortical inhibitory reflex; sensation from non-fixating eye is ignored
- Three clinical types: Central vs peripheral, monocular vs alternating, facultative vs obligatory
- Central vs peripheral
  - Central – image from fovea of deviating eye suppressed to avoid visual confusion
  - Peripheral – image from peripheral retina of deviating eye suppressed to avoid diplopia
- Monocular vs alternating
- Facultative vs obligatory
  - The purpose of suppression is to eliminate central diplopia
  - In esotropia there is a small 5–6 degree nasal scotoma
  - In exotropia there is a large temporal scotoma extending to the hemiretinal line

Abnormal retinal correspondence

- Cortical adjustment in directional values supplied by the retinal neuroepithelium, to permit fusion of similar images projected onto non-corresponding areas peripheral to the area of conscious regard
- Eliminates peripheral diplopia/visual confusion
- May be total (harmonious) or partial (unharmonious)
- Anomalous retinal correspondence is binocular, cw eccentric fixation, which is monocular

Tests

- Red filter test
- Worth 4-dot test
- 4D base out prism test
- Bagolini striated lenses
- After image test
- Lancaster projectors
- Synoptophore test

Red filter test

- Red filter in front of 1 eye, view white light
- Suppression → either red or white
- Normal retinal correspondence with tropia → uncrossed diplopia in eso + crossed diplopia in exo
- Anomalous retinal correspondence with tropia → fusion (pink)

Worth 4-dot test

- Red before right, green before left, view 4 lights

R

G G

W

- Near dots test macular fusion, far dots test extra macular fusion
- Fusion → 4 lights
- Suppression → only green or only red
- Normal retinal correspondence in strabismus → 5 lights
- Anomalous retinal correspondence in strabismus → 4 lights

4D base out prism test

- To distinguish bifixation and monofixation in a patient whose eyes appear straight

Bagolini striated lenses

- Plano lenses with striations → streaks seen when white light is viewed

After image test

- First eye stimulated by vertical filament × 20 secs, second eye by horizontal filament × 20 secs
- Normal retinal correspondence → cross after image, anomalous retinal correspondence → horizontally displaced after image

Lancaster projectors

- Red and green filters, red and green targets; targets superimposed, objective and subjective angles are compared; similar in normal retinal correspondence, dissimilar in anomalous retinal correspondence

Synoptophore test

- Set tubes at objective angle, patient adjusts to subjective angle for superimposition; 2 angles are compared; equal in normal retinal correspondence, dissimilar in anomalous retinal correspondence

Treatment

- No longer treated; now believed results are as good with just surgery alone; following surgery, suppression and anomalous retinal correspondence are spontaneously adjusted → normal retinal correspondence and peripheral fusion
- Suppression
    - Red filter over one eye, learn to recognise diplopia (rapid cover

  - uncover, 15D base-up prism, wriggle prism)
  - Occlude non-suppressing eye between sessions
- Anomalous retinal correspondence
  - Once diplopia is recognised, normal retinal correspondence is taught using the synoptophore or using prisms
  - May experience transient monocular diplopia or binocular triplopia
  - Maintain occlusion between
  - Then align eyes with prisms or surgery

Congenital nystagmus

Classification

- Manifest; compensated by convergence + null point
- Latent
  - Manifest latent; compensated by adduction
  - Latent latent
- Distinguish on EMG

Features

- May occur in association with congenital esotropia; usually it is manifest latent nystagmus
- May adopt abnormal head posture to put eyes into null position

Treatment

- Prisms temporary; move eyes in direction of face turn
- Surgery; move eyes in direction of face turn; defer surgery until 5–6 years of age; base surgery on greatest amount of abnormal head posture measured; do recess-resect surgery bilaterally (Kestenbaum procedure)

Surgery

Recession

- Small errors on large recessions give large errors
- Bilateral MR recessions have a greater effect at near because recessions have their greatest effect in the field of action of that muscle

Resection

- By resecting a piece of muscle or by a 'tuck' (folding the muscle on itself)
- The redundant tucked muscle disappears over time; (benefit of preserving anterior ciliary flow)

Faden

- A suture is placed to secure muscle to sclera, 12–14 mm posterior to the muscle insertion
- Reduces muscle power
- Most useful on the MR
- Usually performed in combination with a recession on the same muscle
- Indications
  - Dissociated verticle deviation
  - Nystagmus blocking syndrome
  - Double elevator palsy
  - High AC/A ratio
  - VI nerve palsy with lateral incomitance
  - Duane's syndrome (hypertropia in adduction)
  - Head turn in congenital nystagmus
  - Incomitant vertical strabismus
  - Medial wall blowout fracture
- Technique
  - Suture rectus muscle belly to sclera
  - Results in selective weakening of the muscle in its field of action, without changing the ocular alignment in the primary position
  - ± Combine with a recession of the muscle

Transposition

- Changing the location of the muscle insertion so that the muscle pulls the eye in a different direction
- To treat a paretic or lost muscle

- For small vertical deviations – vertically offset the horizontal recti in combination with the horizontal recess ± resect (e.g. A + V patterns)
- Anteriorisation of the IO for DVD and IOOA

Chemodenervation

- Botulinum toxin → temporary muscle paralysis
- Can be used in the MR in VI palsy to prevent formation of a contracture

Recti

- Recessions
- Resections
- Adjustable sutures
- Transpositions
  - Knapp procedure
  - Jensen's procedure
  - Hummelsheim's procedure
  - Faden procedure (posterior fixation suture)

Superior oblique

- Tenotomy
- Recession
- Disinsertion
- Tendon tuck
- Harada-Ito procedure
- Silicone expander

Inferior oblique

- Recession
- Anteropositioning
- Disinsertion

Vertical recti recessions

- Limit recessions to 5 mm, to avoid lid retraction
- 1 mm recession → 3D correction

Harada-Ito procedure

- Indication – bilateral superior oblique palsy
- Technique – split tendon, move anterior one-third 5 mm anteriorly + 8 mm laterally

Inferior oblique recession

- Disinsert, resuture to globe at the equator half way between IR + LR

Adjustable sutures

Indications

- To facilitate more accurate ocular alignment and decrease the need for reoperation (30% → 10%)
- Particularly indicated where results of conventional surgery are unpredictable

Pre-operative assessment

- Cotton bud test – instil LA, manipulate conjunctiva with a cotton bud

Technique

- Operate in the morning, make the adjustment in the late afternoon

Inferior rectus recession

- IR is attached to lower lid 15 mm from limbus
- Free this attachment
- This prevents lower lid retraction that occurs following IR recession

Superior oblique weakening

- Isolate SO on nasal side of SR, 10 mm from SR insertion

Surgical complications

Classification of complications of squint surgery

Systemic intra-operative	Oculocardiac reflex Scoline hypersensitivity Malignant hyperthermia
Local intra-operative	Perforation Haemorrahage Lost muscle
Early post-op	Infection Anterior segment ischaemia Lost muscle
Intermediate post-op	Visible scar Ptosis Suture reaction Conjunctival inclusion cyst Lid malposition
Late post-op	Consecutive overcorrection Limited rotations Diplopia Adherence syndromes

Detached rectus muscle

Types

- Snip
  - Muscle cut and lost during squint surgery
  - No Tenon attachments; therefore, poor prognosis for relocation
- Snap
  - Muscle breaks during squint surgery
  - Muscle has had previous surgery or other pathology
- Slip
  - Suture is incorrectly placed through capsule only and not through muscle belly as well; therefore, muscle belly retracts within its capsule
  - There is increasing angle of incomitant squint on first or second day after operation
- Trauma
  - Medial rectus muscle can freely retract into orbit
  - Other recti are all attached to the globe via their adjacent oblique muscles

Management

- CT scan shows position of muscle and presence or absence of any attachment
- Explore as soon as possible
- Use oculocardiac reflex to locate muscle
- Reattach muscle to globe
- If muscle cannot be found, attach adjacent fascia to globe + recess ipsilateral antagonist

Anterior segment ischaemia

Pathogenesis

- Following squint surgery, with removal of more than 2 rectus muscles from the globe
- Anterior ciliary arteries do not recanalise; blood flow returns through the deep collateral circulation with recovery of circulation within 4 weeks
- Risk is greater with vertical rectus muscles
- Risk is greater in older patients

Clinical features

- Usually presents 2 days post-op

- Iritis, keratitis
- Irregular pupil
- Pain
- Hypotony
- Late cataract
- Usually resolves after 2–4 weeks

Treatment

- Systemic steroids
- Possibly anticoagulants

Botulinum toxin (Botox)

Mechanisms of action

- Bound to muscle receptors, blocks calcium cycle in nerve terminal, blocks release of acetylcholine
- Produces denervation-like phenomena
  - Muscle atrophy
  - Increased sensitivity of muscle fibre surface to acetylcholine
  - Sprouting of motor nerve
  - Contracture of antagonist
- Onset after 2–8 days, duration up to several months

Uses

- Blepharospasm
- Hemifacial spasm
- Torticollis spasmodicus
- Orbicularis myokymia (quivering of muscles)
- Lagophthalmos due to VII palsy
- Dysthyroid eye disease
- Spastic entropion
- Ptosis for neurotrophic ulcers
- Nystagmus
- Strabismus
  - VI nerve palsy
  - IV nerve palsy
  - Convergent squint < 40D
  - Non-accommodative component of accommodative esotropia
  - Infantile esotropia
  - Patient unfit for surgery (acute thyroid eye disease, ischaemic anterior segment)

Blepharospasm

- Inject 1–4 ngm under EMG control 4 mm above and below, medially and laterally, ± above brows; do not inject above middle of upper lid (→ superior rectus and levator paresis)
- Repeat every 2–3 months as necessary

Esotropia

- Inject 0.4–2 ngm (maximum 10 ngm) into overacting muscle under EMG control
- 65% reduction in angle can be achieved after 3 injections
- Most useful for angle < 40D
- Can be used for final adjustment following surgery

Paralytic strabismus

- VI nerve palsy – inject into muscle under EMG control
- IV nerve palsy – inject into inferior temporal quadrant under EMG control
- Allows denervation atrophy of injected muscle and contracture of homolateral antagonist

Complications

- Ptosis
- Scleral perforation – 1 in 1 000

10

11

Neuro-ophthalmology

Congenital disc anomalies 307
Swollen disc 309
Optic atrophy 311
Anterior ischaemic optic neuropathy 313
Optic neuritis 315
Multiple sclerosis 317
Traumatic optic neuropathy 319
Nutritional and toxic optic neuropathies 320
Optic nerve tumours 321
Neuro-ophthalmic associations of diabetes mellitus 323
Cerebral aneurysms 323
Brain lesions 324
Cortical blindness 325
Headache and migraine 326
Myopathies 328
Nystagmus and spontaneous eye movement disorders 329
Optic chiasm syndrome 335
Diplopia 336
Third (oculomotor) nerve palsy 338
Fourth (trochlear) nerve palsy 340
Sixth (abducens) nerve palsy 342
Seventh (facial) nerve palsy 344
Combined ocular motor nerve palsies 346
Supranuclear and internuclear gaze palsies 348
Vascular malformations 352
Pupil 353
Visual fields 356
Neuroimaging 360

Congenital disc anomalies

Elevated disc abnormalities – differential diagnosis of papilloedema

- Disc drusen
- Hypermetropia
- Persistent Bergmeister's papilla/glial remnants
- Myelinated nerve fibres
- Epipapillary hamartomas and tumours
- Optic neuritis

Excavated disc abnormalities – differential diagnosis of glaucoma

- Congenital deep cup; large disc area, normal neuroretinal rim area
- Hypoplasia
- Fuch's typical coloboma
- Morning glory disc
- Atypical coloboma/optic pit
- Tilted disc
- Congenital crescent

Disc drusen

- 0.3–1% prevalence
- Deposition of hyaline calcific material in nerve substance
- May be congenital; ? autosomal dominant with incomplete penetrance
- May be associated with acquired eye disease (retinitis pigmentosa, pseudoxanthoma elasticum, Allagille's syndrome)
- Only seen in Caucasians, 75% bilateral

- Autofluorescence
- Usually no loss of vision, but may cause pressure atrophy → field defects
- May be buried within the disc substance early on and only exposed later
- May be associated intraretinal, preretinal and subretinal haemorrhage adjacent to the nerve head
- To differentiate from papilloedema – spontaneous venous pulsation, irregular disc margin outline, no haemorrhages/exudates/cotton wool spots, no peripapillary retinal folds, and no fluorescein leakage

Myelinated nerve fibres

- Male > female, familial, associated field defect

Aplasia (dysplasia)

- Rare, decrease in vision varies nil → total
- A markedly deformed disc that does not conform to any recognisable category

Hypoplasia

- Unilateral or bilateral
- Diminished number of nerve fibres; normal vessels
- Double ring sign of concentric chorioretinal pigmentary changes
- Increased incidence with intrauterine exposure to anti-epileptics, alcohol, quinine
- May be a sign of intracranial tumours e.g. craniopharyngioma, optic glioma
- De Morsier's syndrome → optic nerve hypoplasia, absence of septum pellucidum, endocrine deficiencies
- Neuroimaging essential

Fuchs' typical coloboma

- Isolated disc coloboma
- Excavation within nerve head
- No decreased vision
- Often associated inferior crescent

Morning glory disc

- Non-hereditary (bilateral cases very rare → may be hereditary)
- Typical coloboma, funnel-shaped excavation, disc posteriorly displaced, vessels leave disc at its margin
- Usually unilateral, associated serous retinal detachment in 30%
- Resembles the morning glory flower
- Poor VA
- Systemic associations – frontonasal dysplasia, midfacial abnormalities, basal encephalocoele, neurofibromatosis type 2

Optic disc pit

- Atypical disc coloboma, due to excessive resorption of glial tissue
- Usually temporal, single or multiple, unilateral or bilateral
- Associated field defect in 60%, ± associated inferior chorioretinal coloboma
- Serous maculopathy in 40%, with detachment, oedema, hole formation
- Fluid travels through pit, ? from vitreous, choroid, pit vessels, or CSF
- Treat with photocoagulation

Congenital tilted disc

- Form fruste of typical coloboma
- Inferonasal crescent, pallor of inferonasal fundus, inferonasal staphyloma
- ± Associated superotemporal field defect (pseudobitemporal hemianopia)

Congenital disc crescent

- Inferior, non-progressive, due to malclosure of embryonic fissure
- Compare with acquired crescent, which is temporal, progressive, associated with myopia

Ocular coloboma

Aetiology

- Genetic
  - Single gene disorder with isolated coloboma; sporadic, autosomal dominant usually, autosomal recessive rarely
  - Single gene disorder with multisystem involvement
  - Chromosomal abnormalities e.g. trisomy 21
- Teratogens
  - Thalidomide
- Multisystem disorders of unknown aetiology – e.g. Goldenhar syndrome, Rubinstein-Taybi syndrome

Classification

- Typical – inferonasal, due to failure of fusion of embryonic fissure
- Atypical – e.g. aniridia, ectopic pupil, lid notching, optic pit

Phenotypic expression

- Lid – notching
- Iris – inferonasal, complete or incomplete
- Zonular – associated lens opacities, flattening of lens
- Chorioretinal – inferonasal; retinal detachment may complicate
- Disc – partial (inferior crescent), complete (Fuchs' or morning glory)
- Macula
- Microphthalmos, orbital cyst/anophthalmos
- May be unilateral or bilateral, symmetric or asymmetric
- Systemic associations
  - Chromosomal abnormalities – trisomy 13, 18, 22, Goltz, Goldenhar, etc.

Management

- Complete ophthalmalogical evaluation
- Systemic evaluation
- History of pregnancy, family history
- Genetic counselling
- Follow-up refraction, amblyopia treatment, retinal detachment treatment

Swollen disc

Aetiology

- Congenital – drusen, hyaloid remnants, myelinated fibres, hypermetropia
- Inflammatory – uveitis, sarcoidosis, TB
- Mechanical – papilloedema, ocular hypotony, retrobulbar mass
- Neoplastic – lymphoma, leukaemia, haemangioma, glioma, metastatic
- Metabolic – dysthyroid eye disease, diabetes mellitus
- Vascular – central retinal vein occlusion, proliferative retinopathies, anterior ischaemic optic neuropathy, cranial + collagen arteritis
- Raised intracranial pressure – papilloedema, benign intracranial hypertension

Papilloedema

Pathogenesis

- Increased intracranial pressure → increased CSF pressure in sheath around nerve
- Decreased axoplasmic flow + decreased venous return
- Once established, it takes 6–10 weeks to resolve

Symptoms

- Transient obscurations of vision, due to fluctuations in nerve head perfusion
- Enlarged blind spot
- Field constriction late, especially inferonasally
- Late secondary optic atrophy with loss of central acuity

Signs

- Early – loss of venous pulsation (although absent in 20% of normal, therefore, helpful only if present)
- Blurred superior and inferior disc margins

- Thickening of axons in nerve fibre layer
- Established – oedema of nerve head and surrounding retina
- Venous congestion
- Splinter haemorrhages, hard exudates and soft exudates
- Late – resolution of oedema takes 6–10 weeks
- Glial proliferation, secondary optic atrophy

Benign raised intracranial pressure

- Pseudotumour cerebri/idiopathic intracranial hypertension

Definition

- Increased intracranial pressure not due to a space occupying lesion or hydrocephalus

Aetiology

- Decreased venous outflow – dural sinus thrombosis, neck surgery, chronic obstructive airways disease, right-sided cardiac failure, Pickwickian syndrome
- Metabolic – obesity, Addison's disease, steroid withdrawal, pregnancy, oral contraceptives, galactosaemia, hypoparathyroidism
- Blood dyscrasias
- Drugs – vitamin A excess or deficiency, tetracycline, gentamycin, nalidixic acid
- Idiopathic in 95%

Features

- Young obese female, peak incidence third decade
- Headaches and transient obscurations
- Papilloedema, VI nerve palsy + diplopia in 30%, field changes of papilloedema
- Increased CSF pressure (more than 200 mm of water), normal composition
- Normal or small ventricles on CT scan
- ± Pulsatile tinnitus

Treatment

- Remove the cause
- Weight loss in obesity
- Acetazolamide, furosemide
- Steroids controversial – they decrease ICP but it increases with taper
- Repeated lumbar punctures
- Lumboperitoneal shunt
    - Decreases intracranial pressure, improving headache, VI palsy + papilloedema
    - Potential complications – shunt blockage, infection, migration
    - Re-operation required in > 50%
- Optic nerve sheath fenestration
    - When headache is a lesser component + progressive visual loss occurs
    - Saves the optic nerve but does not lower intracranial pressure + therefore does not treat headache
    - 1–2% risk of blindness – nerve injury, CRVO, CRAO
    - 16% 6 year success + must be repeated
    - Both eyes have to be done, reduction in papilloedema in other eye rare

Prognosis

- Usually good, lasts weeks to months, self-limiting
- 26% develop VA < 6/60 in the worse eye

Causes of transient visual loss

- Seconds
    - Papilloedema from raised intracranial pressure
- Minutes
    - Amaurosis fugax (carotid atheroma with ophthalmic artery embolus)
- Hours
    - Migraine
- Days
    - Optic neuritis

11

Optic atrophy

- Optic nerve shrinkage due to degeneration of retinal ganglion cell axons

Definition

- Pallor ± may be total or segmental (temporal, altitudinal, wedge-shaped); Kestenbaum's sign = < 8–11 vessels crossing temporal disc
- Decreased visual acuity
- Field defects

Pathology

- Degeneration of axons
- Glial replacement
- Cavernous atrophy of Schnabel; no glial replacement (in glaucoma)

Clinical features

- Disc pallor
- ± Accompanying disc swelling
- Thinning of neuroretinal rim
- Retinociliary collateral vessels
- Peripapillary nerve fibre layer defects
- Retinal arteriolar attenuation

Classification of optic atrophy

- Ascending (features of retinal pathology)
- Glaucomatous (cupping)
- Descending (no retinal pathology, no cupping, disc margins well defined, vessels normal)
- Vascular (vessels attenuated)
- Secondary (disc margins blurred, vessels sheathed)

Ascending (features of retinal pathology)

- Retinitis pigmentosa
- Chorioretinitis
- Long-standing retinal detachment
- Retinal degeneration occurring in myopia
- Macular dystrophies

Glaucomatous (cupping)

- Glaucoma
- Chronic anterior ischaemic optic neuropathy (may cause cupping)

Descending (no retinal pathology, no cupping, disc margins well-defined, vessels normal)

- Congenital
    - Recessive – simple\early infantile; complicated\Behr's; with juvenile diabetes mellitus
    - Dominant
    - Indeterminate
    - Leber's optic neuropathy
- Traumatic
    - Post-haemorrhage → haematoma + compression
    - Direct nerve injury
    - Damage from orbital fracture
- Inflammatory
    - Post-retrobulbar neuritis
    - Perineuritis secondary to meningitis, sinusitis, orbital cellulitis, arachnoiditis opticachiasmatica
    - SLE, polyarteritis nodosa, sinusitis, sarcoidosis
- Neoplastic
    - Pituitary adenoma, meningioma, craniopharyngioma metastases, papilloma, optic nerve sheath glioma, lymphoma, optic nerve sheath meningioma
- Bone disease
    - Osteopetrosis, acromegaly
- Toxic
    - Tobacco-alcohol, arsenic, lead, sulphonamides, streptomycin, chloramphenicol, isoniazid, ethambutol
- Demyelinating
    - Multiple sclerosis
    - Devic's disease
    - Syphilis
    - Post-viral

- Metabolic
  - Dysthyroid eye disease → compression
  - Nutritional
- Infiltrative
  - Sarcoid, lymphoma
- Infective
  - Syphilis, TB, Lyme disease, aspergillus, cryptococcus, measles, mumps, chicken pox

Vascular (vessels attenuated)

- CRAO, CRVO
- Arteriosclerosis
- Diabetic microangiopathy
- Syphilitic arteritis
- Other arteritis
- AION – arteritic, non-arteritic

Secondary (disc margins blurred, vessels sheathed)

- Post-papillitis
- Post-papilloedema

Special investigations

- Full blood count, ESR, blood sugar, syphilis serology, serum calcium, serum B12 and folate, collagen screen
- X-ray skull, orbits, optic foramina
- CT scan, MRI → any case without clear cause
- Carotid angiogram

Clinical features of optic neuropathy

- Decreased Snellen acuity, decreased contrast sensitivity
- Field defect – central or caecocentral scotoma
- Colour vision – decreased red and green; hue (red seen as orange) mediated by small myelinated fibres; brightness (red seen darker) mediated by large myelinated fibres
- Afferent pupil defect
  - Pupillary escape = pupil that constricts initially and then dilates on direct light test
  - Relative afferent pupil defect (Marcus Gunn pupil) = pupil that dilates on swinging flashlight test
  - Amaurotic pupil = afferent pupil defect in a NPL eye
- Disc appearance – colour, vessels, cup, border

Optic atrophy in children

- Tumours 30% (glioma, craniopharyngioma, other)
- Inflammation 20%
- Trauma 10%
- Idiopathic 10%
- Central nervous system disease – meningitis, periventricular haemorrhage, cerebral tumours, hydrocephalus
- Chiasmal compression – craniopharyngioma (dissociated vertical nystagmus)
- Optic nerve – optic nerve glioma (in neurofibromatosis), surgery + radiation for chiasmal tumours, post optic neuritis (infectious or idiopathic)
- Orbit – sinus disease, tumours, abnormal bone growth (fibrous dysplasia)
- Ocular – glaucoma, high myopia, primary retinal diseases
- Hereditary – autosomal dominant most common, Leber's, autosomal recessive rare + severe, Wolfram's, Behr's
- Miscellaneous – trauma, non-accidental injury, drugs + toxins

Hereditary optic atrophies

- Recessive
  - Simple/early infantile
  - Complicated/Behr's – severe; associated mental deficiency and ataxia
  - Associated with juvenile diabetes (Wolfram's syndrome) – associated diabetes insipidus and deafness, short stature, mental retardation, endocrine problems
- Dominant (Kjer's syndrome)
  - Less severe than recessive forms
  - Onset at 4–8 years of age
  - Insidious onset, moderate decrease in visual acuity

  - May show some progression at 35–40 years of age
  - Typically shows bilateral wedge-shaped temporal pallor
  - No systemic abnormalities
- Indeterminate/Leber's
  - Associated heredodegenerative neurologic syndromes
  - Combinations of cerebellar degeneration, pyramidal degeneration, deafness, and optic atrophy

Leber's hereditary optic atrophy

Aetiology

- Maternal transition in mitochondral DNA

Clinical features

- Typical Leber's
  - Male > female
  - Onset in second and third decades
  - Family history of male visual loss
  - Subacute painless loss of vision over 2–3 weeks
  - Fellow eye involved after 3–4 months
  - Optic disc shows mild papillitis with telangiectatic vessels
  - Some improvement in vision occurs in 30% of cases
  - Prognosis generally poor, usually < 6/60
- Atypical Leber's
  - 20% are female
  - 45% have no family history
  - 40% have normal discs
  - Visual loss may occur for up to 2 years
  - Final vision may vary 6/18 to NPL
  - Atypia is due to heteroplasmy (mixture of normal and abnormal mitochondria)

Treatment

- Advise to stop smoking and drinking excessive alcohol

Optic nerve injuries

- Direct or indirect
- Indirect → tethered in canal, therefore subject to shearing
- Transection, contusion and tearing, concussion, compression (oedema and haemorrhage)

Management

- Delayed decreased visual acuity = compression; therefore, decompression within 24 hours is imperative
- Neuroimaging
- IV Methylprednisolone
- Surgical optic canal decompression – transcranial, transethmoidal
  - Acute cases – megadose intravenous methyl prednisolone even if NPL
  - If VA improves, change to oral + taper after 48 hours
  - No medical response after 12–48 hours → surgical decompression (controversial)

Anterior ischaemic optic neuropathy

- Arteritic AION (giant cell arteritis) → a necrotising vasculitis affecting primarily the cranial branches of the arteries of the aortic arch
- Non-arteritic AION

Blood supply to anterior optic nerve

- Posterior ciliary arteries supply:
- Surface nerve fibre layer – branches of retinal arterioles
- Prelaminar region – branches from choroidal vessels
- Lamina cribrosa – branches from posterior ciliary arteries direct + circle of Zinn-Haller
- Retrolaminar region – branches from pial vessels (from posterior ciliary arteries); ± branches from central retinal artery

Pathogenesis

- Infarction of anterior part of optic nerve, as a result of compromised posterior ciliary artery circulation
- Temporal arteritis → infarction of medial and lateral short posterior ciliary arteries
- Non-arteritic disease → occlusion of the short posterior ciliary arteries
- Three groups of diseases
  - Local vascular – internal carotid, ophthalmic, posterior ciliary artery; arterio/atherosclerosis 80%; temporal arteritis 12%
  - Systemic – arterial hypotension, embolus, blood dyscrasias
  - Ocular – increased IOP, nerve head drusen, small crowded optic nerve

Features of temporal arteritis

- Systemic disease with ocular involvement in 50%

Ocular features

- AION
- III, IV and VI nerve palsy → diplopia
- Muscle ischaemia → diplopia
- Cilioretinal artery occlusion
- CRAO
- Anterior segment ischaemia (episcleritis, scleritis, uveitis, secondary glaucoma)
- Tonic pupil from ciliary ganglion ischaemia
- Cotton wool spots
- Maximum age incidence 65–70 years, whites > blacks, female > male
- 9% elderly persons subclinically involved
- Second eye involved in 80% within 2 months (one-third within 1 day, one-third within 1 week, one-third within 1 month)

Symptoms

- Usually no prodrome of AION
- Headache, jaw claudication, tender swollen temporal artery, malaise, loss of weight, fever, polymyalgia rheumatica in 50%, euphoria due to cerebral artery involvement
- Four most important diagnostic criteria of giant cell arteritis
  - Jaw claudication
  - Neck pain
  - CRP > 2.45
  - ESR > 47

Features of arterio/atheroscloerosis

Risk factors

- Crowded optic disc
- Hypertension (50%)
- Diabetes (25%)
- Hypercholesterolaemia
- Collagen vascular diseases
- Antiphospholipid antibody syndrome
- Hypotensive events
- Cataract surgery
- Hypermetropia
- Maximum age incidence 60–65, male = female
- Second eye involved in 60–70% within 20 years

Symptoms

- Prodrome transient obscurations of vision
- Other cardiovascular symptoms, hypertension occurs in 50%

Signs of anterior ischaemic optic neuropathy

- Sudden loss of vision; more severe in temporal arteritis; may progress for up to 6 weeks
- Afferent pupil defect
- Pale swollen disc due to infarction of prelaminar nerve head + accumulation of axoplasm
  - Swelling subsides after 10 days → cupping as in chronic glaucoma after 4 months
  - Disc involvement may be diffuse or segmental
  - Second eye involvement → pseudo Foster-Kennedy syndrome

11

  - ± Peripapillary splinter haemorrhages, retinal arteriosclerosis
- Visual field defects
  - Inferior altitudinal
  - Central
  - Arcuate
  - Segmental
  - Contraction of peripheral field
  - Vertical (border through blind spot)
- Fluorescein angiogram → disc hyperfluorescence

Special investigations

- Full blood count and ESR; ESR elevated in temporal arteritis (> 50 in 80% of cases, normal in 20% of cases)
- Blood sugar, collagen screen, syphilis serology
- Temporal artery biopsy (within 3 days of starting treatment), if ESR 20–50
  - Histology shows damage of internal elastic lamina and inflammatory cell infiltrate (± giant cells, variable in extent)
- Three variants of histology
- Remove 2 cm of artery, do serial sections (to avoid skip lesions)
- If negative repeat on other side
- If both negative and ESR normal, assume not temporal arteritis

Treatment

- Early high dose steroids in both (1 gm methylprednisolone daily IVI × 3 days + prednisolone 80 mg orally)
  - Beneficial for involved eye in arteriosclerotic ischaemic optic neuropathy
  - Protects fellow eye in temporal arteritis ischaemic optic neuropathy
- In temporal arteritis, continue tapered oral steroids to maintain normal ESR for 9 months to 1 year

Prophylaxis

- Temporal arteritis
  - High index of suspicion, early diagnosis, long-term steroids to keep ESR normal
  - Most need treatment for 1–2 years, some need indefinite maintenance treatment (may even need steroid sparing agents)
- Arteriosclerosis
  - Avoid systemic hypotension, disprin to improve systemic circulatory haemodynamics, maintain low IOP

Posterior ischaemic optic neuropathy

- Ischaemic damage to the retrobulbar optic nerve

Causes

- Vasculitis (syphilis, SLE, polyarteritis nodosa, irradiation)
- Herpes zoster
- Trauma
- Anaesthetic hypotension/hypoxia
- Severe anaemia

Features

- As above, but discs are normal early

Optic neuritis

Classification

- Papillitis (more common in children)
- Retrobulbar neuritis (more common in adults)

Incidence

- One to 5 per 100 000 per year

Papillitis (one-third)

- All cases are vascular ischaemic (arteritis)
- Some are true inflammatory as for optic neuritis\retrobulbar neuritis

Retrobulbar neuritis (two-thirds)

Demyelinating disease
- Multiple sclerosis
- Neuromyelitis optica (Devic's disease), Schilder's disease, carcinomatosis, post-viral, SLE

Inflammatory
- Para infection
  - Viral (measles, mumps, rubella, chicken pox, glandular fever)
  - Infection – cryptococcal meningitis, cat scratch fever (Bartonella henselae), syphilis (Treponema pallidum), Lyme disease (Borrelia burgdorferi), toxoplasmosis (Toxoplasma gondii), tuberculosis (Mycobacterium tuberculosis), leprosy (Mycobacterium leprae)
- Toxins
  - Toxins – tobacco, alcohol, lead, arsenic, carbon disulphide, bee sting
  - Drugs – chloramphenicol, sulphonamides, isoniazid, streptomycin, ethambutol, indomethacin

Idiopathic
- May develop multiple sclerosis

Contiguous inflammation
- Sinuses
- Orbit
- Meninges
- Uvea

Endocrine
- Dysthyroid eye disease
- Diabetes
- Hyperparathyroidism

Nutritional
- Nicotinic acid
- Hydroxycobalamin
- Thiamine

Hereditary
- Leber's optic neuropathy

Vascular
- Arteritis
- Arteriosclerosis
- Collagen disease

Carcinomatous infiltration

Features
- Papillitis
- Retrobulbar neuritis

Papillitis

- Decreased visual acuity
- Ocular or orbital pain
- Afferent pupil defect
- Cells in vitreous
- Swollen disc and surrounding retinal oedema; perivascular sheathing, gliosis, pallor

Clinical features of retrobulbar neuritis

- 77% female

Symptoms
- Decreased visual acuity, rapid over 2–3 days, stable for 1–2 weeks, recovers over 2–3 months
- Colour desaturation, decreased light intensities, decreased depth perception
- Pain on ocular movements
- Uhthoff's phenomenon in multiple sclerosis
- Auditory evoked phosphenes

Signs
- Decreased visual acuity
- Fields – diffuse loss (48%), central or ceco-central scotoma (8%), altitudinal (15%)
- Dyschromatopsia → decreased colour perception (red-green)
- Afferent pupil defect; pupil escape → Marcus Gunn pupil → amaurotic pupil
- Nil on fundoscopy, later ± pallor

Clinical classification
- Typical
  - Monocular loss of vision in a patient 20–50 years, ± pain on movement, ± multiple sclerosis history

  - Decreased visual acuity, nerve fibre bundle defect, afferent pupil defect, ± swollen disc
  - Course – maximal loss of vision after 1 week, improves over weeks – months
  - Treatment – nil, ± investigate for multiple sclerosis
  - Prognosis – 90% recover to 6/9, no improvement after 6 months
- Atypical
  - Occurs outside 20–50 year span, worsens after 1 week, bilateral, painless, shows other abnormalities
  - Investigate for a cause

Differential diagnosis

- Rapidly expanding space-occupying lesion
- Papilloedema
- Central serous retinopathy
- Ischaemic optic neuropathy
- Leber's
- Benign intracranial hypertension
- Toxic neuropathy

Special investigations

- Typical → no investigations (maybe MRI for prognostic value)
- Blood tests – full blood count, ESR, collagen screen, syphillis serology
- X-rays – orbits, optic canals, sinuses, skull, chest
- Lumbar puncture – cell count, protein, IgG
- CT scan
- Visually evoked potential
- MRI

Treatment

- Oral prednisolone contraindicated → increases rate of relapse
- IV methylprednisolone
  - Faster recovery in first 2 weeks only
  - Reduced conversion to multiple sclerosis for first 2 years, no difference after 3 years
- Methylprednisolone 1 gm daily × 3 days IVI
- Then prednisone orally 1 mg/kg/day for 10 days

Prognosis

- Improves after 1–4 weeks, takes 2–3 months, no improvement after 6 months
- 95% recover to 6/12 or better after 3 months, 87% 6/9 or better
- 90% are aware of a permanent visual defect
- Better with younger age
- Risk of recurrence 20–30% in either eye
- MRI: No brain lesions → 16% risk of progression to multiple sclerosis in 5 years, 3 or more lesions → 51%
- Progression to multiple sclerosis in typical: 30–50% by 5–15 years

Multiple sclerosis

- A demyelinating condition characterised by acute neurological deficit of the Central nervous system with spontaneous exacerbations and remissions

Aetiology

- Unknown
- Autoimmune post viral infection
- Role of heredity; association with HLA B7 + A3
- Exacerbation precipitated by fatigue, trauma, infections, cold, allergic reactions
- Genetic basis → suppressor T-cells (OKT 8) deficient → childhood infection
- B-cells mature to plasma cells to produce autoantibodies against myelin

Epidemiology

- Common in Europe + North America
- Incidence increases with latitude north + south of the equator
- Rare in blacks
- Northern hemisphere 30–50 per 100 000
- Africa 3–5 per 100 000
- South Africa 5–11 per 100 000

11

- Female > male (up to 2 : 1)
- Uncommon in children < 10 years of age
- Highest incidence 25–40 years of age, peak at 30 years, but onset after 50 years not uncommon
- Risk of getting multiple sclerosis twenty times greater in first degree relatives

Pathology

- → Inflammatory demyelination
- Acute lesion – circumscribed area of myelin sheath destruction, little inflammatory reaction
- Chronic lesion – reactive gliosis → glial scar
- Lesions widely scattered, mainly in optic nerves around ventricles, and in spinal cord

Course and prognosis

- Multiple lesions, separated in space and time
- Relapses and remissions, continues for ± 20 years
- ± One-third have a benign disease without serious disability
- 90% slow, remitting course; 10% fast + progressive to total disability in 2 years
- Favourable prognosis – female, early age of onset, relapsing–remitting course, optic neuritis or sensory symptoms at onset, few attacks or minimal disability within the first 2–3 years

11

Clinical features

- Very variable
- Three common presentations
  - Retrobulbar neuritis
  - Corticospinal tract demyelination → weakness + paraplegia
  - Cerebellar dysfunction – intention tremor, ataxia, dysarthria
- Motor symptoms – upper motor neuron deficit with paraparesis, hemiparesis, monoparesis
- Mental changes – depression, labile emotions, dementia (10%)
- Sensory symptoms
  - Parasthesias
  - Lhermitte's sign → electric shock sensation in the limbs and trunk produced by neck flexion
  - Uhthoff's phenomenon → transient deterioration of vision brought on by exercise or elevations of body temperature
- Sphincter disturbances
- Ocular muscle palsies

Optic neuritis

- 30–40% of patients with optic neuritis develop multiple sclerosis
- Increased likelihood if recurrent
- 25% of patients with multiple sclerosis present with optic neuritis
- 75% will have optic neuritis at some point clinically + 90% on visually evoked cortical response
- 90% of females with optic neuritis develop multiple sclerosis by 20 years
- 50% of males with optic neuritis develop multiple sclerosis by 20 years

Prognosis

- 95% end up with VA 6/12 or better
- 3% end up with VA 6/60 or worse
- Subtle visual defects persist in 90%
- 30% develop multiple sclerosis within 4 years
- Presence of ≥ 3 plaques → 43% chance of MS developing
- Normal MRI → 9% chance of multiple sclerosis developing
- Poor correlation between plaque size and number and multiple sclerosis severity
- ± 75% within 15 years develop multiple sclerosis

Treatment

- Oral prednisolone alone contraindicated → increase risk of second optic neuritis
- IV methylprednisolone speeds recovery of vision in first 2 weeks only

- IV methylprednisolone decreases conversion to multiple sclerosis in first 2 years but not beyond

Ocular features

- Optic neuritis, (neuroretinitis very unlikely) chiasmal and post-chiasmal lesions
- Ocular dysmetria and flutter (cerebellar signs), abnormal saccades and pursuit
- Internuclear ophthalmolplegia, often bilateral; also saccadic and smooth pursuit palsies, pontine paramedian reticular formation palsy
- Ocular motility disorders
  - Diplopia common
  - Lesions in the supranuclear, nuclear + fascicular parts
  - Internuclear ophthalmoplegia under 50 years → multiple sclerosis likely
  - Skew deviations
  - Parinaud's dorsal midbrain syndrome
  - Nystagmus – horizontal, rotatory or vertical; pendular or jerk
- Extraocular muscle/infranuclear palsies
- Orbicularis myokymia, pain in V distribution, uveitis, peripheral retinal neovascularisation
- Pars planitis in 10%
- Perivenous sheathing and leaking in peripheral veins
- Posterior + anterior uveitis 10 times more common than general population

Cerebrospinal fluid (CSF)

- Abnormal in 90% cases
- Increased lymphocytes, increased protein, increased IgG : albumin ratio
- IgG is synthetised in Central nervous system → IgG level in CSF > serum level
- Often as an oligoclonal band

Other special investigations

- Visual evoked potential (single flash and pattern) → delay before symptoms are manifest
- Sine wave gratings → decreased VA not evident on Snellen chart
- Eye movement tests → abnormal saccades and pursuit
- MRI → early detection of plaques

Management

- Physiotherapy, occupational therapy
- Steroids for acute exacerbations → no evidence for long-lasting benefit
- Interferons → reduce exacerbations by one-third

Poser's classification for diagnosis

- Clinicaly definite, laboratory supported definite, clinically probable, laboratory supported probable
- Based on history of attacks, objective clinical signs, paraclinical evidence (visually evoked response, CT scan, hot bath test), laboratory evidence (increased IgG in CSF)

Devic's disease (neuromyelitis optica)

- Acute variant of multiple sclerosis, with bilateral optic neuritis and transverse myelitis within 6 weeks, typically occurring in children and young adults
- May actually be a separate disease altogether

Traumatic optic neuropathy

Pathology

- Direct injury → avulsion of the nerve itself or laceration by bone fragments
- Indirect injury → shear forces
- Nerve is tethered in optic canal; therefore, subject to shearing
- Primary lesions → transection, tearing, contusion, concussion, haemorrhage
- Secondary lesions → compression from haemorrhage or oedema, necrosis from systemic circulatory failure or local compression of vessels

Treatment

- No clear benefit of surgical decompression or steroids
- Steroids
  - Anti-inflammatory + neuroprotective effects
  - Dexamethasone 1 mg/kg stat IVI; then 0.25 mg/kg 6-hourly IVI
  - Or: Methylprednisolone 30 mg/kg stat IVI, then 15 mg/kg 6-hourly IVI
  - For 12 hours in patients with delayed onset of visual loss → if no response → decompression; if response → continue treatment
  - For 24 hours in all other patients → if no response → stop all steroids
  - If initial response and subsequent visual loss on tapering → decompression
  - If response occurs → taper after 48 hours → oral steroids
- Optic canal decompression
  - As indicated above
  - Especially if visual loss delayed
  - Transethmoidal approach

Nutritional and toxic optic neuropathies

- Usually retrobulbar
- Earliest presentation → minimal, undetectable signs
- Complaints can be vague and unconvincing

Vitamin deficiency

- Progressive, bilateral visual loss, central or centrocaecal scotomas
- B complex vitamins
  - Thiamine, B1 (beriberi)
  - Riboflavin, B2
  - Pyridoxine, B6
  - Hydroxycobalamin, B12 (pernicious anaemia)
  - Niacin
  - Folic acid
- Hydroxycobalamin deficiency → decreased ability to detoxify cyanide → optic neuropathy
- Treat with vitamin supplements

Tobacco-alcohol amblyopia

- Pipe tobacco usually; 100 g per week × 1 year
- High in cyanide → optic neuropathy (degeneration of papillomacular bundle)
- Associated ethanol excess, vitamin B1 deficiency, zinc deficiency, arteriosclerosis contribute

Treatment

- Stop tobacco and ethanol
- Hydroxycobalamin or cystine; combine with cyanide → cyanocobalamin, excreted
- Hydroxycobalamin 1 000 micrograms IMI weekly
- Zinc supplements
- Thiamine supplements (vitamin B1); 25 mg 8 hourly
- Good prognosis for visual recovery except in the most chronic cases

Toxic amblyopia

- Barbiturates, chlorpromazine, monoamine oxidase inhibitors, perphenazine, chloramphenicol, chloroquine, ethambutol, quinine, streptomycin, sulphonamides, isoniazid, rifampicin, rifampicin, quinine, butazolidine, salicylates, digitalis, chlorpropamide, nicotinic acid, penicillamine, vincristine, cisplatin
- Ethambutol – toxic dosage is 25 mg per kg per day, but is reversible on stopping the drug
- Aniline dyes, arsenic, lead, methanol, carbon disulphide, carbon tetrachloride, ethylene glycol

Methanol amblyopia

- First phase – Narcosis
- Second phase – Metabolic acidosis; lasts 2–3 days, may be fatal, treat with gastric lavage, ethanol and bicarbonate
- Third phase – Retinal and optic nerve toxicity
- Formaldehyde is toxic to ganglion cells
- Retinal oedema and papillitis with loss of vision onset after a few days, lasts a few days, then vision improves
- Then after ± 1 month optic atrophy with chronic loss of vision occurs

Optic nerve tumours

- Two-thirds glioma
- One-third meningioma

Gliomas

- Only 1% of intracranial tumours
- It is unknown whether this is a true neoplasm or a hamartoma

Benign hamartoma of childhood (benign optic glioma)

- Chiasmal more common, orbital less common
- May be associated with von Recklinghausen's disease

Pathology

- Fusiform intradural enlargement of nerve; may grow through canal forming a dumbbell shape

Histology

- Benign pilocytic astrocytoma

Clinically

- 70% discovered in the first decade
- Male = female
- 50% behave as hamartomas, 50% as active neoplasms
- More likely hamartomatous if associated with von Recklinghausen's disease
- Orbital
    - Decreased visual acuity
    - Proptosis
    - Strabismus
    - Nystagmus
    - Disc pallor or papilloedema
    - Afferent pupil defect
    - Hypermetropia
    - Retinal striae
    - Variable field loss
- Chiasmal
    - Decreased visual acuity
    - Strabismus
    - Nystagmus (± seesaw)
    - Disc pallor or papilloedema
    - ± Foster-Kennedy syndrome
    - Afferent pupil defect
    - Disturbance of pituitary and hypothalamic function
    - Hydrocephalus
    - Variable field loss

Special investigations

- X-ray shows enlargement of optic foramen; CT scan shows tumour
- MRI – fusiform or globular enlargement of optic nerve ± kinking
- Biopsy not warranted

Treatment

- No universally accepted management
- No evidence that surgery alters prognosis for life and vision
    - Orbital glioma → excise only if eye is blind and proptosis is progressive
    - Chiasmal glioma → only do shunt surgery for hydrocephalus
- Growth is episodic, recurrences may occur after incomplete excision
    - Aim for complete excision of tumour before chiasm is involved
    - Radiotherapy + chemotherapy for chiasmal tumour

Malignant glioblastoma multiforme of adulthood (malignant optic glioma)

- Rare, presents as acute optic neuritis, rapidly progressive, fatal within a few months
- Treatment rarely successful

Meningiomas

Incidence

- Comprise 15% of intracranial tumours
- 40–50 years peak
- Female : male = 3 : 1; whites > blacks
- Only 1–2% of all meningiomas, but 5% of orbital tumours
- Increases incidence in neurofibromatosis

Aetiology

- Associated with neurofibromatosis
- Increased growth in pregnancy
- Trauma
- Radiation

Pathology

- Macroscopic
  - Orbital circular, envelop nerve
  - Canalicular small
  - Intracranial variable in size; lateral one-third sphenoid wing meningiomas often en plaque
- Microscopic
  - Arise from arachnoid cells
  - Epithelial-like cells arranged in whorls, interspersed by psammomma bodies
- Five histologic types
  - Meningoepitheliomatous
  - Transitional
  - Fibroblastic
  - Angioblastic
  - Sarcomatous

11

Sites

- Orbital – arise from optic nerve sheath
- Intracanalicular – usually extension from orbit or intracranial
- Intracranial – olfactory groove, tuberculum sellae, greater wing of sphenoid (medial third, middle half, lateral third)
- Orbital more common in childhood, intracranial more common in adults

Natural history

- Slow growing, higher growth in pregnancy, more aggressive in children
- Usually locally (bone) invasive but never metastasise

Features

- Slow, painless loss of vision
  - May be intermittent, may improve with steroids
  - Loss of colour vision
  - Field loss – centrocaecal, bitemporal, generalised
- Afferent pupil defect
- Optic atrophy, disc oedema, Foster-Kennedy syndrome
- Optociliary shunt vessels – in any orbital tumour, due to central vein occlusion
- Proptosis and decreased mechanical motility in orbital tumours
- Intractable optic neuritis → intracanalicular tumours
- Intracranial tumours may → I–VI nerve palsy; visual loss early in central tumours, proptosis and late visual loss in lateral one-third tumours
- Other neurologic features – headache, raised intracranial pressure, epilepsy, pituitary – hypothalamic dysfunction, change in mental state

Radiology

- Straight x-ray → enlargement, distortion, hyperostosis, calcification in tumour
- Tomography of canal
- CT scan
- Angiography, pneumoencephalography, ultrasound
- MRI → diffuse optic nerve enlargement

Differential diagnosis

- Tumours – craniopharyngioma, glioma, pituitary tumour, metastases
- Optic neuritis

Treatment

- Surgical excision – severe visual loss
- Orbital – < 40 years remove immediately (because tumour more aggresive), > 40 years remove only when vision is lost

- Intracranial – remove as soon as possible; recurrence rate 10–20%
- Radiotherapy – tumour limited to orbit + useful vision present

Melanocytoma

- Of optic nerve head
- Benign, may grow locally
- Treat conservatively

Neuro-ophthalmic associations of diabetes mellitus

- Optic disc hypoplasia
  - Associated with diabetic mother
  - Varies mild → severe
- Optic atrophy
  - Associated with juvenile diabetes mellitus
  - Wolfram's syndrome – ? autosomal recessive inheritance
  - DIDMOAD (diabetes insipidus, diabetes mellitus, optic atrophy, deafness)
- Chronic open angle glaucoma
- Anterior ischaemic optic neuropathy
- Papillopathy
  - Form fruste of AION
- Decreased corneal sensation
- Cranial nerve palsies (III, IV, VI, VII)
  - Due to micro infarcts within brainstem?

Cerebral aneurysms

Incidence

- 5% of population
- Associated with hypertension, atherosclerosis, trauma, neoplasm, inflammation
- May be developmental
- Can be familial or associated with systemic abnormality: Marfan's, Ehlers-Danlos, etc.

General

- Berry aneurysm most common
- 90% supratentorial, 10% infratentorial
- > 10 mm in size most likely to rupture
- Problems → pressure effects + rupture with sub-arachnoid haemorrhage

Ophthalmic implications

- Aneurysms of internal carotid + basilar arteries → neuro-ophthalmic manifestations
- Ophthalmic artery aneurysm → progressive unilateral optic neuropathy, ipsilateral optic pain
- Anterior communicating aneurysm → optic chiasm or tract compression
- Aneurysm at junction of internal carotid + posterior communicating artery → ipsilateral III palsy (with headache + pupil involvement)
- Intracavernous carotid aneurysms → cavernous sinus syndrome, (confined by walls of sinus, therefore, do not rupture), occasionally isolated VI palsy

Clinically

- Unruptured aneurysms
  - Mass effect → progressive neurological dysfunction
  - Transient ischaemic attack, infarction, seizures
  - Occasional monocular blindness – compression of II by internal carotid artery aneurysm
  - Field defects – giant ophthalmic artery aneurysm
  - May invade the sella + mimic a pituitary adenoma
- Ruptured aneurysms
  - Neurological emergency
  - Symptoms and signs of a subarachnoid or subdural haemorrhage
  - Severe headache, nausea + vomitting, neck stiffness, focal defects
  - Raised intracranial pressure with VI palsies + papilloedema
  - Terson's syndrome

11

Investigations
- Cerebral arteriogram
- Four vessel study important – 10% have more than one aneurysm
- MRI detects > 5 mm size
- High quality MRA detects 3 mm in size
- CT useful acutely to identify blood, not good screening for unruptured aneurysms

Prognosis
- Risk of aneurysm rupture 1% per year
- 50% mortality with rupture
- Survivors have considerable neurological defects
- Interval from warning mass signs to rupture varies from 1 day to 4 months

Treatment
- Ideally treat prerupture
- Lower intracranial pressure → hyperventilate, mannitol
- Surgical clipping or coiling

Dissecting aneurysms

- May develop in the internal carotid or branches
- Traumatic or spontaneous

Clinically
- Severe cerebral ischaemia and coma
- Traumatic dissection
    - Headache
    - Ipsilateral ophthalmic signs and contralateral neurological deficit
- Spontaneous dissection
    - Amaurosis fugax
    - Acute cerebrovascular accident
    - Monocular blindness
    - Ipsilateral Horner's syndrome
    - Cranial neuropathies
- Visual loss → embolic occlusion of the ophthalmic artery, central retinal artery, short posterior ciliary arteries, retinal branch arteries
- Can be a rare cause of ocular ischaemic syndrome

Diagnosis
- MRI
- Angiography

Treatment
- Intracranial – bypass + anticoagulate

Brain lesions

Ocular features of frontal lobe tumours

- Foster-Kennedy syndrome
    - Ipsilateral atrophy and contralateral papilloedema
    - Usually not fully developed
- Field defects – bitemporal, uniocular, homonymous
- Saccadic palsy

Ocular features of temporal lobe lesions

- Tumours
- Anterior cerebral artery cerebrovascular accident 9 : 1
- Field defects
    - Superior homonymous quadrantanopia or complete homonymous hemianopia
- Formed visual hallucinations, olfactory hallucinations, deja vu (psychomotor seizures)
- Ipsilateral III palsy with Hutchinson's pupil, due to uncal herniation
    - Stages of Hutchinson's pupil – miosed, dilated but reacts, dilated and non-reactive, affects other side
- Decreased V sensation
- Upper motor neurone VII palsy

Ocular features of parietal lobe lesions

- Tumours
- Middle cerebral artery cerebrovascular accident 1 : 1
- Field defects
    - Inferior homonymous quadrantanopia or complete homonymous hemianopia

- Absent optokinetic nystagmus on rotating drum to same side
  - Saccadic ipsilateral pursuit
  - Spasticity of conjugate gaze; tonic deviation to opposite side on attempted Bell's
- Visual agnosias
- Alexia, agraphia on dominant side
  - Unawareness of left visual space on non-dominant side
  - Jackson's epilepsy
- Decreased V sensation

Ocular features of occipital lobe lesions

- Tumours
- Vertebrobasilar or posterior communicating artery cerebrovascular accident 1 : 4
- Field defects
  - (Central) homonymous hemianopia, ± macular sparing, ± preservation of temporal crescent, ± tunnel vision
  - Cortical blindness, Anton's syndrome, Riddoch's phenomenon
- (Unformed) visual hallucinations
- Prosopagnosia – inability to recognise faces
- Palinopsia – persistence or recurrence of visual images
- Alexia without agraphia – due to lesion in left occiput + splenium of corpus callosum
- Vertebrobasilar insufficiency → vertigo, nausea, tinnitus, dysarthia, dysphasia, paraesthesia, hemiparesis, visual loss
- Presence of optokinetic nystagmus asymmetry = expanding tumour; lack of optokinetic nystagmus asymmetry = cerebrovascular accident

Ocular features of cerebellar tumour

- Papilloedema → atrophy
- Nystagmus, horizontal, jerk, worse to same side
- Ocular dysmetria, ocular flutter, opsoclonus
- VI palsy

Cortical blindness

Definition

- Bilateral visual loss + normal pupils

Causes

- Children
  - Usually hypoxia
  - Sometimes trauma, epilepsy, infections, drugs, poisons
- Adults
  - Traumatic
  - Injury
  - Post-angiography
- Inflammatory
  - Subacute sclerosing panencephalitis
- Neoplastic
  - Meningioma
  - Glioma
- Vascular
  - Vertebrobasilar or posterior cerebral artery cerebrovascular accident
  - Pre-eclampsia
- Migraine, cerebral oedema, post-ictal
- Toxic
  - Ethanol
  - Methanol
  - Lead
  - Arsenic

Pathogenesis

- Bilateral occipital lobe destruction

Features

- Blindsight
- Anton's syndrome
- Simultanagnosia
- Balint's syndrome
- Visual agnosias
- Riddoch's phenomenon

Blindsight

- A rudimentary visual capacity that survives total destruction of the primary visual cortex

- Persistent visual function in impaired visual hemifield due to occipital pathology
- May be improved by training, which increases conscious awareness of visual function in the hitherto blind area
- Preservation of subcortical visual areas
- No useful visual function

Anton's syndrome

- Denial of blindness in cortical blindness (or any other severely affected part of the visual system e.g. dense cataract)

Simultanagnosia

- In bilateral superior occipital lobe lesions
- Only able to attend to one component of a picture at a time

Balint's syndrome

- Bilateral parieto-occipital infarction → simultanagnosia, optic ataxia (misreading)

Visual agnosias

- Object agnosia = inability to recognise objects
  - Left hemisphere lesion → disruption of internal detail of drawing
  - Right hemisphere lesion → disruption of external configuration
- Prosopagnosia = inability to recognise faces
- Topographic agnosia = inability to find route or objects

Riddoch's phenomenon

- Moving objects may still be perceived but not static objects

Headache and migraine

Headache

- Headaches secondary to ocular causes are very rare (iritis, scleritis, acute glaucoma, orbit)

Mechanism

- Intracranial
  - Pain sensitive structures in head are dura and vessels
  - Dura and vessels above tent supplied by V; pain referred to eye and around
  - Dura and vessels below tent supplied by cervicals I–III; pain referred to neck
- Extracranial
  - Fascia
  - Muscles
  - Mucous membranes
  - Tympanic membrane
  - Extracranial arteries + veins

Characteristics

- Quality, duration, location, periodicity, precipitating and relieving factors, associated phenomena
- Daily pattern, family history
- Eyestrain → headache after using the eyes
- Pain in eye may be due to
  - Local eye disease
  - Part of vascular headache syndrome
  - Referred from intracranial source

Causes

- 90% functional + 10% organic
- Vascular headache of migraine type
- Vascular headache of non-migraine type (systemic infection)
- Hypertension
- Muscle contraction/tension headache
- Delusional/hypochondriacal headache
- Traction/raised intracranial pressure headache (from whatever cause)
- Intracranial inflammation
- Eye disease
- Ear disease
- Nose and sinus disease
- Teeth and temperomandibular joints
- Giant cell arteritis
- Skull disease
- Cranial neuralgias (trigeminal, post-herpetic)
- Cervical spine disease

- Check blood pressure, pulse, neck stiffness, cranial nerves, for homonymous field defect

Painful ophthalmoplegias

- Diabetes (pupil sparing in 80%)
- Aneurysm (posterior communicating artery; pupil involved in 95%)
- Migraine
- Cavernous sinus syndrome
- Parasellar syndrome
- Orbital apex syndrome

Migraine

- Repetitive bouts of headache

Incidence

- Affects 10–20% of the population
- Male > female
- Peak incidence 15–30 years of age
- Childhood migraine → 5% prevalence

Pathophysiology

- Vascular constriction → auras (intracranial)
- Vascular dilatation → headache (extracranial)
- Mediated by kinins, histamine, serotonin
- Five-hydroxytryptamine receptors involved (5-HT produced by platelets)
- Due to deficiency of endorphins
- Prostaglandins and oestrogen also implicated

Classification

- Common
- Classic
- Complicated – cerebral, ophthalmoplegic, ocular/retinal, basilar, acephalgic, abdominal
- Cluster

Common (migraine without aura)

- Vague prodrome, mood change, throbbing headache, fatigue, nausea + photophobia
- ± Conjunctival injection + tearing

Classic (migraine with aura) – 20%

- Prodrome – visual auras (20–40 mins)
  - Scintillating scotoma
  - Fortification spectra (small scotoma near fixation, gradually expanding, bounded by a zig-zag, shimmering image)
  - Others
  - Homonymous field pattern
  - Tunnel vision
  - Altitudinal field loss
  - Heat waves
- Headache – unilateral, throbbing – follows aura
- 80% family history

Complicated

- Cerebral
  - Motor defects
  - Sensory defects
  - Visual field defects
  - Language defects
- Ophthalmoplegic
  - III, IV, VI palsies (usually III), usually transient → diplopia
  - Differentiate other causes of painful ophthalmoplegia
  - Due to swelling of posterior communicating artery or intracavernous carotid artery
  - Occurs in young people, onset < 10 years of age
  - Headache ipsilateral to ophthalmoplegia, occurs at height of pain
- Ocular/retinal
  - Constriction of retinal artery → transient or permanent monocular visual loss
  - Headache may not occur; occurs in young females
  - Repeated episodes may → permanent field loss, AION, CRAO, CRVO
- Acephalgic/acephalic
  - Neurological dysfunction (usually scintillating scotomas), no headache

- Confusion with transient ischaemic attack
- One of the most common forms of migraines seen by ophthalmologists

- Abdominal migraine
  - Children
  - Mesenteric vasospasm → cramps

Cluster

- Severe unilateral throbbing headache with associated facial flushing and tearing, often behind one eye
- Lasts 1–2 hours, ends abruptly
- Common in males in their 30s, usually smokers
- Occur in clusters over days/weeks, then remit for months or years
- May be associated transient Horner's, ? from sympathetic damage from swelling of internal carotid
- Raeder's paratrigeminal neuralgia → painful Horner's syndrome
- May be due to a migranous dilatation of the internal carotid

Management

- Full clinical examination and neurological assessment ± neuroimaging
- Treatment of acute attack
- Prophylaxis

Treatment of acute attack

- Analgesic
  - Paracetomol
  - Asprin
- Antiemetic
  - Metoclopramide
- Ergotamines
  - Give early
  - Contraindicated in cardiac ischaemia, Raynaud's
- Sumatriptan
  - A 5-HT agonist → selective arterial constriction
  - Also contraindicated in ischaemia
  - Fewer side effects

Prophylaxis

- Avoid precipitating factors e.g. prolonged fasting, chocolates, cheese, wine
- Propranolol
- Methysergide (ergot alkaloid); avoid complications by stopping for 1 month every 4–6 months
- Calcium channel blockers
- Amitryptyline
- Lithium carbonate
- Clonidine
- Indomethacin
- Antihistamine
- Anxiolytic

Ocular causes of headache

- Asthenopia
  - Hypermetropia and astigmatism → ciliary muscle contraction
  - Myopia → muscle contraction
    Muscle imbalance
    Especially convergence insufficiency
- Ocular inflammation
  - Uveitis and optic neuritis
- Acute glaucoma
- Disorders of ocular adnexa
  - Lid inflammations
  - Orbital cellulitis
  - Orbital tumour or pseudotumour
  - Zoster

Myopathies

Myasthenia gravis

- An acquired, chronic immunological disorder
- Characterised by muscle weakness as a result of defective neuromuscular transmission
- 50–75% present with ocular signs

Incidence

- Onset at any age
- Rare in childhood or > 70 years
- One in 8 – 20 000
- Female : male = 3 : 2

Pathology

- Acetylcholine receptor sites for neuromuscular junction transmission blocked by immune complexes
- May be caused, unmasked or aggravated by drugs
  - Procainamide
  - Quinine
  - Polymixin
  - Aminoglycosides
  - Steroids
  - Beta-blockers
  - Calcium channel blockers
  - Chloroquine
  - Lithium
  - Phenytoin
  - Cisplatin
  - Magnesium

Clinical

- Ptosis
  - Unilateral or bilateral → variable + fatigueable
  - Cogan's lid twitch – elicited following downgaze back to primary position, – a brief over elevation of the upper eyelid with an upward saccade
- Diplopia
  - Variable + fatiguable → great mimic of CN palsies + supranuclear gaze palsies
  - Variable phorias and tropias
  - Orbicularis weakness
  - No pupil + sensory disturbance
  - Proximal muscle weakness, bulbar weakness – dysphagia, dysarthria, respiratory muscle weakness
  - Graves' disease in 5% (also SLE, RA, Sjögren's, etc.)
  - Thymomas in 12%

Diagnosis

- Clinically
- Pharmacologically
  - Edrophonium chloride/tensilon test – can be false negative
  - Ice test
  - Neostigmine
  - Methylsulphate test
  - Sleep test – resolution of ptosis after 30 mins of sleep
- Serology
  - Acetylcholine receptor antibodies (in one-third)
- Electromyographic repetitive nerve testing
  - Decremental muscle response
- Chest MRI/CT for thymoma

Treatment

- Acetylcholinesterase inhibitors, steroids, immunosuppressives, plasmaphoresis
- Thymectomy
- Monocular occlusion, prisms
- Pyridostigmine
- IV immune globulin

Prognosis

- Ranges
- May be progressive with death within a few years
- Or periods of long remissions

Myotonic dystrophy

Chronic progressive external ophthalmoplegia

Nystagmus and spontaneous eye movement disorders

Definition

- Nystagmus – involuntary rhythmic repeated oscillations of one or both eyes

Pathophysiology

- Multiple factors involved
- Abnormality of tone in one pair of muscles → deviation of eyes
- Saccadic centre then initiates correction
- The slow eye movement is the pathological condition, the jerk is a correction

Description

- Pendular or jerk
- Horizontal, vertical or rotary
- Range of movement – fine < 5 degrees, medium 5–15 degrees, coarse > 15 degrees

Symptoms

- Often asymptomatic
- Decreased visual acuity, due to inability to maintain steady fixation
- Head tilt, to decrease nystagmus
- Oscillopsia (sensation of the world moving → vertigo) in lesions of lower centres
- Head nodding, particularly in congenital nystagmus and spasmus nutans
- Vestibular dysfunction → poor hearing, tinnitus, vertigo

Examination

- Examine first without fixation with Fresnel goggles
- Direct ophthalmoscopy reveals subtle spontaneous globe movements
- Ocular motor recordings → electro-oculogram, infrared tracking, electromagnetic coil recording
- Observe stability in primary and eccentric gaze positions
- Note amplitude, frequency, direction of gaze that induces nystagmus, null point where nystagmus is least evident
- Alexander's law → jerk nystagmus increases in amplitude on gaze in the direction of the fast phase

Important questions

- Congenital or acquired?
- Is the movement characteristic of a specific lesion location?
- True nystagmus or nystagmoid movements (saccadic oscillations)?
- Conjugate (symmetrically affecting both eyes)?
- Slow or fast phases or movements of equal speed?
- Horizontal, vertical, torsional or mixed?
- Mostly conjugate?
- Jerk or pendular (jerk more common)

Classification of nystagmus

■ Physiological	□ End point □ Induced – caloric, rotational, optokinetic, positional
■ Congenital	□ Sensory □ Motor □ Latent □ Monocular nystagmus of childhood □ Spasmus nutans
■ Acquired nystagmus	□ Acquired primary position nystagmus – vestibular □ Seesaw □ Upbeat □ Downbeat □ Gaze evoked □ Periodic alternating □ Dissociated □ Rebound □ Elliptical □ Drug induced □ Oculopalatal myoclonus

11

Induced nystagmus

- Caloric stimulation
  - Unilateral + horizontal; fast component COWS (cold opposite, warm same)
  - Bilateral + vertical; fast component CUWD (cold up, warm down)
- Rotational
  - Fast component in direction of rotation
- Optokinetic
  - Slow eye movement (pursuit) from occipital cortex + fast eye movement (fixation) from frontal cortex
  - Abnormal when asymmetric
- Uses
  - Asymmetric with deep parietal lobe lesions, when drum rotated to side of lesion
  - May be used as a test for hysteria

Congenital nystagmus

- 1 : 6550
- Check for impairment of visual tracking or optic atrophy → imaging if there is
- Conjugate + usually horizontal, small torsional component
- Jerk or pendular
- Commonly a null point
- Head turn or posture to improve vision common
- Fixation usually amplifies the nystagmus
- 15% have strabismus
- Abolishes in sleep
- Present with or without normal acuity
- Horizontal movements consistent in up or downgaze

Sensory (secondary)

- Pendular, erratic, more often vertical
- Often associated with searching eye movements
- Worse if age of onset of visual loss younger, if pathology anterior, visual loss severe
- Develops < 2 years (< 2 years always, 2–6 years sometimes, > 6 years never)
- Afferent pathway defect, does not occur with cortical blindness
- Causes include – cataracts, corneal opacities, chorioretinal colobomas, retinopathy of prematurity, aniridia, optic nerve hypoplasia, albinism, cone dysfunction, achromatopsia, congenital stationary night blindness, Leber's congenital amaurosis

Motor

- Pendular or jerk, remaining horizontal on upgaze
- Attempted distance fixation increases the intensity
- Nystagmus abolished in sleep and anaesthesia
- May be due to brainstem lesion, idiopathic or inherited
- 20% inherited autosomal recessive
- Improve spontaneously up to the age of 10
- Damped by convergence
- Abolished during sleep/voluntary eyelid closure
- May have associated high astigmatism, squint, dissociated vertical deviation, latent nystagmus, worse on attempted fixation, worse with stress

Treatment

- Base-out prisms
- Bimedial rectus recessions with posterior fixation sutures
- Kestenbaum procedure; move eyes in the direction of the head turn, to bring the null zone into the primary position of gaze
- Simultaneous retroequatorial recessions of all four horizontal recti
- Auditory biofeedback training

Latent nystagmus

- Usually a benign entity but can profoundly affect vision
- Elicited by uniocular fixation
- Horizontal jerk nystagmus, fast phase away from the occluded eye

11

- May be cortical in origin
- Almost always associated with esotropia
- Subnormal stereopsis
- Manifest latent nystagmus – a nystagmus characteristic of larent nystagmus but both eyes open
- Amblyopia treatment poorer in larent nystagmus

Treatment
- Cycloplegic refraction
- Strabismus surgery decreases the larent nystagmus

Monocular nystagmus of childhood

- One eye, vertical, small amplitude, rare
- Observed in chiasmal glioma, therefore neuroimaging essential

Spasmus nutans

- Triad of ocular oscillation, head nodding and torticollis; also dissociated nystagmus
- Starts at 4–6 months, better by 3 years
- Cause unknown, may be related to vitamin D deficiency
- Some have perichiasmal tumours
- Nystagmus is asymmetrical, dissociated vertical or horizontal
- Requires neuroimaging because it can be hard to distinguish from monocular nystagmus when monocular

Adult neurological nystagmus

Acquired primary position nystagmus

- Mostly jerk, pendular rare

Peripheral vestibular
- Primary position, horizontal jerk nystagmus
- Often associated vertigo, past pointing, Romberg fall, tinnitus, deafness
- Dampened by fixation
- Maximal early in disease, usually improves, worse with eyes closed
- Hearing good → probably labyrinthitis
- Hearing poor → probably Ménière disease

Central vestibular
- Jerk nystagmus, vertical, horizontal or rotatory
- Unidirectional or bidirectional
- Vertigo, tinnitus + hearing loss less prominent
- Downbeat, upbeat, horizontal

Seesaw nystagmus (chiasmal lesion)

- Disconjugate → one eye elevates and intorts, one eye depresses and extorts
- Slow, pendular nystagmus

Aetiology
- Craniopharyngioma most common pathology

Upbeat nystagmus (cerebellar vermis lesion)

- Lesion somewhere in the posterior fossa
- Fine upbeat nystagmus seen in fourth ventricle lesions

Aetiology
- Multiple sclerosis
- Stroke
- Smoking
- Cerebellar degeneration

Gaze evoked nystagmus (cerebello-pontine angle lesion)

- Coarse jerky nystagmus in one direction, minimal in other direction (low frequency, large amplitude)
- No nystagmus in the primary position
- The most common form of acquired nystagmus
- Patients cannot maintain eccentric gaze
- Caused by a dysfunctional neural integrator

- Advanced age, metabolic, drugs or cerebellar and brain stem posterior fossa lesion, myasthenia

Downbeat nystagmus (cervico-medullary junction lesion)

- Defective vertical gaze holding → eyes drift up, corrective downward saccades
- Common causes are platybasia, Arnold-Chiari malformation, syringomyelia, multiple sclerosis, tumours

Treatment
- Baclofen
- Clonazepam
- Base-out prisms

Periodic alternating nystagmus

- Jerk nystagmus with beats in one direction for 2 mins, slows and then beats in the other direction for 2 mins
- Seen in posterior fossa lesions, especially of the cerebellum, craniocervical junction lesions, and Central nervous system sedatives
- Treatment: Baclofen

Dissociated nystagmus (internuclear ophthalmoplegia)

- Medial longitudinal fasciculus lesions → nystagmus of the abducting eye when gaze is to the side opposite to the lesion
- Asymmetry between the two eyes (in direction or amplitude)
- Causes are spasmus nutans, internuclear ophthalmolplegia, multiple sclerosis, myasthenia gravis, old blind eye, and posterior fossa lesions

Rebound nystagmus

- Induced by peripheral gaze
- Normal patients or cerebellar disease

Elliptical nystagmus

- Pendular nystagmus with a horizontal or vertical component may be oblique/circular/elliptical
- Usually associated with multiple sclerosis

Drug induced

- Barbiturates, tranquillisers, phenothiazines, anticonvulsants
- May cause any kind of nystagmus, often gaze evoked

Oculopalatal myoclonus

- Due to lesion in region of red nucleus, inferior olive and dentate nucleus
- Vertical pendular nystagmus and contraction of soft palate, pharynx or extremity
- Usually occurs several months or years after a brain stem stroke
- Not a true nystagmus

Ocular oscillations

Saccadic intrusions

- Rapid movements of the eye that take it away from fixation
- Square wave jerks
  - An involuntary break in fixation followed by a single refixation movement
  - May be normal in elderly
- Macrosquare wave jerks
  - Larger amplitude
  - Usually multiple
  - Associated with multiple sclerosis
- Macrosaccadic oscillations
  - Occur in runs + increase in amplitude before declining
- Saccadic pulses
  - Saccade away from fixation, rapid drift back
  - Seen in internuclear ophthalmoplegia or normal
- Ocular flutter
  - Saccadic oscillations without intersaccadic interval
  - Equivalent to intention tremor
  - Intermittent + small amplitude
  - Frequently co-exists with ocular dysmetria

- Opsoclonus (saccadomania)
  - Rapid involuntary chaotic eye movements
  - May occur following infectious encephalopathy (benign, self-limiting)
  - Persists during sleep
  - Paraneoplastic effect of neuroblastoma (infants) (may also have myoclonus + ataxia → dancing eyes and dancing feet)
  - Visceral carcinoma (adults)

Ocular dysmetria

- Overshoot or undershoot in saccade followed by several oscillatory movements in the new position before coming to rest in the desired position
- Equivalent to past pointing

Ocular bobbing

- Fast down, slow up (cw downbeat nystagmus)
- Occurs in grave neurological disease → cerebrovascular accident, hydrocephalus, metabolic
- Typical – absence of horizontal gaze = pontine lesion
- Atypical – full horizontal gaze; seen in metabolic encephalopathy

Ocular dipping

- Slow downward movement with rapid return
- Poor localising value
- Seen in unconsciousness

Ping-pong gaze

- Horizontal ocular deviations that reverse every few seconds
- Bilateral hemispheric damage
- Seen in unconsciousness

Superior oblique myokmia

- Isolated monocular intermittent superior oblique contraction
- Aetiology benign; occasionally in multiple sclerosis
- Treat with carbamazepine, SO tenotomy + IO recession

Convergence retraction 'nystagmus'

- Rostral/posterior midbrain
- Elicited by attempted elevation
- Features of Parinaud's syndrome
- Contraction of the horizontal extraocular muscles on attempted upgaze
- Not a true nystagmus

Roving eye movements (searching)

- Blind children

Cerebellar eye signs

- Ocular dysmetria
- Ocular flutter
  - Disease of the pause cells in the pons unleash burst of saccades → horizontal, small amplitude, high frequency movements
  - Seen in children with neuroblastoma, adults with carcinoma of lung, breast, ovary (paraneoplastic)
- Opsoclonus; if the above movements are multidirectional
- Nystagmus
- Skew deviations

Aetiology of neurological nystagmus

- Structural lesions (tumours, etc.)
- Metabolic disease
- Leukodystrophies
- Neurodegenerative disorders
- Trauma

Management of nystagmus

- Refraction and spectacles, if appropriate
- Schooling arrangements
- Medical
  - Rarely useful

- Baclofen
- 5-hydroxytryptophan
- Optical – biofeedback
- Contact lenses
- Prisms, to move null point to primary position

- Surgical
  - Correct strabismus
  - Recess all four recti to reduce muscle power
  - Move null point to primary position by appropriate recess-resect (Kestenbaum/Anderson procedure)
  - Retrobulbar botulinum

Optic chiasm syndrome

Causes of chiasmal lesions

- Congenital
  - chiasmal dysplasia
- Traumatic
- Inflammatory
  - Chiasmal neuritis
  - Basal meningitis/arachnoiditis optica chiasmatica (syphilis, TB, sarcoid)
- Neoplastic
  - Pituitary adenoma
  - Craniopharyngioma, meningioma, glioma, pinealoma, metastases, meningioma
  - 25% of all brain tumours occur in chiasmal area
- Vascular
  - Aneurysms of internal carotid artery
  - Thrombosis, arteriosclerosis, arterial compression
- Demyelination
- Miscellaneous
  - Empty sella syndrome
  - Hydrocephalus
  - Suprasellar arachnoid cysts
  - Pituitary apoplexy (sudden increase in size of pituitary tumour, often secondary to haemorrhage)
- The inflammatory lesions cause third ventricle dilation + pressure effects

Symptoms

- Headache, features of pituitary dysfunction, epilepsy
- Decreased visual acuity, field loss, loss of depth perception, diplopia (± with free floating nasal hemifields, hemifield slide phenomenon), post-fixational blindness, seesaw nystagmus

Signs

- Colour loss occurs first
- Field loss
- Usually bitemporal hemianopias; may be homonymous hemianopia, prechiasmal field loss
- Optic atrophy, papilloedema in only 5%, afferent pupil defect, seesaw nystagmus, III, IV, V, VI pareses
- Optic atrophy occurs 2 years after onset of visual loss; initially it is temporal pallor, later bow tie, later total

Radiology

- Plain skull x-ray – double floor of sella; enlarged sella; erosion of clivus
- Tomography
- Angiography – to exclude aneurysm
- CT Scan and MRI scan

Pituitary adenoma

- Constitute 10% of all intracranial tumours
- Chromophobe adenoma – most common, they enlarge the sella and expand above dural roof
- Eosinophil adenoma – produce growth hormone or prolactin; seldom expand above sella
- Basophil adenoma – rare, small, do not enlarge sella

Treatment

- Radiotherapy
- Surgery
  - Transsphenoidal or transfrontal
- Bromocryptine
  - For treatment of all micro prolactin adenomas (within sella turcica)

11

  - For treatment of macro prolactin adenomas (extended beyond sella turcica)

Craniopharyngioma

- More common in children
- Slow growing tumour → develops from remnants of Rathke's pouch along pituitary stalk
- Affects chiasm from above

Empty sella syndrome

- In 30% of people, an arachnoid diverticulum extends through the foramen where the pituitary stalk passes
- If this enlarges, it compresses the pituitary and produces enlargement of the sella on x-ray

Parasellar meningiomas

- Middle-aged females
- Asymmetrical bitemporal visual field loss
- May enlarge during pregnancy

Chiasmal gliomas

- Mostly in children
- Complex field defects

Diplopia

Definition

- Subjective sensation
- Due to simultaneous perception of two images of one object as a result of similar images stimulating non-corresponding retinal areas (cw visual confusion, where dissimilar images stimulate corresponding retinal areas)

Classification

- Physiological
- Pathological
  - Monocular
  - Binocular – horizontal, vertical, torsional, or combination
- Horizontal diplopia is crossed in exotropia, uncrossed in esotropia

Physiological diplopia

- Occurs in front of and behind Panum's fusional area, where objects project on to non-corresponding retinal points
- In front of Panum's area → crossed diplopia, beyond Panum's area → uncrossed diplopia

Causes of diplopia

- Monocular
- Binocular

Monocular (25%)

- Any beam splitting opacity in optical axis
- Corneal – irregular astigmatism, scarring, keratoconus
- Iris – iridectomy
- Lens – subluxation, tilting, vacuoles, lens opacities
- Vitreous – gas bubbles
- Retina – macular cysts
- Central nervous system – scotoma bisecting fixation of one eye
- Psychogenic

Binocular (75%)

- Orbital – mass displacing globe (tumour, mucocoele, haematoma, pseudotumour)
- Muscle – restrictive myopathy, myasthenia gravis, broken down phorias; overcorrected squint (hemiretinal trigger activation), dysthyroid eye disease
- Ocular motor nerves – III, IV, VI palsies
- Central nervous system supranuclear – convergence insufficiency, divergence paralysis, skew deviation, superior oblique myokymia, cerebral diplopia, any cause of raised intracranial pressure, internuclear ophthalmolplegia, multiple sclerosis
- Primary overaction syndromes – primary oblique overaction, convergence spasm, superior oblique myokmia (intermittent, repetitive firing of the SO), ocular neuromyotonia (failure of III or IV to relax), oculogyric

crisis (tonic supraduction with neck hyperextension, seen in phenothiazine overdose)
- Drugs – > 250 drugs described as causing diplopia (psychiatric, antibiotics, anti-inflammatory, antiTB)

Clinical approach
- History
  - True diplopia or not
  - Horizontal, vertical, oblique
  - Monocular or binocular
  - In which gaze position is it worst (= field of action of palsied muscle)
  - Distance and near different
  - Duration
  - Intermittency
  - Progression
  - Associated symptoms
  - General health
  - Medications
- Examination
  - Signs that suggest restriction; proptosis, injection, enophthalmos, ptosis, etc.
  - Abnormal head posture; ocular motility; measure deviation with prisms and Maddox rod
  - Bielschowsky head tilt
  - Diplopia fields with red filter; Hess chart; single binocular vision field; forced duction test; tensilon test
  - IOP measurement with eccentric gaze (> 4 mmHg increase suggestive of restriction in the opposite muscle)

Management
- Monocular
  - Define and treat the cause
  - Refraction and contact lens; add + 0.50 or –1.00 to eliminate light splitting and reduce visual acuity slightly
  - Miotics → pin hole effect
- Binocular
  - Define and treat the cause
  - Relief from symptoms – monocular occlusion
  - Ground-in prisms – maximum of 7–8D
  - Fresnel prisms (will not eliminate torsional diplopia) – more dioptre possible but blurred vision as prism increases
  - Squint surgery ± adjustable sutures – Primary goal → alignment in primary position and down reading gaze, secondary goal fusion in horizontal gaze
  - Botulinum toxin – injection of the ipsilateral agonist to prevent muscle contracture

Diplopia following unilateral cataract

- Long-standing unilateral cataract or uncorrected aphakia → loss of central fusion with intractable diplopia following vision restoration
- Prevention – correct as soon as possible after onset of cataract

Treatment
- Not possible to test binocular potential before surgery
- Therefore, do not do primary IOL implant but fit a contact lens and defer secondary IOL implant until binocular potential is confirmed
- If diplopia is confirmed
- Correct any residual refractive error
- Adjustable sutures
- Prisms, orthoptic training

Central fusion disruption

Aetiology
- Head injury, cerebrovascular accident, midbrain neoplasm, viral infection
- Area of damage somewhere in the midbrain

Clinical features
- Diplopia in all directions of gaze
- Second image is constantly moving (bobbing)

Treatment
- Monocular occlusion

11

Third (oculomotor) nerve palsy

Anatomy

- Nucleus
  - Ventral to aqueductal grey matter, at level of superior colliculus
  - Warwick's model
  - Single nucleus for both levators
  - Superior rectus supplies contralaterally
  - Oculomotor + accessory oculomotor (Edinger-Westphal) nuclei
- Within brainstem
  - Fibres pass ventrally through red nucleus and medial cerebral peduncle (pyramidal tract)
- Within posterior cranial fossa
  - Passes under origin of posterior cerebral artery
  - Runs parallel with and lateral to posterior communicating artery
  - Runs between edge of tentorium cerebelli and uncus of temporal lobe
- Within cavernous sinus
  - Pierces dura
  - Runs in roof of cavernous sinus
- Within orbit
  - Divides into superior and inferior divisions in superior orbital fissure
  - Superior division → levator + superior rectus
  - Inferior division → medial rectus, inferior rectus, inferior oblique and parasympathetic root of ciliary ganglion

Causes of III palsy

■ Nuclear	□ Daroff's rules – nuclear lesion must include contralateral superior rectus palsy + bilateral ptosis □ Uncommon
■ Within brain stem	□ Cerebrovascular accident, tumour, demyelination □ Benedikt's syndrome – in association with red nucleus → contralateral ataxia + intention tremor □ Weber's syndrome – in association with pyramidal tract → contralateral hemiplegia
■ Within posterior cranial fossa	□ Traumatic – three sites of injury are emergence from brainstem, against tent, entry into superior orbital fissure □ Inflammatory – basilar meningitis (TB and syphilis) □ Neoplastic □ Posterior communicating artery (or posterior cerebral, superior cerebellar, or basilar artery) aneurysms □ Uncal herniation with raised intracranial pressure – tumour (Hutchinson's pupil), cerebrovascular accident
■ Within cavernous sinus	□ Traumatic – carotid-cavernous fistula □ Inflammatory – Tolosa-Hunt syndrome, herpes zoster, temporal arteritis, syphilis

11

- Neoplastic – nasopharyngeal carcinoma, sphenoid ridge meningioma, lymphoma, metastases, multiple myeloma, neurofibroma
- Carotid artery aneurysm (characteristically superior division 3 only)

- Within orbit
  - Inflammatory – pseudotumour, cellulitis, myositis
  - Neoplastic
  - Dysthyroid eye disease
- Pupil sparing III palsy
  - Pupillomotor fibres run in outer layer of nerve nearer blood supply; therefore, spared in 80% of ischaemic III paresis and affected in 90% of compressive III paresis
  - Pupil sparing may also occur in cavernous sinus syndrome
  - Common causes of ischaemic III palsy – diabetes mellitus, collagen diseases, temporal arteritis, syphilis, migraine
- Other causes of III palsy
  - Congenital – always pupil sparing; extraocular muscle involvement variable; ? due to developmental defect of III
  - Toxic neuritis – lead, arsenic, alcohol, carbon monoxide
  - Viral neuritis – Guillain-Barré syndrome, Fisher's syndrome, herpes zoster
- Causes of painful III palsy
  - Not a very helpful sign because it occurs in – diabetes (pupil sparing) and aneurysms (not pupil sparing)
- Congenital III palsy
  - Rare, but account for half of congenital ocular palsies
  - ± Associated neurological deficits
  - Aberrant regeneration common
  - Pupil involvement variable
- Ophthalmoplegic migraine

Features of palsy

- Partial or complete
- Limited ocular motility
- Incomitant squint – eye is exotropic and hypotropic with ptosis (down + out)
- Diplopia, ± abnormal head posture
- ± Dilated pupil

Pupil involved vs pupil sparing

- Complete III palsies → nerve compression by posterior communicating artery aneurysm → do an MRA
- Pupil sparing palsies
  - Complete loss of somatic function → usually benign
  - Partial loss of somatic function → not always benign → may be an evolving compressive lesion

Aberrant regeneration

- Weeks to months after III palsy recovery
- Slow, progressive damage of III may allow some fibre regeneration

11

- The sprouting fibres may innervate muscles other than those they originally innervated
- Mechanism ? aberrant regeneration, ? ephaptic transmission, ? central reorganisation
- Seen after compressive or traumatic III palsy, never after ischaemic III palsy
- Lid retraction on adduction (inverse Duane's)
- Lid retraction on depression (pseudo von Graefe's sign)
- Pupil constriction on adduction, elevation, depression
- Lid retraction and adduction on attempted upgaze
- Persistent vertical gaze limitation caused by co-contraction of SR + IR

Investigations

- Ischaemic work-up (if pupil sparing and > 45 years)
  - BP
  - Full blood count
  - ESR
  - Syphilis serology
  - Blood sugar
  - Collagen screen
- Radiology work-up
  - If a pupil sparing III does not show significant recovery in 3–4 months
  - Vessel angiography – if MRA negative but clinical suspicion high
  - CT, MRI, MRA (with attention to the Circle of Willis, can detect aneurysms as small as 3 mm, which is usually enough)
- Lumbar puncture
  - May be helpful if neuroimaging normal → inflammation/neoplasia/ haemorrhage

Treatment

- Identify and treat the underlying cause
  - If ischaemic (pupil sparing), do only ischaemic work-up and straight x-rays
  - If negative, > 50 years, isolated, history of diabetes hypertension or migraine, watch for 2–3 months
  - Proceed to CT scan and angiography if it fails to improve or shows signs of aberrant regeneration
- Wait 6 months for recovery; use alternate occlusion if necessary
- Surgery
  - Lateral rectus recession + medial rectus resection for exotropia
  - Superior oblique (loop) recession for hypotropia
  - Frontalis sling for ptosis; before of weak Bell's phenomenon
  - ± Superior oblique resection + insertion at medial rectus insertion if no recovery (Scott procedure)

Fourth (trochlear) nerve palsy

Anatomy

- Longest and thinnest cranial nerve, only nerve to emerge from the dorsal aspect of the brain
- Nucleus at caudal end of III nucleus, at level of inferior colliculus
- Fascicles cross at anterior medullary velum, emerge dorsally
- Winds around tectum, between superior cerebellar and posterior cerebral arteries; reaches free edge of tentorium, enters dura
- Runs through cavernous sinus, superior orbital fissure
- Runs above cone → superior oblique

Causes of palsy

- Congenital – 50%
- Acquired – 50%
  - 40% Trauma – may have been trivial, bilateral IV always due to trauma (contusion of anterior medullary velum)
  - 30% Miscellaneous or undetermined – surgery, zoster, multiple sclerosis, encephalitis, decompensated congenital

11

- 20% Ischaemic – diabetes mellitus, arteriosclerosis
- 10% Neoplasms – posterior fossa tumours, metastases, nasopharyngeal carcinoma
- 1% Aneurysms – posterior cerebral artery aneurysm
- May be mimicked by myasthenia, dysthyroid eye disease

Features
- 88% unilateral, 12% bilateral (10–30%)

Symptoms
- Vertical diplopia
- Worse in field of action of superior oblique (depression, adduction, intorsion)

Signs
- Abnormal head posture
- Chin down, face turn to opposite side, head tilt to opposite side
- Check old photos
- Hypertropia, worse on adduction
- Superior oblique underaction + inferior oblique overaction later, with V pattern eso on downgaze
- Excyclotorsion; measure with Maddox rods; worse on downgaze; torsional cyclotropia < 5 degrees → no symptoms, > 8 degrees always → symptoms
- Positive Bielschowsky head tilt – hypertropia increased on tilt to same side
- Hess chart, single binocular field
- To check for IV palsy in a patient with III palsy – abduct good eye and look down; intorsion of involved eye confirms IV function
- Bilateral SO palsy → left hypertropia in left gaze and right hypertropia in right gaze

Investigations (very low yield)
- If isolated – full blood count, CT, chest x-ray, blood sugar, tensilon test
- If negative, 90% will spontaneously improve within 6 months

Treatment
- Congenital – treat as soon as possible to permit development of single binocular vision and avoid abnormal head posture
- Acquired – treat conservatively × 6 months with occlusion or prisms

Surgery
- Unilateral incomitant < 10 D hypertropia
  - Ipsilateral inferior oblique weakening (disinsert, resuture to globe on equator half way between inferior rectus and lateral rectus)
- Unlilateral incomitant > 15 D hypertropia (= contracted ipsilateral superior rectus)
  - ± Ipsilateral superior rectus adjustable suture recession
  - Or contralateral inferior rectus adjustable suture recession
- Unilateral comitant
  - Contralateral inferior rectus adjustable suture recession
- Bilateral
  - Harada-Ito tuck procedure
  - Split tendon, tighten anterior third; this avoids vertical disturbance and corrects torsion only
  - Do only on one eye; move anterior third 5 mm anteriorly and 8 mm laterally

Superior oblique myokymia

- Intermittent repetitive firing of the superior oblique muscle

Aetiology
- Unknown, ? inflammatory or vascular lesion of IV nucleus

Features
- Benign, self-limiting, occurs in healthy young adults
- Intermittent episodes of vertical or torsional oscillopsia

Treatment
- Reassure, carbamazepine

- ± Superior oblique + inferior oblique recessions

Sixth (abducens) nerve palsy

Anatomy

- Nucleus in pons, beneath floor of fourth ventricle; facial nerve fibres loop around
- Fibres course ventrally, exit at ponto-medullary junction
- Nerve ascends ventral face of pons
- Crossed by posterior communicating artery
- Pierces dura of clivus, runs up against clivus
- Traverses inferior petrosal sinus, runs under petroclinoid ligament, enters cavernous sinus
- Enters orbit within annulus at superior orbital fissure
- Innervates lateral rectus

Causes of VI palsy	
■ Congenital	□ Rare □ Due to hypoplasia or aplasia □ Almost never occur in isolation □ Möbius syndrome – bilateral VI + VII
■ Idiopathic	□ Up to 30% of cases □ Transient, benign, ? viral
■ Increased intracranial pressure	□ False localising sign □ Seen in 30% of cases of benign increased intracranial pressure
■ Brainstem syndromes	□ Cerebrovascular accident, tumour, demyelination □ May involve – any of the following: □ Ipsilateral V, VI, VII, VIII palsies □ Cerebellum → cerebellar signs □ Oculosympathetic central neurone → ipsilateral Horner's □ PPRF → ipsilateral conjugate gaze palsy □ Medial longitudinal fasciculus → ipsilateral INO □ Pyramidal tract → contralateral hemiparesis (Millard-Gubler syndrome) □ Raymond's syndrome: VI paresis, contralateral hemiparesis □ Foville's syndrome: horizontal conjugate gaze palsy, ipsilateral V, VII, VIII, ipsilateral Horner's
■ Cerebellopontine angle tumour	□ Acoustic neuroma, meningioma □ Triad of decreased hearing, V palsy, VI palsy, gaze evoked nystagmus
■ Clivus	□ Nasopharyngeal carcinoma □ Clivus chordoma □ Basal meningitis

11

- Gradenigo's syndrome
  - Localised inflammation or extradural abscess secondary to complicated otitis media at tip of petrous bone → pain in V distribution, VI palsy, decreased hearing
  - Pseudo-Gradenigo's syndrome – due to nasopharyngeal carcinoma
- Cavernous sinus
  - Traumatic: Carotid – cavernous sinus fistula
  - Inflammation: Tolosa-Hunt syndrome, herpes zoster, temporal arteritis, syphilis
  - Neoplastic: Nasopharyngeal carcinoma, sphenoid ridge meningioma, lymphoma, metastases, multiple myeloma, neurofibroma
  - Vascular: Carotid artery aneurysm
- Orbital apex
  - Inflammatory: Pseudotumour, cellulitis, myositis
  - Neoplastic
  - Dysthyroid eye disease
- Isolated ischaemic (microvasculopathy) VI palsy
  - Up to 30% of cases – most common cause
  - Diabetes mellitus
  - Collagen disease
  - Temporal arteritis
  - Syphilis
- Toxins
  - Lead, arsenic, alcohol, carbon monoxide

Features
- Uncrossed horizontal diplopia, worse for distance
- Esotropia, abduction weakness, worse for distance
- Abnormal head posture – head turn
- ± Pain

Special tests
- Hess chart
- Red filter
- Maddox rod
- Forced duction test
- Electrooculogram

Approach
- Isolated VI in older adults → usually benign, resolve spontaneously (microvascular or idiopathic)
- Lack of spontaneous recovery → neuroimaging
- Under the age of 40 → neuroimaging ± tensilon test
- Young adults + adolescents → multiple sclerosis
- Children → remember leukaemia, post-viral (4-month resolution)

Investigations
- Blood pressure
- Full blood count
- Blood glucose
- ESR
- Syphilis serology
- Antinuclear antibodies
- MRI

Causes of abduction weakness
- VI palsy
- Duane's syndrome
- Möbius syndrome
- Myasthenia gravis
- Dysthyroid eye disease
- Spasm of near reflex
- Old blowout fracture + restrictive myopathy

First 6 months
- Occlusion of involved eye and 6 D base-out Fresnel prism in front of uninvolved eye

- Forced adduction fixation of uninvolved eye → decreased innervation and tonus to medial rectus of involved eye
- Therefore, decreased medial rectus contracture

- Occlusion of involved eye and temporal hemiocclusion of uninvolved eye
  - Same principle
- If possible, base-out prism in front of both eyes → single binocular vision
- Botulinum in medial rectus of involved eye to relax it, if there is no sign of recovery within 1 month
- 50% show spontaneous recovery

After 6 months/recovery static

Surgery

- If some LR function – ipsilateral LR resection + bilateral MR recession
- No LR function
  - Recess MR behind equator (15 mm) with adjustable suture + resect LR (10–12 mm) to hold eye in midline
  - Recess contralateral MR (9 mm), to prevent long-term contracture
  - This achieves alignment + central 25 degrees SBV
- Transposition of vertical recti + MR adjustable suture recessions
- Hummelscheim procedure
  - Temporal halves of vertical recti transpositioned to LR insertion + MR recessed/botulinum to MR
  - This achieves central 50–80 degrees single binocular vision
- Jensen's procedure
  - Loops of temporal halves of vertical recti secured to loops of halved LR + MR recessed
  - This achieves central 40 degrees single biocular vision

11

Seventh (facial) nerve palsy

Anatomy

- A motor + sensory nerve
- Facial muscles, taste, secretomotor fibres
- Seventh nerve
  - Main motor nucleus in lower pons (also parasympathetic + sensory nuclei)
  - Fibres emerge from anterior surface of the brain stem, passing laterally in the posterior cranial fossa, enter the internal acoustic meatus with VIII, then the facial canal, running through the inner ear, emerge from skull through stylomastoid foramen
  - Pass through parotid, divides into five branches: temporal, zygomatic, buccal, marginal mandibular, cervical
- Nervus intermedius
  - Tearing, salivation, taste
  - Visceral motor + sensory
  - Fibres run with VII, join VII after posterior bend
  - Gives off greater petrosal nerve + tympanic branches, continues as chorda tympani
  - Greater petrosal nerve travels forward and medially through petrous temporal, passes under trigeminal ganglion in Meckel's cave
  - Deep petrosal nerve joins it at foramen lacerum
  - Passes into pterygoid canal and pterygopalatine fossa as Vidian nerve, enters pterygopalatine ganglion
  - Lacrimal post-ganglionic fibres join maxillary nerve, enter orbit in zygomatic branch, pass up lateral wall of orbit, join lacrimal nerve

Disorders of underactivity

- Supranuclear lesions
  - Lesion of facial portion of precentral gyrus → contralateral facial weakness, lower face

  - Tarsorrhaphy not usually required
  - Extrapyramidal disorders (Parkinson's, progressive supranuclear palsy) → minimal spontaneous facial expression, reduced blink rate, normal volitional movements
- Brain stem lesions
  - Ipsilateral facial weakness, upper + lower face
  - Vascular lesions + tumours
  - Other signs of pontine lesions also present
  - Möbius syndrome – aplasia of VII nuclei in the brainstem, with bilateral VI palsies, deafness, lingual palsy, extremity defects
- Peripheral lesions
  - Lower motor neurone lesions – numerous causes
  - Ipsilateral facial weakness

Bell's palsy

- Most common facial neuropathy
- Diagnosis of exclusion
- Sudden onset facial paresis ± pain

Aetiology

- Autoimmune, viral, ischaemia
- Progressive facial weakness > 3 weeks → investigate for neoplasia
- 84% spontaneous recovery, usually within 3 months

Treatment

- Prednisolone orally

Ramsay-Hunt syndrome

- Geniculate ganglionitis
- Herpes zoster involving VI + VIII → Bell's palsy

Neoplasms

- Acoustic neuroma, meningioma, nasopharyngeal carcinoma
- At cerebellopontine angle, in facial canal, parotid gland
- MRI with contrast

Infectious agents

- Meningitis
- Lyme disease
- Herpes zoster
- HIV seroconversion
- Guillain-Barré

Sarcoidosis

- The cranial nerve most commonly involved, usually at parotid
- Usually bilateral

Trauma

- Battle's sign → ecchymosis over the mastoid

Congenital

- Birth trauma

Melkersson-Rosenthal syndrome

- Recurrent unilateral or bilateral facial nerve paralysis accompanied by paralysis and furrowed tongue
- Idiopathic, starts in childhood.

Crocodile tears

- Aberrant VII regeneration → tearing when eating

Treatment

- Corneal exposure
  - Tears, lubricants
  - Lid taping
  - Moisture chambers
  - Tarsorrhaphy
  - Botulinum toxin inducing ptosis
- Neurotrophic keratitis → treat aggressively (presence of V palsy)
- Surgery
  - Gold eyelid weights → ptosis
  - Reinnervation with hypoglossal to facial anastamosis

Disorders of overactivity

- Essential blepharospasm
  - Episodic contraction of orbicularis

- Onset 40–60 years of age
- Idiopathic, ? basal ganglia dysfunction
- Meige's syndrome → facial grimacing + other movements associated with blepharospasm
- Rule out causes of reflex blepharospasm e.g. dry eyes, meningeal irritation
- Treatment: Haloperidol, clonazepam, bromocriptine are rarely helpful
- Botulinum toxin into orbicularis

- Hemifacial spasm
  - Unilateral, episodic spasm of facial musculature
  - Lasts seconds to minutes
  - Aetiology: previous VII injury, cerebellopontine angle tumour, anomalous angle vessels
  - Treatment: Medical as above, Botulinum toxin, facial neurectomy, myectomy
- Facial myokmia
  - Signifies intramedullary lesions of the pons
  - Pontine glioma (children), multiple sclerosis (adults)

Combined oculomotor palsies

Causes

- Cavernous sinus syndrome
- Superior orbital fissure syndrome
- Orbital apex syndrome
- Guillain-Barré syndrome
- Fisher's syndrome
- Myasthenia gravis
- Dysthyroid eye disease

Causes of painful ophthalmoplegia

Common	Diabetes mellitus, aneurysm, migraine
Intracranial	Inflammatory – petrositis, basal meningitis (TB, sarcoid, syphilis)
	Neoplastic – pituitary adenoma, meningioma, nasopharyngeal carcinoma, craniopharyngioma, metastases, clivus chordoma
	Vascular – cranial arteritis, aneurysm, diabetes mellitus, migraine
Cavernous sinus and superior orbital fissure	Inflammatory – sarcoidosis, herpes zoster, sphenoid sinus mucocoele, Tolosa-Hunt syndrome
	Neoplastic – nasopharyngeal carcinoma, lymphoma, metastases
	Vascular – carotid cavernous fistula, aneurysm, thrombosis
Orbit	Inflammatory – contiguous sinusitis, cellulitis, mucormycosis, pseudotumour
	Neoplastic – glioma, meningioma, lymphoma, metastases

11

Cavernous sinus syndrome

Causes

- Traumatic
- Inflammatory – mucormycosis, herpes zoster, contiguous sinusitis, Tolosa-Hunt syndrome
- Neoplastic – nasopharyngeal carcinoma, pituitary adenoma, meningioma, sphenoid sinus carcinoma, lymphoma, metastases
- Vascular – carotid cavernous fistula, thrombosis, aneurysm

Features

- III, IV, VI, Vabc (posterior)
- III, IV, VI, Vab (middle)
- III, IV, VI, Va (anterior)

Superior orbital fissure syndrome

- Causes: As above
- Features: III, IV, Va, VI, + proptosis

Orbital apex syndrome

Causes

- Inflammatory – contiguous sinusitis, cellulitis, myositis, pseudotumour, dysthyroid eye disease, mucormycosis
- Neoplastic – glioma, lymphoma, meningioma, metastases

Features

- II, III, IV, Va, VI + proptosis

Tolosa-Hunt syndrome

Aetiology

- Unknown
- Part of pseudotumour spectrum
- Aseptic thrombosis of cavernous sinus

Pathology

- Non-specific granulomatous inflammation of cavernous sinus and/or superior orbital fissure

Features

- Painful cavernous sinus syndrome; diagnosis of exclusion
- II and VII may also be involved
- Dramatic response to steroids (48 hours prednisone test)
- No age or sex preponderance
- whites > blacks
- Acute onset, spontaneous remissions, recurrences

Special investigations

- Diagnosis of exclusion, after:
- Full blood count, ESR, syphilis serology, collagen screen
- CSF cytology and chemistry
- X-ray skull
- Angiogram, CT scans
- ENT consultation

Treatment

- Systemic steroids

Prognosis

- Good – remains localised, recurrences occur

Carotid cavernous fistula

Aetiology

- Congenital rare
- Arteriosclerotic 25%
- Traumatic 75%

Pathology

- Carotid artery ruptures into cavernous sinus
- Rupture of small meningeal arterial branches supplying dural wall of cavernous sinus

Features

- Carotid rupture → pulsating proptosis, bruit, conjunctival chemosis, dilated episcleral veins, elevated IOP, hypoxic ocular sequelae
- Meningeal artery rupture – occurs in middle-aged females, → unilateral red eye with minimal proptosis, ± antecedent VI palsy + headache

Treatment

- Surgical – embolisation, carotid ligation, balloon angioplasty

Supranuclear and internuclear gaze palsies

Anatomy

- As a general rule
  - Vertical eye movements → midbrain
  - Horizontal eye movements → pons
- Frontal eye field and frontomesencephalic pathway
  - Centre located in area 8 frontal premotor cortex, at posterior end of second frontal convolution
  - Pathway passes through internal capsule, crosses in lower midbrain, descends in contralateral pontine paramedian reticular formation to level of 6 nucleus
  - Stimulation → conjugate saccadic gaze to opposite side
- Occipital eye field and occipitomesencephalic pathway
  - Centre located in area 19 parieto-occipital visual association cortex
  - Pathway connects bilaterally with both fields, passes through internal sagittal striatum medial to optic radiations
  - Does not cross, reaches ipsilateral pontine paramedian reticular formation
  - Stimulation → smooth pursuit to same side
- Vestibular mechanism
  - Horizontal semicircular canals orientated 30 degrees to the horizontal with capsule anterior
  - Movement of endolymph towards ampulla → stimulation of that ampulla
  - Connected with ipsilateral vestibular nucleus, then to contralateral pontine paramedian reticular formation
  - Stimulation/disturbance of tonic balance → deviation of eyes to opposite side
- Vergence mechanism
  - Convergence or divergence, stimulated by retinal image disparity
  - Reflex originates in area 19, descends direct to 3 nucleus
- Vertical eye movements
  - Precise pathway incompletely understood
  - Corresponding areas in area 8, pretectal area + 3 and 6 nuclei
- Pontine paramedian reticular formation
  - Final common pathway for horizontal eye movements
  - Connects with ipsilateral 6 nucleus + contralateral 3 nucleus via medial longitudinal fasciculus
- Cerebellar role
  - Vermis concerned with control of saccadic and vestibulo-ocular reflexes
  - Hemispheres concerned with control of smooth pursuit and fixation

Classification of conjugate horizontal eye movements

- FEM (Fast Eye Movements)
  - 300–700 degrees/second
  - Saccadic/voluntary
  - Originate in area 8
- SEM (Slow Eye Movements)
  - 20–50 degrees/second
- Pursuit SEM
  - Originate in area 19
- Vergence SEM
  - Originate in area 19
- Vestibular SEM
  - Originate in horizontal semicircular canals

11

Function of eye movements	
Saccades	To bring object of interest onto fovea
Nystagmus	Reset the eyes during prolonged rotation
Smooth pursuit	Hold image of a small moving target on fovea
Optokinetic	Hold images steady on the retina during sustained head rotation
Vestibular	Hold images steady during brief rotation
Vergence	To move the eyes in opposite directions so that the images of a single object are placed on both foveas

Testing for eye movements

- FEM
  - Command right, left, up, down
  - OKN strip to opposite direction
  - Corrective phase in Báràny chair rotation and calorics
- SEM pursuit
  - Follow finger right, left, up, down
  - OKN strip to same side
- SEM vestibular
  - Doll's eye movements; rotate head to the same side + rotation of eyes to opposite side
  - Báràny chair rotation; rotate chair to same side → rotation of eyes to opposite side + compensatory FEM to same side (therefore, also tests saccades)
  - Calorics
- SEM vergence
  - Converge and diverge on accommodative target

Classification of gaze palsies

- Horizontal
- Vertical

Horizontal

- Conjugate
  - Supranuclear gaze palsies – saccadic; smooth pursuit
  - Pontine paramedian reticular formation lesion
  - Chronic progressive external ophthalmoplegia
- Disjugate
  - Internuclear ophthalmoplegia
  - Infranuclear ophthalmoplegia/palsy (III, IV, VI)
  - Myopathy (myasthenia gravis, dysthyroid eye disease)

Vertical

- Parinaud's syndrome
- Progressive supranuclear gaze palsy (Richardson-Steele-Olszewski syndrome)
- Oculogyric crisis
- Skew deviation

Supranuclear gaze palsies

Saccadic palsy

Causes

- Destructive
  - Acute cerebrovascular accident
  - Tumour
  - No voluntary FEM to opposite side; eyes deviate to same side; in cerebrovascular accident, after 3 days the contralateral area 8 assumes control for both sides
  - Therefore, bilateral voluntary movements are re-established with gaze paretic nystagmus during recovery

- Irritative
  - Tumour
  - Seizure focus
- Features are vice versa

Features unilateral
- Deviation of eyes to ipsilateral or opposite sides
- No voluntary fast eye movements
- Asymmetric optokinetic nystagmus testing
- Intact pursuit SEM and vestibular SEM

Features bilateral
- Loss of saccades in all directions
- Spasm of fixation due to release of latent occipital fixation

Smooth pursuit palsy

Causes
- Unilateral – cerebrovascular accident or tumour
- Bilateral – sedatives, fatigue, diffuse cerebral disease, inattention

Features
- Absent SEM pursuit; saccadic pursuit substitutes
- Intact FEM and vestibular SEM

Congenital ocular motor apraxia

- Deficient voluntary and pursuit horizontal gaze, vertical movements normal, vestibular SEM normal, random and pursuit horizontal movements seen
- Voluntary horizontal gaze achieved by head thrust toward desired direction + eyelid closure, to utilise opposite vestibular SEM effect

Acquired ocular motor apraxia (Roth-Bielschowsky syndrome)

- Features as above
- Due to extensive bilateral cerebral and upper brainstem disease
- Causes include
  - Balint's syndrome
  - Huntington's chorea
  - Multiple sclerosis
  - Wilson's disease
  - Lipidosis
  - Spinocerebellar degeneration
  - Wernicke's encephalopathy

Pontine paramedian reticular formation lesion/pontine conjugate gaze palsy

Causes
- As for internuclear ophthalmoplegia
  - Multiple sclerosis
  - Cerebrovascular accident

Features
- Absent voluntary FEM, pursuit SEM and vestibular SEM to same side (vestibular SEM involved if lesion is at level of VI nucleus, spared if lesion is above VI nucleus)
- Intact SEM vergence

Internuclear ophthalmoplegia

Causes
- Lesion of medial longitudinal fasciculus
  - Multiple sclerosis – young patients; bilateral internuclear ophthalmoplegia
  - Cerebrovascular accident – elderly patients; unilateral internuclear ophthalmoplegia

Features
- Deficient adduction on same side; but can converge
- Abducting nystagmus of opposite side; due to simultaneous interruption of inhibitory fibres to ipsilateral III medial rectus sub-nucleus
- Subtle internuclear ophthalmoplegia → less nystagmus with optokinetic nystagmus to same side
- Anterior internuclear ophthalmoplegia – lesion superior near III nucleus, therefore, affects also SEM convergence
- Posterior internuclear ophthalmoplegia – lesion inferior away from III nucleus, therefore, SEM convergence unaffected

- Bilateral internuclear ophthalmoplegia may also have nystagmus on upgaze and skew deviation

WEBINO syndrome

- Wall-eyed bilateral internuclear ophthalmoplegia; indicates long-standing condition
- One and a half syndrome – lesion of pontine paramedian reticular formation and ipsilateral medial longitudinal fasciculus → pontine conjugate gaze palsy to same side + internuclear ophthalmoplegia on gaze to opposite side – only able to abduct opposite eye with nystagmus; but can converge both eyes
- Paralytic pontine exotropia – seen in first few days after onset of one and a half syndrome; opposite pontine paramedian reticular formation is unopposed, therefore, opposite eye remains in tonic abduction/exotropia

Parinaud's syndrome (also known as dorsal midbrain syndrome, pretectal syndrome, Sylvian aqueduct syndrome)

Pathogenesis

- Lesion is in periaqueductal grey matter in rostral midbrain
- Features are due to desynchronisation of excitation and inhibition

Causes

- Age
    - 0 – Congenital aqueductal stenosis
    - 10 – Pinealoma
    - 20 – Head trauma
    - 30 – Vascular malformation
    - 40 – Long-standing multiple sclerosis
    - 50 – Basilar artery stroke

Features

- Vertical upgaze palsy; vertical voluntary FEM and pursuit SEM deficient, SEM vestibular intact
- Normal downgaze + eyes straight in primary
- Paresis of convergence, spasm of near reflex
- Convergence retraction nystagmus on attempted upgaze (due to impaired facilitation of agonist elevators and failure of suppression of antagonist depressors); elicited with downward rotation of optokinetic nystagmus tape
- Lid retraction (Collier's sign)
- Light near dissociation of pupil
- ± Skew deviation, III palsy and IV palsy
- ± Papilloedema

Progressive supranuclear gaze palsy (Richardson-Steele-Olszewski syndrome)

- Degenerative disease, affects older people, progressive dementia, dead within 5 years
- Features similar to Parkinson's, but no resting tremor
- Affects vertical gaze initially, mostly downgaze, later also horizontal, eventual global paralysis of gaze
- SEM vestibular better than FEM voluntary and SEM pursuit

Oculogyric crisis

- Upward
    - Causes– Parkinson's (post-encephalitic), phenothiazine toxicity
    - Features – tonic vertical deviation of eyes, overcome with vestibular SEM
- Downward
    - Causes – Neonates, coma, metabolic encephalopathy, hydrocephalus

Skew deviation

- An acquired vertical + torsional ocular deviation from supranuclear dysfunction
- Comitant or noncomitant
- May be seen with internuclear ophthalmoplegia and/or vertical gaze-evoked nystagmus

Aetiology

- A lesion anywhere in the midbrain
- Pons
- Medulla
- Vestibular nerve or inner ear

Vergence abnormalities

- Spasm of near reflex
    - Seizure
    - Head injury
    - Parinaud's syndrome
    - Craniocervical junction lesion
    - Hysteria
- Convergence paresis
    - Senescence
    - Multiple sclerosis
    - Cerebrovascular accident
    - Encephalitis
- Divergence paresis
    - Following trauma
    - Lasts a few months, diplopia for distance

Parkinson's disease

- Degenerative disease of extrapyramidal system, with imbalance between dopaminergic and cholinergic systems within the basal ganglia
- Triad of tremor, rigidity and akinesia
- Ocular signs – blepharospasm, decreased blinking
- Cogwheel saccades; initially for upgaze, later for horizontal gaze and down gaze
- Smooth pursuit replaced by micro saccades
- Convergence paresis
- Oculogyric crisis

Wernicke's encephalopathy

- Due to thiamine deficiency (especially in alcoholics)
- Ophthalmoplegia, mental confusion, gait ataxia
- Ocular motor
    - Abduction weakness
    - Gaze-evoked nystagmus
    - Internuclear ophthalmoplegia
    - Upbeat nystagmus
    - Impaired vestibule-ocular reflex
    - Horizontal and vertical gaze palsies that may progress to total ophthalmoplegia
- Bilateral but may be asymmetric
- Lesions occur throughout brainstem, thalamus, hypothalamus and cerebellum
- Treatment: Thiamine replacement
- Korsakoff's syndrome
    - A more severe thiamine-deficiency encephalopathy with memory loss and permanent oculomotor abnormalities

Vascular malformations

Incidence

- Usually congenital + familial
- Male > female slightly

General

- 90% supratentorial
- 70% cortical
- 20% deep
- 10% posterior fossa or dura

Clinically

- Intracranial bleed usually the first presentation
- Seizures, headaches, focal deficits
- Intracranial bruit

Neuro-ophthalmic manifestations

- Depend on location
- Occipital lobe – visual symptoms + migraine-like headache
- Hemispheric – homonymous field defects
- Brain stem – non-specific diplopia, nystagmus, gaze palsies, anisocoria, motor nerve palsies

Diagnosis

- Ruptured – unenhanced CT
- MRI – small arterovenous malformations
- Cerebral angiography

11

Treatment

- Surgical resection, ligation of feeder vessels, embolisation

Prognosis

- 20% mortality with bleeding

Pupil

Anatomy

- Parasympathetic → accommodation + constriction (fibres 30 : 1)
- Sympathetic → dilatation

Parasympathetic pathway

- Retinal photoreceptors → optic nerves → optic tract → brachium of colliculus superior → pretectal nuclei → intercalated neurones → ipsilateral + contralateral Edinger-Westphal nuclei; rostral accomodation, caudal pupil constriction
- Cranial nerve III (fibres superficial in nerve) → inferior division → inferior oblique branch → ciliary ganglion
- Ciliary ganglion → short ciliary nerves → sphincter pupillae + ciliary muscles

Sympathetic pathway

- Posterolateral hypothalamus → tegmentum of mesencephalon + pons → lateral medulla → ciliospinal centre of Budge C8–T2
- Ciliospinal centre → ventral nerve roots (T1 mainly) → white rami communicantes → paravertebral sympathetic chain → inferior + middle cervical ganglia → superior cervical ganglion
- Superior cervical ganglion → plexus around carotids → cavernous sinus →
  - Va → nasociliary nerve → long ciliary nerves → dilator pupillae
  - III → inferior division → ciliary ganglion → short ciliary nerves → orbital vasomotors

Near synkinesis pathway

- Occipital area 19 → III nuclei → accommodation, miosis, convergence

Pharmacology

- Parasympathetic end plate – acetylcholine
- Sympathetic end plate – noradrenaline
- Miotics/parasympathomimetics
  - Direct action on sphincter receptor site – pilocarpine
  - Cholinesterase inhibitors – physostigmine, neostigmine, edrophonium – phospholine iodide
- Mydriatics
  - Parasympatholytics: Competitive binding with acetylcholine receptors – atropine, homatropine, scopolamine, cyclopentolate, tropicamide
  - Sympathomimetics: Act directly on muscle – phenylephrine, epinephrine

Physiologic anisocoria

- Hippus = physiologic pupillary unrest
- Pupil size varies from 0.5–9.0 mm
- Physiologic (simple, essential) anisocoria present in > 20% of people, usually < 1 mm difference
- Anisocoria is the same in light and dark
- Tadpole pupil – benign, sectoral dilatation, seen in migraine sufferers
- Midbrain corectopia – oval pupils in midbrain disease

Baseline pupil size

- Most important influence → ambient light
- Sleep → less sympathetic, smaller pupils
- Increasing age → smaller
- Excitement, arousal → sympathetic, larger
- Raised IOP → pupil enlargement, ischaemic iris
- Anoxic brain injury → midbrain ischaemia, pupil dilation

- Extremely small pupils → pontine infarct, narcotic abuse
- Extremely large pupils → pharmacological blockade

Afferent pupil defect

- Relative afferent pupil defect (Marcus Gunn pupil)
- Amaurotic pupil = Marcus Gunn pupil in a NPL eye
- Kestenbaum's number = difference in size of pupils in mm with light shone in each eye + other eye covered

Tonic pupil (Holmes-Adie pupil)

Aetiology

- Ciliary ganglion/post-ganglionic parasympathetic pupillomotor damage – trauma, surgery, inflammation e.g. viral (zoster, others), grant cell arteritis, diabetes, alcoholism, syphilis, amyloidosis

Features

- Young healthy females 70%, unilateral in 80–90%
- Dilated pupil, poor response to light, slow response to near with slow redilatation (tonic)
- Sluggish, segmental pupillary responses to light
- Slow accommodation for near and slow relaxation of accommodation
- Vermiform movements of iris border, seen on slit lamp
- Lentiform astigmatism (same side where vermiform movements seen)
- ± Areflexia – diminished deep tendon reflexes (Holmes-Adie syndrome); ± decreased corneal sensation
- ± Other autonomic dysfunction (orthostatic hypotension, familial dysautonomia)
- 0.125% pilocarpine → intense constriction due to denervation hypersensitivity

Treatment

- Pilocarpine drops for cosmetic purposes as necessary

11

Argyll-Robertson pupil (light-near dissociation)

Aetiology

- Neurosyphilitic lesion rostral to III nucleus, involving light pathway but not accommodation pathway
- 20% of patients with neurosyphilis have Argyll-Robertson pupil
- Also seen in diabetes, multiple sclerosis, chronic alcoholism and midbrain tumours

Features

- Seeing eye, bilateral, asymetrical
- Small irregular pupils
- Poor dilatation in response to mydriatics and in dark (poor dilatation differentiates from pseudo Argyl-Robertson pupil)
- Variable iris atrophy

Horner's syndrome

- Any lesion along the oculosympathetic pathway
- Ipsilateral ptosis and miosis

Aetiology

- No cause found in 40% cases
- Most common causes are tumours (metastases and carcinoma bronchus), cluster headaches, surgery
- First order neurone
  - cerebrovascular accident
  - Tumours
  - Demyelinating diseases
  - Syringobulbia/myelia
  - Cervical disc disease
- Second order neurone
  - Pancoast's tumour
  - Lymphoma
  - Secondaries
  - Trauma
  - Surgery
- Third order neurone
  - Carotid artery degeneration
  - Cluster headache
  - Nasopharyngeal carcinoma
  - Lymphoma

- Thrombosis
- Aneurysm in cavernous sinus

Features

- Ptosis (mild – due to palsy of Muller's muscle)
- Miosis (mild, more apparent in dim light)
- Light + near pupillary reactions intact
- Upside-down ptosis (lower lid)
- Conjunctival congestion
- Anhidrosis (= lesion central, first order lesion – cervical spinal cord to superior cervical ganglion)
- Iris heterochromia (if congenital)
- Slowed accommodation for distance
- Transient ocular hypotony
- Increased skin temperature
- Increased flushing
- Epiphora and nasal stuffiness

Pharmacologic tests

- Wait 45 mins for the effect
- Cocaine 10%
  - To diagnose whether or not there is a Horner's pupil
  - Increases noradrenaline by decreasing its uptake → pupil dilation
  - Dilates a normal pupil, but fails to dilate a Horner's pupil
- Hydroxyamphetamine 1%
  - To diagnose whether the lesion is pre-or post-ganglionic
  - Releases noradrenaline from the nerve
  - Preganglionic → nerve intact → pupil dilates
  - Post-ganglionic → nerve damaged → fails to dilate
- Phenylephrine 2–5%
  - → Marked dilatation on denervated side due to denervation supersensitivity

Sweat tests

- Starch and iodine
- Friction test
  - Clean forehead and prism bar with alcohol
  - Stroke prism bar down forehead
  - Anhydrosis → less friction

Special investigations

- Chest x-ray (lordotic views)
- Angiography
- X-ray cervical spine and base of skull
- CT + MRI

Treatment

- ± Phenylephrine drops
- Treat the cause

Congenital Horner's syndrome

Aetiology

- Birth trauma → brachial plexus injury
- Neuroblastoma → arising in the sympathetic chain in the chest
- Irritative sympathetic lesion, which may precede Horner's syndrome → Claude Bernard syndrome
  - Pupil dilatation
  - Lid retraction
  - Conjuctival blanching

Raeder's syndrome

Definition

- Painful post-gangliotic Horner's syndrome

Features

- Group 1 – associated multiple para sellar cranial nerve palsies (III, IV, V, VI)
- Group 2 – typical cluster headache history
- Group 3
  - Atypical cluster headache history, ± Va paraesthesia
  - Common – unilateral headache and Horner's

Management

- Group 1 – complete work-up to exclude tumour
- Group 2 – treat headache
- Group 3 – exclude hypertension + sinusitis; treat headache; watch for other signs

11

Mydriasis

Causes

- III nerve palsy (Note: Hutchinson's pupil in uncal herniation)
- Claude-Bernard syndrome
- Trauma
  - Contusion paresis of sphincter
  - Sphincter tears
  - Damage to short ciliary nerves
- Tonic pupil
- Instillation of mydriatic

Pharmacologic tests

- Pilocarpine 0.125% → constriction in tonic pupil
- Pilocarpine 1% → constriction in III palsy, no constriction in mydriatic use

Causes of light near dissociation pupil

- Argyll-Robertson pupil – loss of pretectal light input to Edinger-Westphal nucleus
- Parinaud's dorsal midbrain syndrome
- Adie pupil – ciliary ganglion
- Aberrant III regeneration, therefore, pupil constricts with adduction
- Severe afferent visual deficit
- Amyloidosis
- Myotonic dystrophy

Hutchinson's pupil

- Comatose patient with unilaterally dilated, poorly reactive pupil
- Due to ipsilateral, expanding, intracranial mass (e.g. tumour, subdural) → uncal herniation → III entrapment → pupillomotor fibre damage

Disorders of accommodation

- Inadequate
  - Ageing
  - III palsy
  - Anticholinergic treatment
  - Local ocular injury or disease
- Spasm
  - Parinaud's syndrome
  - Functional
  - Drugs – sulphonamides, tetracycline, chlorpromazine, promethazine

Visual fields

- The first consideration in patients complaining of visual loss but with normal VA

Definition

- Portion of space where objects are visible to the steadily fixating eye
- Traquair's 'island of vision surrounded by a sea of blindness'
- Kinetic (isopter) perimetry → horizontal section
- Static (profile) perimetry → vertical section
- Visual acuity at fixation 6/6
  - 2 degrees from fixation 6/9
  - 5 degrees from fixation 6/24
  - 20 degrees from fixation 6/60

Terminology

- Absolute field defect – no stimulus perceived in the affected area
- Relative field defect – bigger, brighter stimuli seen; smaller, dimmer not seen
- Scotoma – area of depressed visual function surrounded by normal
- Arcuate area – the part of the field arching from the blind spot, above + below fixation to end at the horizontal raphe
- Central scotoma – involves fixation only
- Cecocentral scotoma – extends from fixation to blind spot
- Paracentral – region next to fixation
- Pericentral – region symmetrically surrounding fixation
- Ring scotoma – seen in retinitis pigmentosa
- Nasal step scotoma – glaucoma
- Temporal crescent scotoma – occipital lobe pathology

- Arcuate – corresponds to and represents nerve fibre bundle loss
- Altitudinal – a more extensive arcuate defect involving two quadrants in the superior or inferior hemifield
- Quadrantinopia – one quadrant of visual field involved
- Hemianopia – one half of visual field involved (nasal or temporal)
- Homonymous – same side of visual space affected in each eye
- Bitemporal – opposite temporal sides
- Complete – entire visual field
- Incomplete – a portion of visual field spared
- Congruity – a tendency for homonymous defects to be symmetrical, same size, location, shape in each eye's field

Examination
- Confrontation
- Instruments

Confrontation

- Red confrontation
- Simple confrontation
- Simultaneous double stimulation (two hands)
- Out line perimetry

Instruments

Kinetic
- Goldmann perimeter
  - Primarily for peripheral field
  - Standardisation
  - Use test object just detectable at temporal horizontal meridian in 25 degree isopter, 15 degrees above and 15 degrees below
  - 12e usually used for central field + 14e for peripheral field

Amsler grid
- Qualitative assessment of central 10 degree field
- When held 30cm from patient, each square subtends 10 degrees

Normal field

Monocular
- Temporal 100 degrees
- Inferior 75 degrees
- Superior 60 degrees
- Nasal 60 degrees
- Blind spot 15.5 degrees temporal to fixation, 1.5 degrees below horizontal, 5.5 degrees wide × 7.5 degrees high
- Central field < 30 degrees
- Peripheral field > 30 degrees

Binocular
- Central circular binocular field extending 60 degrees around fixation
- Temporal 30-degree crescent on either side

Factors affecting size of field
- Age, pupil diameter, media opacities, refractive error, aphakia

Localisation of fibres in visual pathway

- First order – bipolar cells
- Second order – ganglion cells → lateral geniculate nucleus
- Third order – lateral geniculate nucleus → occipital cortex

Retina (optic fibre bundle)
- Field + retina → inverted + reversed relationship
- Three types of nerve fibre bundles → three types of nerve fibre bundle defects
  - Arcuate superior + inferior – Bjerrum arcuate scotoma – 15 degrees from fixation; Seidel scotoma – comma-shaped extension of the blind spot (defect in proximal nerve fibre bundle); nasal step of Ronne – respects horizontal meridian (defect in distal nerve fibre bundle); isolated scotoma within Bjerrum scotoma – defect in intermediate nerve fibre bundle

11

- □ Papillo macular bundle – central; caecocentral; paracentral scotoma (65% of total fibres)
- □ Radiating superior + inferior → edge-shaped temporal scotoma

Nerve

- Fibres grouped in same pattern
- Macular bundle occupies temporal sector

Chiasm

- Anterior knee of Willebrand – inferior nasal fibres
- Posterior knee of Willebrand – superior nasal fibres
- Macular fibres cross mainly posteriorly

Optic tract

- Superior fibres medial
- Inferior fibres lateral

Lateral geniculate nucleus

- Superior fibres medial
- Inferior fibres lateral
- Macular fibres in posterior two-thirds
- Crossed fibres in layers 1, 4, 6
- Uncrossed fibres in layers 2, 3, 5

Optic radiation

- Traverses temporal, parietal and occipital lobes
- Inferior fibres loop into temporal lobe in Meyer's loop
- Superior fibres pass straight through parietal lobe

Striate cortex

- Area 17; identified macroscopically by stria of Gennari on calcarine sulcus
- 83% central 30 degrees
- Macular fibres on posterior 2.5 cm pole
- Upper fibres above, lower fibres below
- Temporal crescent is represented most anteriorly
- Blood supply of macular area is a watershed area, with dual blood supply – terminal branches of posterior cerebral artery + deep optic branch of middle cerebral artery

Abnormal visual fields

Optic nerve lesions

- Classic defect is central/centrocecal scotoma due to susceptibility of central small calibre papillomacular bundle fibres
- Nerve head pathology e.g.papilloedema, myelinated fibres → enlarged blind spot
- Due to disruption of peripapillary elements, ? due to Stiles-Crawford effect, ? due to peripapillary hypermetropia
- Vascular lesions → altitudinal hemianopia
- Three main nerve fibre bundle defects
  - □ Arcuate – superior + inferior: Bjerrum arcuate scotoma –15 degrees from fixation; Seidel scotoma – comma-shaped extension of the blind spot (defect in proximal nerve fibre bundle); nasal step of Ronne – respects horizontal meridian (defect in distal nerve fibre bundle); isolated scotoma within Bjerrum scotoma – defect in intermediate nerve fibre bundle
  - □ Papillo macular bundle → central, caecocentral or paracentral scotoma (65% of total fibres)
  - □ Radiating superior + inferior → edge-shaped temporal scotoma

Factors suggestive of optic nerve problem in a visual field defect

- Decreased VA
- Light brightness – less bright with optic nerve lesions
- Colour desaturation
- Light stress test – decreased recovery in macular defect
- Afferent pupil defect – optic nerve
- Visually evoked potential
- Disc evidence

Chiasmal lesions

- Bitemporal hemianopias
- Below
  - □ Pituitary tumours – chromophobe adenoma, acidophil adenoma, basophil adenoma

- Above
  - Anterosuperior – meningioma
  - Posterosuperior – craniopharyngioma
- Anterolateral (anterior junction syndrome, involving anterior knee) – meningioma of tuberculum sellae
- Posterolateral (posterior junction syndrome, involving posterior knee) – posteriorly expanding pituitary tumour
- Quadrantinopias will not extend to the blind spot in chiasmal lesions but will in optic nerve lesions

Binasal haemianopia

- Due to glaucoma, retinoschisis, optic nerve disease, multiple sclerosis, ectatic internal carotids

Post-chiasmal lesions

- Occipital lobe > parietal lobe > temporal lobe > optic tract > lateral geniculate nucleus
- Contralateral homonymous hemianopias
- May be total
- May be partial
  - Congruous – posterior/optic radiation, where fibres are close together
  - Incongruous – anterior/optic tract, where fibres are far apart (the more posterior the lesion, the more congruous)
- Optic tract – incomplete incongruous homonymous heminaopia with macular splitting
- Lateral geniculate nucleus – lesions are rare
- Optic radiation
- Internal capsule
  - Congruous homonymous hemianopia with macular splitting
  - Other features are contralateral hemiplegia (i.e. same side as hemianopia)
  - Lesions – vascular, of lenticulostriate and lenticulo-optic branches of middle cerebral artery
- Temporal lobe
  - Meyer's loop involvement → superior quadrantanopia (pie in the sky); usually incongruous or complete homonymous hemianopia with macular splitting
  - Other features – formed visual hallucinations, olfactory hallucinations, déjà vu, ipsilateral III palsy
- Parietal lobe
  - Involves superior fibres → inferior quadrantanopia; usually complete homonymous hemianopia with macular splitting

Other features

- Dominant left visual agnosias (alexia, agraphia, apraxia)
- Non-dominant right neglect of left visual space
- Absent optokinetic nystagmus on rotating drum to same side
- Contralateral decreased sensation from cranial nerve V (corneal)
- Lesions – tumour : vascular (middle cerebral artery) = 1 : 1

Occipital lobe and cortex

- Congruous homonymous hemianopia, ± macular sparing (macular sparing = at least 5 degrees spared; majority do not have macular sparing)
- Superior quadrantanopia – inferior lip of calcarine fissure
- Inferior quadrantanopia – superior lip of calcarine fissure
- Other features
  - Riddoch's phenomenon (perception of motion in a field blind to form)
  - Anton's syndrome (denial of any visual defect)
  - Tunnel vision
  - Unformed visual hallucinations
  - Optokinetic nystagmus asymmetry = tumour, not ischaemia
  - Mechanism of macular sparing – ? only apparent due to shift of fixation, ? dual blood supply
  - Lesions – vascular : tumour 4 : 1

11

Causes of tunnel vision

- Glaucoma
- Retinitis pigmentosa
- Optic atrophy – post-papilloedema
- Hyaline bodies of optic disc – disc drusen
- Bilateral occipital infarct with macular sparing
- Hysteria (true tunnel vision)
- Chronic papilloedema

Neuroimaging

CT

- With contrast, improves visualisation of most tumours, large vessels + inflammation

MRI

- Imaging of choice for intracranial soft tissue
- Signal intensity related to tissue water content (magnetically alterable proton density)
- Contrast between white and grey matter considerably greater than CT
- Air, cortical bone, fast flowing fluids (e.g.blood in an artery) → give no signal → black (unless special pulse sequences used)
- Magnetic field causes tissue protons to align parallel with field
- Field switched off, protons return to position, releasing energy
- T1 – the spin-lattice time: Time taken for 63% of tissue protons to realign with the main magnetic field
- T2 – the spin-spin relaxation time: Time taken for 63% of protons to align perpendicular to magnetic field
- Different tissues have different T properties
- T1 weighted scans
    - Excellent anatomical detail, poor on pathology
    - White matter → bright
    - Water, CSF, vitreous → dark
    - Orbital fat → bright (can be 'fat suppressed')
    - Optic nerve + muscles → darker
- T2: CSF, water, vitreous → bright
- Contrast enhancement: Gadolinium – inflammation, tumour, broken down blood brain barrier enhanced

MRI vs CT

- Advantages of CT
    - Images faster, good for children, brain abscess
    - Better for bone, calcification, acute intracranial haemorrhage
    - Cheaper
- Disadvantages of CT
    - Poor soft tissue contrast
    - Cannot scan sagitally
    - Side effects of IV contrast
    - Accumulated radiation dose

12

Trauma

Chemical burns	361	Orbital fractures	365
Blunt trauma	363	Intraocular foreign bodies	367
Penetrating eye injuries	363	Uveal trauma	369
Stabbed orbit	365	Traumatic retinopathy	371

Chemical burns

Alkali burns

Agents

- Important alkalis: Ammonium hydroxide (most damaging), sodium hydroxide, potassium hydroxide, magnesium hydroxide and calcium hydroxide (least damaging)
- Ammonium hydroxide is biphasic; therefore, it penetrates rapidly and a rise in aqueous pH occurs within seconds

Biochemical changes

- Saponification of fat components of cell membranes → cell death in all layers (epithelium to lens)
- Degradation of collagen and proteoglycans – by hydroxide, which is fixed in the stroma; ulceration therefore continues indefinitely

Burn severity

- Depends on – degree of chemical penetration (nature of chemical and time of exposure) + area of chemical exposure
- Grade 1 – Clear cornea + no limbal ischaemia
- Grade 2 – Hazy cornea but visible iris details + < one-third limbal ischaemia
- Grade 3 – No iris details + one-third to half limbal ischaemia
- Grade 4 – Opaque cornea + > half limbal ischaemia

Clinical stages

Acute (0–1 week)

- Disruption of cell membranes → loss of cells (epithelium to ciliary body and lens)
- Thrombosis → ischaemia
- Trabecular damage → rise in IOP

Early reparative (1–3 weeks)

- Corneal ulceration starts
- Epithelial regeneration
- Corneal vascular and fibroblast invasion

Late reparative (> **3 weeks)**

- Continued corneal ulceration
- Progressive corneal vascularisation and scarring
- Complications
  - Symblepharon
  - Tear film deficiency (obstruction of lacrimal secretory ducts, destruction of glands of Krause and Wolfring, destruction of goblet cells, destruction of meibomian and tarsal glands)
  - Neurotrophic keratitis (loss of corneal innervation)

- Persistent corneal oedema from endothelial destruction
- Trabecular injury → glaucoma, ciliary body injury → phthisis bulbi, cataract

Treatment

- First aid
- Medical treatment
- Surgical treatment

First aid

- Irrigation with any non-toxic liquid for 30 mins minimum

Medical treatment

- Topical steroids
  - Decrease inflammation + decrease neutrophil infiltration
  - Decreased collagen synthesis + decreased keratocyte migration → decreased healing
  - Use for 7–10 days, then stop
- Ascorbic acid
  - Normally secreted by ciliary epithelium, necessary for collagen production, inhibits neutrophil activity
  - Administer topically (10% drops 2 hourly) + orally (2 g four times daily)
- Tetracycline
  - Inhibits collagen and neutrophil activity
  - Administer topically (ointment) + orally (doxycycline 100 mg 12 hourly)

Surgical treatment

- Early
  - Advancement of Tenon's capsule
  - Amniotic membrane grafting
- Late
  - Division of symblephara and conjunctival bands
  - Conjunctival or mucous membrane grafts
  - Correction of eyelid deformities
  - Keratoplasty; delay for at least 6 months
  - Keratoprosthesis
  - Limbal stem cell transplantation

Acid burns

Agents

- Sulphuric acid (most damaging)
- Chromic acid
- Hydrochloric acid
- Nitric acid
- Acetic acid

Biochemical changes

- Effect of H+, heating effect, explosive effect → coagulation and precipitation of proteins (collagen and proteoglycans)

Burn severity

- Less than alkalis, due to coagulation of epithelium → barrier to penetration + buffering action of corneal stroma

Clinical stages

Acute (0–1 week)

- Coagulation and opacification of surface epithelium
- Stromal penetration → stromal, iris, lens injury
- Elevated IOP may occur due to collagen shrinkage

Early reparative (1–3 weeks)

- Vessel and fibroblast invasion
- Stromal ulceration in more severe burns

Late reparative (> 3 weeks)

- Usually recovered by 3 weeks
- ± Progressive vascularisation and scarring
- Complications as for alkali burns

Treatment

- As for alkali burns

12

Blunt trauma

- Eyelid ecchymosis
- Conjunctival haemorrhage
- Corneal abrasion
- Corneal endothelial injury
- Hyphaema
- Angle recession (tear between medial + circular fibres of ciliary muscle; risk of subsequent glaucoma is 6–9% if > 2 quadrants are recessed)
- Cyclodialysis
- Iridodialysis
- Iris sphincter tears
- Vossius ring
- Corneoscleral rupture
- Scleral rupture
- Cataract
- Lens subluxation or dislocation
- Vitreous haemorrhage
- Retinal oedema
- Retinal dialysis
- Retinal haemorrhage
- Horseshoe retinal tear
- Choroidal rupture
- Optic nerve injury
- Blowout fracture

Penetrating eye injuries

Epidemiology

First World (UK, Europe, USA)

- Male : female 80 : 20
- Most common in third, second and first decades
- Left eye > right eye
- Accidental – industrial accidents, domestic accidents and sport injuries
- Assaults – knives, bottles

Clinical assessment

Classification

- Sharp
- Blunt
- Missile (IOFB)
- Grade 1 injury – anterior segment without lens involvement
- Grade 2 injury – anterior segment with lens involvement
- Grade 3 injury – posterior segment without anterior segment involvement
- Grade 4 injury – posterior segment with anterior segment involvement
- Anterior segment = cornea ± sclera adjacent to limbus without vitreous presentation or prolapse
- Posterior segment = sclera with vitreous presentation or prolapse

Predictors of final visual outcome

- Grade of injury
  - 1 > 2 > 3 > 4
  - Anterior scleral > posterior scleral
  - Shorter laceration > longer laceration
- Type of injury
  - Sharp > blunt
- Initial VA
  - Better > worse; if ≥ or = 5/200, 97% chance that the final visual acuity will be as well
- Afferent pupil defect
- Type of lens injury
  - Subluxation or loss of lens through the wound has a worse prognosis
- Vitreous haemorrhage
  - Absent > present, mild > severe (obscuring view with indirect)
- Ultrasound appearances
  - (Better) normal → vitreous haemorrhage → limited retinal detachment → extensive retinal detachment → haemorrhagic retinal detachment (worse)
- ERG
  - Normal > diminished > absent
- VEP
  - Normal > diminished > absent
- Two most important predictors of final visual outcome in posterior segment injuries
  - Presence or absence of afferent pupil defect

12

  - Diminished or absent visually evolved potential

Pathology of scleral rupture following blunt injury

- Usually superior + anterior, usually superotemporal quadrant
- Predictors – VA PL or NPL, IOP < 10 mmHg, hyphaema, chemosis

Pathology of posterior segment injuries

- ± Retinal and vitreous incarceration or loss in the wound
- Immediate vitreous haemorrhage
- Posterior vitreous detachment after 10–14 days
- Fibroblast invasion from the wound + glial proliferation after 4 weeks
- Traction retinal detachment after 7–11 weeks; this may become rhegmatogenous

Management of anterior segment injuries

- Primary corneoscleral repair immediately
- If < 8 hours old, iris is not ischaemic or infected, then reposit iris; otherwise excise
- Corneal sutures should be deep, interrupted, not too tight (astigmatism), not too loose (watertight)
- Corneal wound < one-third of corneal diameter → low incidence of astigmatism
- Corneal wound > one-third of corneal diameter → high incidence of astigmatism
- Anterior synechiae predispose to vascularisation of corneal wound
- Anterior synechiae in periphery may be prevented by peripheral iridectomy
- If there is a cataract with intumescence, rupture of the capsule, subluxation, or dislocation, remove the lens either at the primary repair or after 3–5 days
- Otherwise the timing of the lens extraction is not important, except in young children
- ± Capsule supported IOL, irts fixated lens, suture
fixated IOL, contact lens, or uncorrected aphakia following lens removal
- Only implant IOL when blood-aqueous barrier has returned to normal; this may take up to 2 years; but usually within 4 months
- Penetrating keratoplasty is indicated if a corneal scar involves the visual axis
- Children < 8 years may develop suppression, amblyopia, and squint

Management of posterior segment injuries

- Primary scleral repair as soon as possible; no prophylactic cryotherapy, as this worsens the vitreous traction
- Vitrectomy at 10–14 days; this timing is important; it allows time for the posterior vitreous detachment, it decreases the risk of intra-operative haemorrhage and it intervenes before traction retinal detachment occurs
- The purpose of vitrectomy is to remove the fibrous scaffold and to prevent the development of traction retinal detachment
- ± Prophylactic encircling scleral band
- ± Retinal detachment repair if necessary
- ± Drugs to decrease fibroblast activity in the vitreous – steroids, 5-fluorouracil

Intraocular foreign body

- Vitrectomy + removal ASAP

Endophthalmitis

- Incidence after penetrating injury 2–12%
- Prophylaxis

12

  - Subconjunctival antibiotics at the time of the primary repair
  - Oral antibiotics
- Treatment
  - as for endophthalmitis

Excision of eye – indications

- Immediately – NPL + massive globe disruption
- Delayed
  - Persistent NPL + less massive disruption
  - Persistent PL only + massive globe disruption
  - Endophthalmitis → NPL

Stabbed orbit

Incidence

- 12% of stab orbits have intracranial involvement
- Of those, 50% show no fracture on x-ray but do show fracture on CT scan

Complications

- False aneurysm of Circle of Willis (30% of cases; 80% mortality)
- Carotid cavernous sinus fistula
- Frontal lobe contusion
- CSF fistula
- Meningitis, brain abscess

Management

- If suspected, do a CT scan
- If CT scan shows a fracture
  - Prophylactic triple antibiotics
  - Carotid angiogram (? at 14 days, ? earlier)
  - Refer neurosurgery

Orbital fractures

Classification

- External (involving rim)
  - Inferolateral
  - Inferomedial
  - Superior
- Blowout
  - Floor
  - Medial wall
- Orbital apex + optic canal

External

Midfacial fractures

- Involve the maxilla; often complex + asymmetric; extend posteriorly through the pterygoid plates
- Treatment: Dental stabilisation + open reduction
- Le Fort I: Low transverse maxilla – no orbital involvement
- Le Fort II: Pyramidal configuration, involving nasal, lacrimal + maxillary bones, including floor of orbit
- Le Fort III: Entire facial skeleton detached from skull; orbital floor, medial + lateral orbital walls

Zygomatic fractures

- Usually involve the orbital floor, but may not involve the orbit at all
- Can cause a downward displacement of the lateral canthus
- Treatment: May not be required, or open reduction + internal fixation

Orbital apex fractures

- Usually occur in conjunction with fractures of the rest of the skull
- May involve optic canal, superior orbital fissure
- Damage to optic nerve through ischaemia, bone compression, oedema

Treatment

- Steroids ivi – pulsed over 3 days
- Medial wall decompression within 5 days
- Anecdotal evidence of benefit

Orbital roof fractures

- Uncommon
- Blunt trauma or missiles
- Brain + frontal sinuses may be involved

- Complications: CSF rhinorrhoea, pneumocephalus, intracranial injuries, ptosis, EOM imbalance

Treatment

- Neurosurgical decompression

Medial orbital fractures

- Often have a traumatic telecanthus → transnasal wiring
- Surgery seldom necessary unless the MR is entrapped

Mechanism of blowout fractures

- Blunt injury → increased intraorbital pressure (hydraulic theory)
- Trauma to inferior orbital rim → temporary distortion, transmitted to orbital floor (buckling force theory)

Anatomy

Floor

- Thinnest posteriorly, weakened by groove
- Fracture → IR + IO entrapment
- III inferior division injury (IO branch most vulnerable)

Medial wall

- Thinnest over ethmoid plate (lamina papyracea)
- Fracture → MR entrapment rarely
- Disruption of medial canthal tendon
- Lacrimal sac and duct injury

Clinical presentation

- Diplopia and limitation of movements
  - Due to muscle injury, muscle entrapment or nerve injury
  - IR and IO limitation results from entrapment or damage
  - SR limitation results from IR entrapment
  - Forced duction test differentiates palsy and entrapment
- Enophthalmos – due to prolapse of fat and tissues, fat necrosis, and muscle fibrosis
- Infraorbital nerve sensory disturbance
  - If absent, the fracture may be medial or lateral to groove
  - Zygomatic nerve sensory disturbance may occur in lateral fractures
- Unilateral epistaxis
- Surgical emphysema, more usually with medial wall fractures
- Loss of vision, commotio retinae

Orbital floor (blowout) fractures

Clinical findings

- Eccymosis + lid oedema
- Diplopia with limitation upgaze +/or downgaze
- Vertical diplopia
- Enopthalmos + ptosis – may be initially masked by orbital oedema
- Hypoaesthesia – infraorbital nerve distribution
- Orbit + eyelid emphysaema
- Loss of vision – ON injury

Special investigations

- Hess charts, single binocular field
- X-ray orbits shows
  Prolapse of orbital contents,
  Into maxillary sinus,
  Fragmentation of orbital floor,
  Opacity of sinus,
  Orbital emphysaema
- Forced duction test – IR tendon is grasped and moved
- CT scan – may be helpful
  - To assess size of fracture = degree of orbital herniation
  - To assess depth of surgical exploration

Management

- Very early treatment (within 1–2 hours)

- Early treatment (within 2–3 weeks)
- Late treatment (after 3–6 months)

Very early treatment (within 1–2 hours)

- Contraindicated, as swelling and haemorrhage can cause limitation and 50% of small fractures recover spontaneously

Early treatment (within 2–3 weeks)

- Indications
  - Enophthalmos > 3 mm
  - Diplopia
  - Obvious fracture with herniation into antrum
  - Incarceration with positive forced duction test
- Medial wall fracture rarely requires repair
- Optimum time is 10–14 days, before union occurs
- May be via Caldwell-Luc approach (canine maxillary) or lower lid approach
- Tissues freed and integrity of floor restored with silicone graft/silastic plate
- May be complicated by optic nerve injury, either directly by graft or indirectly by fat traction

Late treatment (after 3–6 months)

- Contraindicated due to increased complications and poorer results
- If presents late with restricted vertical movements, do the following
  - Orthophoria in the primary position but diplopia in elevation → either nil or recess contralateral SR
  - Orthophoria in the primary position but diplopia in depression → contralateral IR Fadens or contralateral SR + IR recession
  - Hypophoria in the primary position → ipsilateral IR recession on an adjustable suture, to align in the primary position; wait 6 months, then transpose ipsilateral MR and LR
  - Hypertropia in the primary position → ipsilateral SR recession, ipsilateral IR resection, ? contralateral IR recession or transposition down of MR and LR (< 10 D hypertropia, to IR insertion; > 10 D hypertropia, to 3 mm posterior to IR insertion)
  - The aim of treatment is to achieve binocular single vision in the primary position and in downgaze
- If present late with a medial wall fracture, do the following
  - Forced duction test positive – ? Free up subperiosteal tissue, recess MR, wait 6 months, transpose SR and IR to MR insertion
  - Forced duction test negative – transpose SR and IR to MR insertion; or treat LR with botulinum

Intraocular foreign bodies

Types

- Metallic
  - inert – silver, gold, platinum
  - Incite purulent reaction – nickel, aluminium, mercury, copper > 85%
  - Long-term metallosis – iron, copper < 85%
- Organic – wood
- Other – glass, plastic, gunpowder

Detection and location

- High index of suspicion
- Slit lamp + indirect examination; 90% are visible
- Straight x-ray – anteroposterior + lateral, look up + look down
- Ultrasound B scan
- CT scan

Treatment

- Primary repair, if necessary

- Chemoprophylaxis – systemic + local; tetanus prophylaxis
- Remove foreign body
  - This depends on the relative risks of leaving it cw risks of surgery, nature of foreign body, site of foreign body
  - Remove immediately to minimise the risks of endophthalmitis

Removal of magnetic foreign bodies

- Anterior chamber – via limbal incision, with forceps or a magnet
- Lens – await cataract formation, then remove the lens; if the lens remains clear, then leave the intraocular foreign body
- Posterior segment
  - Free in vitreous – pars plana vitrectomy, remove with vitreous forceps
  - Embedded in retina – choroid-sclera – sclerotomy over foreign body + remove directly; or via vitrectomy; following sclerotomy, apply cryo ± buckle

Removal of non-magnetic foreign bodies

- Anterior chamber – as for magnetic
- Lens – as for magnetic
- Posterior segment
  - ± Lensectomy, ± vitrectomy, remove with vitreous forceps
  - It is advisable to wait 10–14 days for posterior vitreous detachment to occur
- Large foreign bodies may be removed anteriorly following lensectomy
- Fibreoptic monocular endoscope may be used when the view is inadequate

Siderosis

Definition

- Long-term metallosis occurring following intraocular foreign body containing iron

Pathogenesis

- Retained iron foreign body may cause no reaction, severe purulent reaction, migration, expulsion, dissolution or siderosis
- Onset and severity of siderosis depends on size, iron content, location, duration
- Fe^{2+} is oxidised to Fe^{3+}
- Fe^{3+} combines with glycosaminoglycan, diffuses around the eye and binds to intracellular enzymes → cell death
- First affects peripheral retina, affects ganglion cells + RPE cells, later affects central retina and rods + cones
- Onset is after months to years

Symptoms

- Gradual loss of vision, night blindness, constricted field

Signs

- Rusty staining of peripheral cornea
- Brown yellow staining of iris, mydriasis
- Glaucoma
- Lens anterior peripheral brown subcapsular opacities
- Vitreous diffuse brown spots
- Retinal obliterative sclerosis, retinitis pigmentosa picture, macular degeneration, gliotic atrophy

Electroretinogram

- Normal a + b → elevated a + normal b → elevated a + diminished b → diminished a + b → flat ERG
- Reversible up to elevated a + diminished b

Treatment

- Early removal of foreign body
- Desferroxamine – chelates Fe^{3+} and prevents progression

Chalcosis

Pathogenesis

- Retained copper alloy containing < 85% copper

12

- Cu^+ oxidised to Cu^{2+}, diffuses, fixed to limiting membranes
- Onset after days to years

Symptoms
- Less severe loss of vision

Signs
- Kayser-Fleischer ring in peripheral descemet membrane
- Anterior subcapsular green sunflower cataract
- Stained zonules
- Metal particles in aqueous + vitreous
- Greenish iris
- Retinal changes – gold leaf like particles on retinal surface + around veins

Treatment
- Early removal of foreign body
- Penicillamine

Uveal trauma

Iris

- Iritis – contusion to stroma → flare and cells; treat with cycloplegics
- Pigment dispersion – Krukenberg's Spindle, Vossius ring, on trabecular meshwork
- Haemorrhage – into iris stroma, hyphaema
- Sphincter injury – miosis and mydriasis, irritative or paralytic; sphincter tears
- Iridoschisis – anterior mesodermal leaf detaches, may atrophy
- Iridodialysis – usually associated hyphaema
- Only treat if there is monocular diplopia; either suture or do a sector iridectomy

Ciliary body

- Angle recession
  - Tear in ciliary body between circular and longitudinal muscle, beginning at scleral spur
  - 70–80% of traumatic hyphaemas have angle recession
  - Secondary glaucoma develops in 10%, usually if > 180 degrees
  - There is an initial increase in IOP due to the hyphaema, then a drop, then a secondary rise after 2 months to 15 years
- Cyclodialysis – if around 360 degrees, the iris lens diaphragm is mobile

Choroid

- Haemorrhage
- Tears – in posterior pole; crescentic in shape

Traumatic hyphaema

Aetiology and epidemiology
- Stones, squash balls, fists
- Children > adults
- Male > female
- Left > right

Pathology
- Penetrating injury → uveal laceration
- Blunt injury
  - Tear in ciliary body (angle recession)
  - Iridodialysis
  - Iris tear
- Red blood cells block trabecular meshwork → transient rise in IOP
- Small bleeds do not clot, clear in 5 days
- Larger bleeds clot, clear in 7–10 days
- Lysis and clot retraction occurs at 2–7 days, which is when secondary bleed occurs

Complications
- Secondary bleed
  - At 2–7 days
  - In 25% of cases; higher in children, higher in blacks
  - When clot lysis and retraction occurs
  - More likely if the initial hyphaema is > 3 mm
- Glaucoma – occurs in 33% of cases

- Early rise in IOP due to trabecular clogging by red blood cells or macrophages → normal/decreased IOP due to traumatised ciliary body → elevated IOP → normal IOP
- Pupil block from blood clot
- ± Late glaucoma from angle recession; angle recession occurs in 70–80%; glaucoma occurs in 10% after 10 years

- Corneal blood staining – stromal impregnation by haemaglobin products
  - Associated with elevated IOP
  - May take 2–3 years to clear
- Posterior synechiae and peripheral anterior synechiae
- Ischaemic optic neuropathy

Management

- Principles
  - Prevent secondary haemorrhage
  - Control secondary glaucoma
- Hospitalisation
  - Unnecessary if small, uncomplicated, compliant for follow-up
  - Otherwise admit for 4–5 days
- Bed rest and sedation
  - Does not alter rate of secondary haemorrhage
  - Does increase rate of absorption of blood from the eye
  - Elevate the head 30 degrees + allow bathroom privileges
- Padding
  - Provides comfort
  - Does not influence rebleed rate or rate of absorption of blood
- Analgesia
  - Paracetamol
  - Avoid aspirin (increased risk of secondary haemorrhage)
- Topical corticosteroids and mydriatics
  - To treat uveitis and prevent posterior synechiae
  - Does not decrease the risk of secondary haemorrrhage or increase the rate of resorption of blood
- Systemic steroids
  - Prednisone 40 mg daily
  - As effective as aminocaproic acid in preventing secondary haemorrhage
  - Cheaper than tranexamic acid
- Systemic antifibrinolytics
  - Amino caproic acid – 50 mg/kg 4 hourly × 5 days; → significant decrease in the rate of secondary haemorrhage
  - Tranexamic acid – 25 mg/kg 8 hourly × 5 days; → significant decrease in the rate of secondary haemorrhage; fewer systemic side effects; sudden clot dissolution with rise in IOP may occur after stopping the drug
- Medical treatment of glaucoma – beta blocker, acetazolamide
- Surgery
  - Indications – IOP > 50 for 2 days, IOP > 30 for 5 days, corneal blood staining, sickle cell haemaglobinopathy
  - Techniques – limbal paracentesis, ± viscoelsatic, ± saline irrigation, ± expression of clot

Causes of spontaneous hyphaema

- Bleeding from abnormal vessels in anterior chamber – juvenile xanthogranuloma, rubeosis iridis, iris melanoma, retinoblastoma, previous scleral section
- Bleeding from fibrovascular membranes in anterior vitreous – retinopathy of prematurity, persistent hyperplastic primary vitreous, retinoschisis
- Complication of severe uveitis, microbial keratitis
- Complication of blood dyscrasias

Traumatic retinopathy

Commotio retinae

- Blunt trauma → reflex vasodilatation → oedema
- Usually white retina and cherry red spot; variable haemorrhage and exudation
- Deterioration in visual acuity, variable recovery
- Residual retinal pigment epithelial disturbance, atrophy, macular cyst, macular hole

Purtscher's retinopathy

- From distant trauma
- Arterial – emboli (usually fat) → haemorrhage and exudates
- Venous – valsalva → haemorrhages

Traumatic macular cyst and macular hole

- Cyst formation in outer plexiform layer, following oedema
- Rupture of inner internal limiting membrane covering → hole formation

Chorioretinal rupture

- Splits in Bruch's membrane concentric to disc; may involve macula
- Subretinal neovascularisation may develop later

Rupture of posterior ciliary vessels

- Retinal and optic atrophy

Retinitis sclopeteria

- Traumatic chorioretinopathy, secondary to concussion, usually secondary to nearby passage of a missile

Foveomacular retinitis

- Solar lesion from sun gazing
- Early
  - Oedema and central scotoma; may have appearance of yellow spot in centre of fovea
- Later
  - Macular lesion varying nil → scarring of retina, RPE, and choroid → lamellar hole
- Resolves over 2 months, 75% achieve 6/9+

Radiation retinopathy

- Ischaemic retinopathy, as for diabetes mellitus, due to endothelial injury

13

Refractive error and refractive surgery

Refractive error 372
Anisometropia 376
Abnormalities of accommodation 377
Optical aberrations 378
Astigmatism of oblique incidence .. 379
Asthenopia 379
Aphakia 380
Spectacles 381
Power and notation of lenses 383
Toric lenses 383
Prisms 384
Contact lenses 385
Basic principles of refractive surgery 387
Classification of corneal refractive surgery 389
Intraocular surgery 389
Photoablation 390
Thermokeratoplasty 392
Incisional and inlay corneal surgery 392
IOL power calculation after refractive surgery 393
Presbyopia 393
Refractive surgery in ocular and systemic disease 395

Refractive error

Classification of refractive error

Emmetropia

- Far point at infinity
- 60% of people in developed countries wear glasses
- Emmetropia is an optical ideal, not a biological average
- The eye is made up of 14 optical components
- Each has a statistical distribution; most fall within the emmetropic range

Hypermetropia

- Far point virtual, behind the eye
- Clinical classification
  - Physiological
  - Simple
  - Pathological
- Optical classification
  - Axial – eyeball too short (1 mm = 3D)
  - Lens displaced backwards
- Refractive classification
  - Aphakia
  - Change in refractive index (aqueous or lens decreased, vitreous increased)

Myopia

- Far point nearer than infinity
- Clinical classification
  - Simple
  - Pathological
- Optical classification
  - Axial – eyeball too long
  - Lens displaced forwards
- Refractive
  - Keratoconus
  - Nuclear sclerosis
  - Change in refractive index (aqueous or lens increased, vitreous decreased)

Astigmatism

- Refractive power varies in different corneal meridia
- Clinical classification
  - Compound hypermetropic
  - Simple hypermetropic
  - Mixed
  - Simple myopic
  - Compound myopic
- Optical classification
  - Regular – principal axes at right angles
  - Bioblique – principal axes not at right angles
  - Irregular

Optical correction of ametropia

Principle

- Myopia with –
- Hypermetropia with +
- Astigmatism with cylinder
- The correcting lens is placed with its second principal focus at the far point of the eye; it deviates parallel rays so that they appear to come from the far point

Effective lens power

- This depends on the power of the lens and its distance from the eye
- A spectacle lens is usually placed 12–15 mm from the eye
- + Lens is stronger further from the eye
- – Lens is weaker further from the eye
- $F2 = \frac{F1}{1-dF1}$ F2 – power of lens in dioptres; F1 – power of original lens; d – distance moved in metres

Back vertex distance

- Between the lens and cornea
- This must be given in any lens > 5D
- The power of the new lens can then be calculated

Spectacle magnification

- $M = \frac{\text{corrected retinal image size}}{\text{uncorrected retinal image size}}$
- Relative spectacle magnification $= \frac{\text{corrected retinal image size}}{\text{uncorrected retinal image size}}$
- + Lens moved away from the eye → increased image size
- – Lens moved away from the eye → decreased image size

Hypermetropia

Definition

- The far point is virtual and behind the eye
- The image is formed behind the retina when the eye is at rest; parallel rays are focussed behind the retina

Aetiology

- Physiological
  - Age variations
  - 85% of neonates are hypermetropic → 50% of adolescents are hypermetropic

13

- Simple
  - Axial – variant of normal (1 mm = 3D)
  - Backward displacement of the lens
- Pathological
  - Flattening of the cornea (cornea plana, scarring)
  - Orbital mass, retinal fold, retinal detachment
- Accommodation in hypermetropia
  - Latent – up to 1D overcome by ciliary tone
  - Manifest – facultative, overcome by accommodative effort
  - Manifest – absolute, cannot be overcome
  - 50% of accommodation must be left in reserve for comfort

Symptoms

- Nil
- Accommodative asthenopia
- Transient failure of accommodation → blurring
- Excess accommodation, spasm of accommodation → artificial myopia
- Covergent squint

Ocular features

- Small eye, small cornea, shallow anterior chamber, shot silk retina, small + engorged disc
- Large positive angle alpha → pseudoexotropia

Treatment

- Children
  - Cycloplegic refraction, deduct 1D if > 6 years of age; 1.5–2.0D if < 6 years of age
  - < 6 years – correct if high or squint present
  - > 6 years – correct if > 3D, wear glasses continually; if < 3D, wear glasses for reading
  - Check annually

Myopia

Definition

- Far point is nearer than infinity
- Parallel rays are focussed in front of the retina when the eye is at rest

Aetiology

- Axial
  - Increased anteroposterior diameter – physiologic variant (simple);
  - Pathologic; developmental defect of posterior segment
  - 1 mm = 3D in the phakic eye, 1 mm = 2D in the aphakic eye
- Curvature
  - Increased corneal curvature – keratoconus (1 mm = 6D)
  - Increased lens curvature – anterior + posterior lenticonus; spherophakia; ectopia lentis
- Index
  - Increased lens nucleus refractive index in nuclear sclerosis

Classification

- Physiologic/simple/refractive – all refractive component values fall within the normal range, but there is a mismatch of the components
- Axial/intermediate – excessive enlargement of the posterior segment, with retinal features and complications
- Pathological – axial + staphyloma

Epidemiology

- 25% of Caucasians + 50% of Asians have myopia
- The prevalence is increased with increased family income + increased educational level
- Female > male
- Simple
  - Physiologic variant
  - Inheritance may be autosomal dominant, autosomal recessive, x-linked recessive or multifactorial
- Pathologic/degenerative
  - Male > female

- Common in Chinese, Japanese, Arabs and Jews
- Inheritance may be autosomal recessive or multifactorial
- May be associated with other ocular or systemic anomalies

Pathogenesis

- A visually dependent feedback mechanism is necessary for emmetropisation; deprivation of this → myopia, since there is no control of ocular growth
- Mesodermal dysgenesis → defective scleral development → weakening + distension
- ? Role of accommodative effort over a prolonged period

Progress

- Simple – Onset 3– years of age, slow steady progression, stabilises at 21 years of age, final error around 6D
- Pathologic – rapid progression, never stabilises, final error 20–30D

Symptoms

- Poor distance vision
- Floaters
- Asthenopia
  - Screwing up of lids
  - Accommodative changes over short ranges

Ocular features

- Large eye, large cornea, deep anterior chamber, large sluggish pupil, early vitreous liquefaction and collapse, typical fundal features of high myopia
- Negative angle alpha → pseudoesotropia
- Associated glaucoma, associated lens opacities

Treatment of myopia

- Low myopia – children
  - Full correction, wear constantly
- Low myopia – adults
  - Full correction, for distance only
- High myopia (> 8D)
  - Undercorrect by 1–3D
  - Prescribe tint + best form lenses
  - Prescribe contact lenses if feasible

Surgical correction of myopia

- Refractive keratoplasty
  - Photorefractive keratectomy (excimer laser)
  - Laser in situ keratomileusis (lasik) (excimer laser)
- Intraocular implants
  - Aphakic IOL
  - Phakic IOL

Astigmatism

Definition

- Refractive anomaly in which no point focus is formed, owing to unequal refraction by the eye in different meridia

Types

- Regular
  - Simple myopic/hypermetropic
  - Compound myopic/hypermetropic
  - Mixed
- Oblique
- Bioblique
- Irregular

Aetiology

- Curvature astigmatism of anterior corneal surface
  - Most common cause
  - With the rule – vertical curvature greater; seen in early childhood
  - Against the rule – horizontal curvature greater; seen in old age
  - Irregular – secondary to scarring
- Curvature astigmatism of posterior corneal surface
- Curvature astigmatism of both surfaces of the lens
- Astigmatism from decentering of the lens
- Refractive astigmatism of the lens

Optics
- Two focal lines at the focal points of the meridia of greatest and least curvature, separated by the focal interval

Symptoms
- Decreased visual acuity
- Asthenopia; in low degrees of astigmatism, due to accommodative effort

Treatment
- With toric lens
- Low astigmatism
  - No treatment if asymptomatic
- High astigmatism
  - Correct as far as possible
  - Add spherical equivalent if necessary
- Undercorrect cyl, add half cyl power deducted from the sphere e.g. +10.00/–2.00 = +9.00

Anisometropia

Definition
- Refraction of two eyes is different

Classification
- Simple hypermetropic/myopic – one eye emmetropic
- Compound hypermetropic/myopic – both eyes hypermetropic/myopic
- Mixed – one eye hypermetropic + one eye myopic
- Simple + compound astigmatic

Problems
- Aniseikonia
- Anisophoria

Aniseikonia

Definition
- Size and shape of the images in two eyes is unequal

Features
- Occurs in 20–30% of people who wear glasses
- Knapp's rule – the magnification difference is 2% per dioptre (plus → increase, minus → decrease)
- The maximum tolerable difference is 5% in adults + 8% in children
- Symptoms include visual disturbance, diplopia, squint and eye strain
- Amblyopia potential if
  - > 2D hypermetropic anisometropia
  - > 4D myopic anisometropia

Treatment
- Undercorrect the refractive error; up to the maximum tolerable difference
- Contact lenses – these result in less magnification effect
- Iseikonic lenses – the magnification of a lens depends on the front curve, the thickness and the back curve; the power depends on the back curve
- Increased front curve → increased magnification
- Increased thickness → increased magnification
- Increased back curve of + lens → increased magnification
- Decreased back curve of – lens → increased magnification
- In general, increase the magnification for the more myopic eye + decrease the magnification for the more hypermetropic eye
- Iseikonic lenses may be used to adjust the image size up to 5%

Anisophoria

Definition
- Difference in the effective ocular alignment when the eyes move away from the primary position, due to the prismatic effects of lenses of different power

Treatment
- Horizontal
  - Instruct the patient to move the head, not the eyes

  - The fusional amplitude is large therefore they can often compensate
- Vertical
  - Correct with a slab of prism in the lower portion of minus lens → base up prism effect → correction of prismatic effect without changing the power of the lens

Abnormalities of accommodation

Fatigue of accomodation

Refractive errors

- High hypermetropia
- High myopia; the far point and the near point are close, therefore, the total amplitude of accommodation is used over a small range
- Hypermetropic or mixed astigmatism
- Anisometropic error, especially if small
- Convergence, in exophoria

General factors

- Ill-health
- Anaemia
- Diabetes

Presbyopia

Pathogenesis

- Lens sclerosis + decreased elasticity of capsule + decreased elasticity of choroid with age → decreased amplitude of accommodation
- At 40 years of age, 4D of amplitude of accommodation remains, therefore, symptoms develop for near work at 30 cm (one-third of the amplitude is required in reserve to avoid symptoms)
- 4D of accommodation is required to read at 25 cm
- Hypermetropes develop symptoms earlier
- Myopes develop symptoms later
- Myopes of > 4D never develop presbyopia
- Amplitudes of accommodation
  - 14D at birth; near point 7 cm
  - 11D at 20 years of age
  - 4D at 40 years of age; near point 25 cm
  - 1D or less at 60 years of age (and part of this is due to depth of field)
  - Amplitude of accommodation $= 18 - \text{age} \times \frac{1}{4}$

Symptoms

- Difficulty with near work
- Asthenopia

Treatment

- + Correction $\frac{\text{age} - 30\text{D}}{10}$

Causes of paralysis of accommodation

- Cycloplegic drugs
- III nerve palsy
- Ciliary muscle disease – cyclitis, glaucoma
- CVA
- Encephalitis
- Multiple sclerosis
- Old age

Causes of spasm of accommodation

Functional

- Hypermetropia
- Prolonged near work
- Early cataracts
- Early presbyopia
- Anxiety

Organic

- Miotics
- Intraocular inflammation
- Seizure
- Head injury
- Parinaud's syndrome
- Craniocervical junction lesion
- Sulphonamides

Symptoms

- Pseudomyopia (up to 10D)
- Asthenopia

Diagnosis

- Subjective and objective refraction → varying results
- Range of accommodation decreased
- Weak cycloplegics are ineffective
- Discrepancy between refraction with and without cycloplegic

Treatment

- Treat the underlying cause
- Atropine cycloplegia
- Cycloplegic refraction; prescribe –1D

Optical aberrations

Diffraction

- Interference of light waves with each other at the edge of a wave front
- As a result, the edges of images are never sharp
- This limits the amount of magnification that can be attained without losing sharpness

Chromatic aberration

- Unequal refraction of light rays of different wavelength producing a blurred image with fringes of colour
- Shorter wavelengths are deviated more
- Achromatic lenses – composed of elements of varying material that neutralises the dispersion, while maintaining the overall refractive power
- Ocular chromatic aberration – total dispersion red → blue is 1.5–2D; yellow-green is focussed by the emmetropic eye

Duochrome test

- Two ranks of black Snellen letters, mounted on red glass and green glass
- Red and green are used because their wavelengths straddle the emmetropic yellow-green by equal amounts – 0.4D on either side
- Myopic eye sees red clearly, hypermetropic eye sees green clearly
- Colour blindness does not negate the test

Spherical aberration

- Causes night myopia/night blindness post-refractive surgery by
  - Focus of rays not stigmatic
  - Focus of rays are shifted anteriorly → myopia
- This is caused by
  - Prismatic effect of peripheral lens → rays passing through periphery are deviated more
  - Marginal focus is the point at which the peripheral rays converge
  - Paraxial focus is the point at which the central rays converge
  - Circle of least confusion is quarter the distance from the marginal to the paraxial focus
- Correction in optical systems is achieved by
  - Occlusion of periphery using 'stops'
  - Adjustment of lens form; aplanatic/ aspheric lens, with less peripheral curvature
  - Use of doublets; these comprise a principal lens + a weaker opposite power lens of different refractive index
- Ocular spherical aberration is reduced naturally by
  - Anterior corneal surface is flatter peripherally
  - Iris acts as a stop; the optimum pupil size is 2–2.5 mm
  - Lens nucleus has a higher refractive index than the lens cortex
  - Cones are more sensitive to paraxial than to oblique light (Stiles Crawford effect)

13

- In post-refractive surgery patients, very small changes in pupil size can dramatically increase the spherical aberration and accounts for the fluctuating vision seen in some

Coma

- Also a spherical aberration – light from points not on the principal axis → unequal magnification from different zones of the lens – elongated, comet-like instead of circular
- Avoid by limiting rays to the axial area
- Ocular coma is not of practical importance

Image distortion

- Prismatic effects of lens periphery → uneven magnification
- Extended images
    - Concave lens → barrel distortion
    - Convex lens → pin-cushion distortion

Curvature of field

- Plane object → curved image
- Due to curvature of lens surface
- Compensated for in the eye by curvature of the retina + accommodation

Astigmatism of oblique incidence

- Occurs when rays of light traverse a spherical lens obliquely
- Obliquely incident light rays → toric effect with interval of Sturm, Sturm's conoid, and circle of least confusion
- Worse with higher power lenses
- Less with meniscus lenses
- Reduced in spectacles by a pantoscopic tilt – lens tilted slightly towards the cheek because we spend most of out time looking slightly down
- Ocular oblique astigmatism reduced by God by
    - Aplanatic curve of cornea
    - Retina is curved and not flat, therefore the circle of least confusion falls on the retina
    - Astigmatic image falls on the peripheral retina, therefore its appreciation is limited

Asthenopia

Definition

- Eye strain
- A vague but real sense of ocular fatigue
- Symptoms due to effort to achieve clear vision
- Weakness or easy fatigue of the eyes, headache, dimness of vision, etc.

Causes of asthenopia

Environmental	Illumination Nature of the object Computer vision syndrome
Ocular	Uncorrected ametropia Accommodative difficulties Heterophorias – common Convergence insufficiency Aniseikonia
Physical	General ill-health
Functional	Ocular neurasthenia

Symptoms

- Visual – transient blurring, diplopia
- Ocular – due to increased muscle work; eyes feel painful and tired
- Referred – headache, usually associated with use of the eyes; vertigo
- Functional

Near asthenopia

- May be due to
  - Convergence insufficiency; treat with convergence exercises
  - Hypermetropia; treat with accommodative exercises if low + correction if high
  - Convergence and accommodative exercises should be done for 2 mins 10 times daily

Computer vision syndrome

- Causes asthenopic symptoms and ocular surface-related symptoms
- Eye strain, tired eyes, irritation, redness, blurred vision, double vision
- Mostly due to dry eye
- Prolonged computer use → diminished power of accommodation + phoria deviation
- Transient myopia
- Usually transient + return to normal after holiday/weekend
- Treatment: Lubricating drops, work breaks, proper lighting, antiglare filters

Aphakia

Optics of uncorrected aphakia

- The lens is absent, the eye is hypermetropic, parallel rays are focussed 31 mm behind the cornea
- Shift of the principal points → reorientation of the visual axis → loss of angle kappa → eyes converge for near an extra 5 degrees
- Accommodation is absent
- Astigmatism may be induced by the surgery
- There is increased glare and the retina is unprotected from UV light

Optical problems of spectacle correction of aphakia

Magnification

- +10D lens at 12–15 mm → 1.33 × magnification
- This results in aniseikonia → inability to fuse the images; tolerable aniseikonia is 5% in adults and 8% in children (0.5D → 1% aniseikonia)
- Magnification also results in
  - Enhanced Snellen acuity performance
  - Difficulty in judging distances

Field reduction

- The field is reduced by 20–30% (cw magnification); a clear image is only seen through the axial part of the lens

Image distortion

- Pin-cushion effect
- Due to unequal refraction of the central and peripheral rays (prismatic effect of the periphery of the lens)

Ring scotoma and Jack in the box

- Due to prismatic effect of the lens periphery → prismatic displacement
- A 10-degree wide scotoma surrounds the central 60 degrees
- The scotoma moves centrally when the eye moves peripherally
- Prentice's formula
  - Prismatic displacement

$$= \text{Radius of lens} \times \frac{\text{Dioptric power}}{10}$$

Chromatic aberration

- Of the lens periphery
- This is not usually a problem due to the effect of the pupil

Spherical aberration

- Of the lens periphery
- This is not usually a problem due to the effect of the pupil

Oblique astigmatism

- Of the lens periphery
- This is not usually a problem due to the effect of the pupil

Coma

- This is not a significant problem

Curvature of field

- This is normally compensated for by accommodation which is lost

Base-out prismatic effect

- With convergence for reading, resulting in convergence insufficiency

Aphakic spectacle design

Problems

- Heavy, ugly, uncomfortable
- Slip down nose → increase in effective power
- Peripheral prismatic effects
- Glare

Solutions

- Plastic lenses are lighter, but they scratch more easily and they have to be thicker because the refractive index is less
- Lenticular lenses are lighter, but have decreased field
- Aspheric lenses; the peripheral power is decreased by 3–4D → decreased peripheral effects
- Added tint + UV filter

Prescribing aphakic spectacles

Back vertex distance

- Place the lens as close as possible to the eye and give the back vertex distance with the prescription
- Power of new lens =

$$\frac{\text{Power of old lens}}{1 - \text{Distance moved in metres} \times \text{Power of old lens}}$$

Centration

- Good centration is important
- Give the interpupillary distance for near and far
- Prentice's formula
  - Prismatic effect = Decentration in cm × Dioptric power of lens

Tilt

- Avoid, as this results in unwanted spherocylindrical effects

Near correction

- Usually +1.75 to +2.25 is sufficient add, because of the magnification effects
- Avoid overplussing
- The reading add must be decentred by 3.5–4.0 mm per eye, to avoid base-out prism effect on convergence
- Distance and near corrections are usually given as separates, to avoid the prismatic effects of the bifocal interface

Stipulations

- Plastic aspheric with UV filter

Spectacles

Materials

- Glass
  - Crown
  - Flint
- Plastic

Tints

- Vacuum coating or polychromatic
- Brown or grey

Best form lenses

- Designed to eliminate oblique astigmatism + peripheral aberrations
- Two types: Meniscus lenses and toric lenses
- Meniscus lenses

    - Correct aberrations in spherical ametropia
- Toric lenses
    - Correct aberrations in astigmatic ametropia

Decentration and prismatic effects

- Prismatic effect = decentration in cm × power of lens
- Uses
    - Correction of heterophoria
    - To overcome deficient or excess convergence
    - To avoid prismatic effects when essential direction of gaze is not in the primary position

Bifocal and multifocal lenses

Indications

- Presbyopia
    - Normal age 45
    - Earlier in hypermetropia, later in myopia, never in myopia > 4D
    - Earlier if there is decreased amplitude of accommodation
- Accommodative esotropia
    - If there is hypermetropia > 6D
    - High AC/A ratio
- Aphakia

Designs

- May be
    - Glass or plastic
    - One piece or fused
- One piece – more plus ground into reading area
- Fused – two pieces of glass of different refractive index; flint glass has a higher refractive index and is used in the near segment
- The size and height of the segment is variable, according to the patient's needs
- The near segment height in adults is usually at the lower lid in adults and in the midpupil in children

Optics

- Near visual point
    - The near visual point is 2 mm nasal + 8 mm below the distance visual point
- Image jump
    - Occurs as the visual axis sweeps over the distance-near interface
    - It is worse with round top, where the near and distance visual points are furthest; and least with flat top, where the near and distance visual points are closest
    - It is worse with high power lenses; separate glasses may then be appropriate
- Image displacement
    - Occurs due to prismatic effects; base down for minus, base up for plus; add induces base down prism; reduced by incorporating a base up prism in the reading segment
- Decentration
    - Of the near segment medially, to compensate for a near exophoria

Trifocals

- These incorporate a third segment of intermediate power (usually half the near add) for middistance (40–100 cm); suitable for musicians, typists and bridge players
- The types are as for bifocals

Invisible bifocals

- These incorporate an invisible zone between the near segment and the distance zone; the vision is blurred through this

Progressive addition lenses

- There is a uniform distance portion, an intermediate 12 mm zone of increasing plus, and a uniform near portion
- Lateral distortion of field occurs in the intermediate portion

Special multifocals

- Look unders (for presbyopic myopes)
- Librarians
- Golfers
- Artists

Power and notation of lenses

Dioptre

- Unit of lens power
- Unit of vergence power
- Dioptre = $\frac{1}{\text{focal length (metres)}}$

Prescription of lenses

- Example: + 2.00/–1.00 × 45

Transposition of lenses

Simple transposition of cylinders

- Example: +4.00/+1.50 × 90 = +5.50/–1.50 × 180
- Add cylinder and sphere power
- Change sign of cylinder
- Change axis of cylinder by 90 degrees

Identification of lenses

- + Moves opposite, – moves with
- Neutralise with lenses from the trial set

Focimeter

- Comprises a focussing system + an observation system
- The focussing system comprises an illuminated target + a collimating lens
- The test lens is placed at the principal focus of the collimating lens
- The target is moved until the light entering the observation pupil is parallel, when the observer sees the focussed image of the target
- The distance the target is moved is proportional to the dioptric power of the test lens (back vertex power of the test lens)
- To measure an astigmatic lens
  - Read 1 set of line foci, adjust and read the second set
  - The first reading gives the sphere, the second reading gives the cylinder axis
- The cylinder power is calculated from the difference
- To measure a prism
  - Mark the centre of the lens on the patient
  - Place the lens in the focimeter; the centre is displaced towards the base; read off the prism dioptres on the circles

Toric lenses

Types

- Cylindrical
- Toric

Cylindrical lenses

- One axis forms part of a sphere + one axis is plane
- The axis lies in the line of zero vergence power
- It forms a line image of a point axis parallel to the axis

Maddox rod

- This is a series of convex lenses mounted side by side
- Light rays parallel to the axes are undeviated and focussed by the eye
- Light rays at right angles to the axes are focussed in front of the eye, too near to be seen clearly on the retina
- Therefore, a distant point white light source is focussed as a line at 90 degrees to the axis of the rod

Toric lenses

- Both meridia are curved, but to a different degree
- They may be thought of as a spherical lens with a cylindrical lens superimposed

- The principal meridia are the meridia of maximum and minimum curvature
- They form separate line foci at right angles to each other
- They are separated by the interval of Sturm, in which the rays form Sturm's conoid
- The circle of least confusion is the plane where the two pencils of light intersect

Cross cylinder

- Toric spherocylindrical lens, in which cyl power = 2 × sphere power,and is of the opposite sign
- This is equivalent to superimposing two cylindrical lenses of equal power but opposite sign, with their axes at right angles to each other

Prisms

Basic optics

- Rays are deviated towards the base
- Chromatic dispersion occurs
- D = alpha ÷ 2
- 1 dioptre prism → displacement of 1 cm of an object situated at 1 m
- 1 dioptre prism produces an angle of apparent deviation of 0.5 degrees
- 1 dioptre = 0.5 degrees; 1 degree = 2 dioptres (for thin glass prisms of RI 1.5)

Prismatic effect of thick lenses

- A thick lens may be considered as a series of prisms, of increasing power peripherally; and therefore, resulting in increasing deviation peripherally
- The Prentice rule gives the prism power of any point on a lens
- Prismatic effect (dioptres) = power of lens × decentration in cm
- The prismatic effect of thick lenses is responsible for ring scotoma, Jack in the box and spherical aberration

13

Prismatic effect of bifocal lens interface

- This is responsible for image jump when the visual angle sweeps over the junction, resulting in a scotoma around the bifocal segment
- A plus distance segment results in a base-up prismatic effect in the lower field, which is countered if the bifocal segment has its optical centre lower down
- Vice versa for a minus distance segment

Uses of prisms in ophthalmology

Diagnostic

- Assessment of squints and heterophorias
    - Prism cover test, measurement of fusional reserve
    - 4D base-out prism test for micro-tropia, measurement of AC/A ratio
- Assessment of simulated blindness

Therapeutic

- Treatment of suppression and abnormal retinal correspondence
- Treatment of convergence insufficiency – base-out for exercises to build up fusional reserve base in for treatment (usually give half)
- Relief of diplopia – in decompensated heterophorias, small vertical squints, some paralytic squints
- Treatment of VI nerve palsy – to prevent medial rectus contracture, base-out in front of unaffected eye
- Treatment of nystagmus – to prevent head tilt, to encourage convergence

Optical instruments

- Used as reflectors of light
- Used in slit lamp, applanation tonometer, keratometer, indirect ophthalmoscope

Prescribing prisms

- May be given as Fresnel or permanent wear
- Correction is usually split between both eyes
- Fresnel prisms are made of polyvinyl chloride
- They are thin and cheap and cause minimal chromatic aberration and distortion

Contact lenses

Types of contact lenses	
■ Hard	□ Polymethylmethacrylate (PMMA) (gas impermeable) (not used anymore) □ Cellulose acetate butyrate (gas permeable) □ Silicone (gas permeable) □ Fluorocarbon (gas permeable) □ They have a low water content and a clinical life of 3 years
■ Soft	□ Hydroxymethylmethacrylate □ Polyvinylpyrrolidone □ Silicone hydrogol □ They have a high water content (25–70%) □ Some soft lenses may be worn as extended wear lenses (30 days)

Optics of contact lenses

Hard lens

- Lens floats on the tear film
- The refractive index of the tears and cornea is about equal therefore corneal astigmatism is corrected
- Total power = contact lens power (determined by ACC) + lacrimal lens power(determined by PCC)

Soft lens

- Lens conforms to the cornea, therefore there is no correction of astigmatism + no lacrimal lens

Optical advantages over glasses

- Correction of corneal astigmatism (hard lenses)
- Less magnification/minification (caused by the vertex distance in glasses)
- Less peripheral aberration and distortion
- Greater field (glasses decrease field of vision by 20 degrees)

Contraindications to contact lenses

- Insufficient motivation
- Patient unable to handle lens
- Uveitis
- Keratitis
- Scleritis
- Conjunctivitis
- Blepharitis
- Abnormal lid position
- Pterygium
- Dry eye syndrome
- Corneal anaesthesia

Problems with contact lenses

- Poor fit – apical touch → epithelial abrasion

- Too tight fit → peripheral abrasion + diminished tear exchange → hypoxia
- Too loose fit → excessive movement with epithelial abrasion
- Trapped air, foreign bodies, dirt
- Allergy (type 4) to thiomerasol preservative
- Allergy (type 1) to protein deposit on lens → giant papillary conjunctivitis
- Corneal neovascularisation, from chronic corneal hypoxia
- Corneal oedema, from hypoxia (build-up of lactic acid)
- Permanent corneal endothelial changes (toxic effect of lactic acid accumulation)
- Infection, from contaminated lens
- Dry eye, from decreased blinking
- Corneal anaesthesia
- Corneal warpage

Care of contact lenses

- Stored in soaking solution
- Cleaned with cleaning solution
- Prepared with wetting solution
- Disinfected with disinfecting solution
- Regular check for damage and protein build-up

Therapeutic uses of contact lenses

- Protective corneal bandage
- Treatment of dry eye syndromes
- Drug delivery system
- Cosmesis (corneal scars, iris defects)

Optical indications for contact lenses

- Myopia (90%)
- Hypermetropia, astigmatism
- Uniocular aphakia (magnification 1.12 cw 1.33)
- Anisometropia
- Accommodative esotropia

Contact lens intolerance

- External disease problems
  - Dry eye
  - Allergic disease (hay fever conjunctivitis, vernal conjunctivitis, atopic and contact dermatitis)
- Non-external disease factors
  - Blepharitis
  - Infrequent blinking
  - Environmental factors (dryness, hair sprays, grease and oil)
  - Loss of patient motivation
- Problems related to contact lens solutions
  - Giant papillary conjunctivitis
  - Sensitivity to preservatives
  - Contact lens deposits

Advantages and disadvantages of hard and soft lenses

Hard lenses

- Advantages
  - Mask corneal astigmatism
  - Less expensive
- Disadvantages
  - Lid edge sensation
  - Tend to fall out with sport

Soft lenses

- Advantages
  - Easier to fit
  - Better tolerated
- Disadvantages
  - More protein build-up

Giant papillary conjunctivitis

Treatment

- Discontinue lens for 1 month
- Use aggressive lens care
- Change to a different lens polymer
- Replace lenses frequently
- Disodium cromoglycate
- Use steroids sparingly

Presbyopia in contact lens wearers

- Monovision (use the dominant eye for distance)
- Bifocal lenses
- Simultaneous vision bifocal contact lenses (progressive power change from centre to periphery)

Basic principles of refractive surgery

Refractive procedures

- Corneal
  - Radial keratototmy (RK)
  - Arcuate keratotomy (AK)
  - Limbal relaxing incisions
  - Tranverse keratectomy
  - Photorefractive keratectomy (PRK)
  - Laser-assisted in situ keratomileusis (LASIK)
  - Laser subepithelial keratomileusis (LASEK)
  - Epikeratoplasty
  - Intrastromal corneal ring segments (Intacs)
  - Keratophakia
  - Laser thermal keratoplasty
  - Conductive (radiofrequency) keratoplasty (CK)
- Lenticular
  - Cataract surgery
  - Clear lens extraction + IOL
  - Phakic IOL
  - Accomodative IOL
  - Piggyback IOL

Corneal topography

- Placido disc based and elevation based
- Placido power maps do not represent the peripheral cornea very well
- Accurate topography can be influenced by several factors e.g. tear film abnormality

Wavefront analysis

- Most effective method to date for describing irregular astigmatism
- Low base laser beam focussed on the retina
- Light emerges from the eye to a sensor
- In the perfect eye, all the light travels at the same speed and the wavefront is flat
- In a non-perfect eye, light travels at different speeds through different parts → wavefront not flat

Aberrations

Low order

- Zero order
  - Piston (non-visually significant)
- First order
  - Prism – vertical + horizontal
- Second order
  - Defocus – myopia (positive defocus)
  - Defocus – hyperopia (negative defocus)
  - Regular astigmatism

High order

- Third order: Coma
  - Rays at one pupil edge get to the retina before rays from the opposite pupil edge
  - Object image resembles a comet
  - Occurs in decentred ablations, grafts, keratoconus
- Third order: Trefoil
  - Less detrimental than coma
- Fourth order
  - Spherical aberration – when peripheral rays focus in front of more central rays

- Causes night myopia
- Common after LASIK + PRK
- Secondary astigmatism
- Quadrafoil

Corneal optics

Corneal zones

- The cornea is aspheric → central cornea 3D steeper than periphery
- Central zone: 3–4 mm
- Paracentral: 4–7 mm
- Peripheral: 7–11 mm (area of greatest flattening)
- Limbal 11–12 mm
- Central + paracentral = apical zone (important in contact lens fitting)
- Optical zone: overlies the pupil
- Vertex: Centre of the keratoscopic image, corresponds with fixation

Shape/curvature/power

- A keratometer measures the corneal power of four points in the central zone, thus estimating vertex power
- Average central corneal power = 43D (anterior surface power of 49D – posterior surface power of 6D)

Topography

- Corneal power increases to the periphery because of the angle of incident light out here
- Spherical aberration – aspheric power that increases to the periphery
- Corneal shape is mapped from anterior + posterior surface perspective

Biomechanics

Incisional effect

- Radial incisions – flattening in the meridian of the incision + 90 degrees away
- Tangential incisions – linear or arcuate → causes coupling i.e. flattening in the meridian of the incision + steepening 90 degrees away
- The closer the lesions are to the visual axis, the greater the effect
- Incisions should be 85–90% thickness for maximal effect

Collagen shrinkage

- Heating collagen to 55 degrees causes it to shrink
- Thermatokeratoplasty – midperipheral → causes peripheral flattening + central steepening for correction of hyperopia

Corneal wound healing

- RK requires initial weakening, followed by permanent healing + replacement of epithelial plugs with collagen
- PRK – requires rapid healing + minimal keratocyte stimulation to avoid scar and haze
- There is increased haze with increased depth of ablation
- Mitomycinc (MMC) has been used to modify healing + prevent haze
- Lamellar surgery – typical stromal healing only occurs in the peripheral wound + the lamellar interface can always be broken + the flap lifted

Lasers

- Photothermal
  - Holmium:YAG → heat → collagen shrinkage
  - Thermal keratoplasty for high myopia
- Photodisruption
  - Picosecond Nd: YAG → tissue vaporisation
  - No clinical use yet
- Photoablation
  - Excimer laser (excited dimer)
  - Breaks C-N or C-C bonds
  - Capable of precision with very little thermal effect

Pre-op evaluation

- Stable refractive error essential
- Contraindications

- Conditions likely to elevate IOP
- Conditions likely to require chronic topical corticosteroid use
- Collagen vascular disease
- Pregnancy + nursing
- Keratoconus + form fruste keratoconus
- Recent contact lens wear

Classification of corneal refractive surgery

Lamellar keratoplasty

- Keratomileusis
  - The cutting of a corneal disc
  - Microkeratome with suction cup
  - Eximer or femtosecond laser
- Keratomileusis in situ
  - Carving corneal bed
- Epikeratoplasty
- Intracorneal lens/ring
  - Hydrogel lens
  - Human donor lens
  - Lamellar pocket
  - Annular lamellar dissection with corneal ring or adjustable gel injection
- Lamellar keratotomy/keratoplasty

Keratotomy

- Radial
- Transverse
  - Isolated straight or arcuate cuts
  - Customisation of cataract surgery incisions
- Circumferential

Keratectomy

- Laser – photorefractive keratectomy (PRK)
- Mechanical

Thermokeratoplasty

- Holmium:YAG
- Deep stromal hot needle thermocoagulation

Intraocular surgery

Phakic IOL

Advantages

- Can treat larger range of myopia, hyperopia
- Similar skills to cataract surgery
- Equipment less expensive
- Lens removable
- No loss of contrast sensitivity
- Low in aberrations

Disadvantages

- Intraocular surgery → risks
- Each type has its own risks
- Difficult to refine refractive outcome as in LASIK
- If cataract develops, need to explant before surgery

Indications

- –20D to +10D
- An alternative to LASIK, PRK when they are not possible e.g. 250 μ rule
- Age 20–50

Contraindications

- Pre-existing ocular diseases – iritis, rubeosis, cataracts, glaucoma, low endothelial counts
- Risk of retinal detachment low
- Angle width < 30 degrees, AC depth < 2.8 mm
- Endothelial cell count < 2 200
- Systemic diseases that may interfere with the eye in future e.g. diabetes, sarcoid
- Corneal disease, uveitis

Complications

- AC PIOL
  - Night glare + haloes
  - Oval pupils
  - Endothelial loss – ? rate

- Pupil block low because of peripheral iridotomy
  - AC depth must be > 3.2 mm, endothelial cell count > 2 000
- Iris fixated
  - Glare – 3%
  - Hyphaema and iris trauma
  - Iritis
  - Glaucoma
  - Mild endothelial cell loss
  - Pupil block rare
- PC IOL
  - Cataract
  - Pigment dispersion, especially if undersized
  - Lens decentration
  - Mild endothelial loss

Bioptics

- PC PIOL plus LASIK 1 month later → for patients with very high myopia

Clear lens extraction

- Controversial
- Only if alternative refractive procedures are not feasible + there is strong reason why spectacles or contact lenses are unacceptable alternatives
- Loss of accomodation
- Substantial risk of retinal detachment in myopia – 0% over 7 years (most occur at 1–4years post-op)
- 3D myopia → four times increased risk of retinal detachment
- > 3D → ten times increased risk of retinal detachment
- Avoid silicone IOLs
- Safety is not really established but offer it on an individual basis

Toric IOL

- 15–30% of cataract patients have astigmatism → 1.5D
- eg. Alcon Acrysof Toric IOL
- Two and 3.5D cylinder powers available
- 2D → corrects 1.4 D of astigmatism
- 3.5D → corrects 2.3D
- Indications: 1.5–3.5 D of regular corneal astigmatism
- Complications
  - IOL rotation + cyl misalignment
  - 10 degrees off axis → reduces correction 33%
  - 20 degrees off axis → reduces correction by 66%
  - > 30 degrees → increases the cylinder!

Multifocal IOL

- Diffractive or refractive
- Complications
  - Glare + haloes
  - Decreased contrast sensitivity

Photoablation

PRK + LASEK

- For low to moderate myopia, astigmatism + low hyperopia
- Contraindicabed in connective tissue diseases due to unpredictable wound healing and corneal melts
- Good for
  - Deep set eyes where microkeratome will not fit
  - Epithelial basement membrane dystrophies
  - Previous buttonholes
- Epithelium removed with sharp blade, blunt spatula, rotating brush, 20% ethanol
- In LASEK the epithelium is preserved, loosened with ethanol and folded back
- Supposed to reduce post-op pain, speed recovery of VA, decrease haze
- Mitomycin c 0.02% can be used intra-op or post-op to reduce haze, ? value of topical steroids
- Bandage contact lens post-op
- Healing within 72 hours
- Pain ranges from minimal to severe
- Myopic, spherical PRK – greater amounts of ablation associated with decreased predictability, increased haze,

loss of best corrected VA, increased regression
- Toric PRK – not as predictable but laser technology improving
- Hyperopic PRK – tissue removed from midperiphery
- Complications
  - Overcorrection
  - Undercorrection
  - Central islands
  - Optical aberrations
  - Decentred ablation
  - Corneal haze
  - Epithelial defect
  - Infiltrations
  - Steroid-induced complications
  - Dry eye
  - Endothelial defects
- Manifest and cycloplegic refractions usually differ by 0.25–1.0 D due to accommodative tone and the effect of the peripheral cornea when the pupil is dilated
- To select the best refraction, the duochrome test can be used
  - A chart with red and green letters is used
  - Red has a longer wavelength and rays fall slightly beyond the green rays
  - Overminus → red letters will be less clear
  - Overplussed → green letters will be less clear

LASIK

- Most popular refractive procedure
- Limit –8 to +4
- Very similar visual results to PRK, one study of patients with PRK in one eye and LASIK in the other showed twice as many highly satisfied with the LASIK eye than the PRK eye
- Flap created with a microkeratome or femtosecond ND:YAG laser (Intralase)
- Pre-op
  - Check for dry eyes, basement membrane dystrophies, forme fruste keratoconus, pellucid marginal degeneration, contact lens warpage
- Steep corneas > 48D – thin flaps + buttonholes
- 250 μm minimal residual corneal bed
- Predictability decreases with high myopia
- Myopia with astigmatism, hyperopic LASIK
- Retreatments can be done earlier than in PRK
- ± 10% retreatment rate
- Complications
  - Microkeratome – advances in technology have decreased these complications; irregular, thin, free cap, buttonhole, corneal perforation
  - Epithelial erosion – microkeratome friction
  - Striae
  - Traumatic flap dislocation – especially on day one
  - Dry eye – 33% – improves with corneal innervation
  - Central islands + decentration
  - Interface inflammation – DLK – sterile interface inflammation (Sands of the Sahara)
  - Keratitis
  - Epithelial ingrowth
  - Interface debris
  - Ectasia

Wavefront guided PRK + LASIK

- Theoretical resolution of the eye 6/1.5 (distance between photoreceptors)
- Conventional photoablation treats lower order (spherocylindrical) aberrations, which comprise 90% of all aberrations
- Higher order aberrations exists in the normal population and are produced by eximer laser ablation (there are ± 30 higher order aberrations)
- Wavefront guided customised ablations to decrease existing and induced higher order aberrations, as well as the lower order

- Shown to give better contrast sensitivity + decreased higher order aberrations compared to conventional
- They may still have more aberrations than they did pre-op
- Technology still evolving

Thermokeratoplasty

Laser thermokeratoplasty (for LTK)

- For hyertropia
- Holmium:YAG
- Laser in a set pattern around the corneal periphery
- Problem: Even heating of the cornea not possible
- Can cause epithelial necrosis, visual fluctuation + regression

Conductive keratoplasty (CK)

- For hyperopia +0.75D to +3.0D and up to 0.75D astigmatism
- Has largely replaced LTK
- Radiofrequency method of heating the cornea
- A ring pattern around the peripheral cornea
- Takes 5 mins under topical anaesthesia
- Being evaluated for the treatment of astigmatism after LASIK + phaco
- Safer than LASIK + LTK
- Efficacy results similar to hyperopic LASIK
- Long-term stability good – comparable to hyperopic LASIK

13

Incisional and inlay corneal surgery

Incisional

Radial keratotomy

- Radial corneal incisions, 85–95% depth
- Wound gape → corneal flattening
- No longer performed
- For –1 to –4
- Many complications
  - Corneal weakening + rupture, keratitis, intra-operative perforation, endophthalmitis, unstable refraction, starbursts, scar vascularisation

Astigmatic surgery

- Transverse keratotomy – no longer performed, replaced by LASIK, PRK
- Arcuate keratotomy – mostly post-PK
- Limbal relaxing incisions – mostly during cataract surgery
- 95% depth with a diamond knife

Onlays + inlays

Keratophakia

- A + power lens placed intrastromally
- Increases anterior corneal curvature for correction of hyperopia
- Homoplastic – from donor cornea
- Alloplastic – synthetic material e.g. hydrogel (promising technology)

Epikeratoplasty

- Suturing donor cornea
- Poor results

Intrastromal corneal ring segments

- Intacs
- 2 × 180 degree segments
- Displaces lamellar bundles, shortening corneal arc length
- PMMA circular rings in the midperipheral stroma
- The thicker the ring the greater the corneal flattening
- Reversible + titratable
- Cornea maintains a prolate shape, fewer visual disturbances
- Requires specialised equipment and training
- Cannot correct astigmatism

- Under investigation to correct corneal ectasias like keratoconus
- Complications: Perforation, keratitis

Orthokeratology

- Contact lens at night changes the shape of the cornea temporarily by day
- For –0.5 to –6, up to 1.75 astigmatism

IOL power calculation after refractive surgery

- Current IOL formulas rely on axial length + k readings
- Post-refractive surgery the keratometer reading is inaccurate because
  - Keratometers take readings of the corneal curvature several millimetres from the centre of the cornea and the centre has a different power post-surgery
  - Anterior + posterior corneal surfaces differ post-surgery
- K-readings read too high; if standard IOL techniques are used → post-op hyperopia
- Several methods can be used to estimate the true corneal power post-refractive surgery
- Clinical history method
  - When you have the pre-LASIK refraction + k readings
  - Example: Pre-op k readings – 44D
  - Pre-op SE: –8D with 12 mm vertex distance, –7.3D at the corneal plane
  - Post-op SE: –1.00D vertex 12 mm, –0.98D corneal plane
  - Change in manifest refraction: 6.32D
  - Post-op K power: 44D – 6.32D = 37.68D
- Do a normal IOL calculation, but use the pre-op refraction as the desired IOL outcome
- Take 20% of the difference between the pre- and post-op refractions, subtract this from the post-op keratometer readings to get the 'true' post-op K reading
- Hard contact lens method
  - When there is no pre-op information
  - Use a plano hard contact lens of known K power
  - Refract with the hard contact lens and without
  - Example: Current refraction: –1D
  - With hard contact lens of 37D power: +2D
  - Difference is 3D
  - Therefore, current corneal power is 37 + 3 = 40D
- There is a nomogram (Feiz) that can be applied if the prerefractive surgery refraction is known; least accurate method
- If one tries several methods, use the lowest K power calculated
- Use third generation IOL formulas
- Can use several of these formulas and select the highest calculated IOL power from these
- Scheimpflug topography K reading far more accurate
- New IOL formulas increasingly accurate

Presbyopia

Theories of accommodation

Helmholtz's capsular theory

- Distance vision – relaxed ciliary muscle, zonular fibres under resting tension
- Accommodation – ciliary muscle contraction, moves forward, releases zonular tension, lens capsule contracts, increased lens surface curvature
- Presbyopia – caused by loss of lens capsule elasticity

Schachar's theory

- Accommodation – ciliary muscle contraction, selective increase in zonulat tension, only equatorial

13

zonules, pulls lens equator towards sclera

- Presbyopia – due to increase lens size, therefore decreased lens-ciliary muscle distance, therefore decreased zonular tension
- No good evidence for this theory

Catenary (hydraulic support) theory

- Lens, zonules + anterior vitreous form a diaphragm
- Ciliary muscle contraction, pressure gradient from posterior to anterior, diaphragm moves forward, causes a steepening of the anterior lens curvature
- Presbyopia – increasing lens volume with age causes a reduced response of the anterior lens curvature

Non-accommodative treatment

Monovision

- Mild myopia of –0.50–1.50D in the non-dominant eye (modified monovion because you cannot get too large an anisometropia)
- Only a mild decrease in distance vision, very good stereopsis, very good intermediate vision
- Could go up to –1.50D to –2.50D in some
- Can be achieved in LASIK, PRK, cataract surgery
- Consider a trial with contact lenses first

Conductive keratoplasty

- Induce a mild myopia after hyperopia treatment
- Simple, safe, non-invasive

IOL implants

- Multifocal IOL
- Patient selection crucial
- Make sure of accurate biometery
- Must have astigmatism < 1D

Custom or multifocal ablations

- Creating a multifocal cornea
- Various possible ablation patterns
    - Small, steep central zone; central – near, midperiphery – distance
    - Inferior – near
    - Central – distance, intermediate – near
- Data limited but so far good

Corneal inlays

Accommodative treatments

Scleral surgery

- Objective of increasing zonular tension by weakening or altering the sclera over the ciliary body in order to allow for passive expansion
- Based on the Schachar's theory
- Anterior ciliary sclerotomy – does not work
- Scleral expansion bands – PMMA bands in scleral tunnels overlying the ciliary body, acting as stents to pull the sclera and expand the space between the ciliary body and the equator
- Erbium:YAG – scleral incisions aimed at expansion
- No evidence

Accommodating IOL

- Vertex phenomenon
- Designed to maximise the anterior movement of the IOL
- Has hinges
- 1D power generated for near
- Long-term capsular fibrosis does not seem to be a problem

Contact lenses

- Bifocal contacts
- Monovision
- Especially relevant with extended wear lenses

Refractive surgery in ocular and systemic disease

Dry eye

- Relative contraindication
- Often seek surgery because of contact lens intolerance
- Normal tear film important for post-op wound healing
- Tear replacements + punctal plugs
- Pre-op steroids or cyclosporin
- Shown to have slower recovery, but selective patients can be suitable

Herpes simplex virus

- Relative contraindication
- May incite herpes simplex recurrence – not enough information yet
- Pretreat with oral acyclovir
- Absolute contraindications – pronounced loss of corneal sensation + corneal anaesthesia, vascularisation, recent attack

Keratoconus

- Contraindication
- Loss of best corrected VA + need for subsequent corneal graft
- Poor predictability

Post-corneal graft

- They get irregular astigmatism + anisometropia
- 10–30% of patients post-PK need a contact lens – this is often not possible because of the corneal curvature
- Compression sutures, AK + wedge resections have been shown to decrease cylinder by an average of 5.5D (56%) in one study
- Sometimes these results are unpredictable
- LASIK increases the chance of being able to fit a contraindications
- Wait 2 years post-graft + at least 6 months after suture removal
- The suction ring can cause stress on the interface
- Can be done in a two-stage procedure – creating the lamellar flap alone can change the astigmatism
- 54–88% decrease in astigmatism
- But 42% need an enhancement
- 35% lose one line of best corrected VA
- Rejection has been reported

Glaucoma

- Frequently higher in the myopic population
- Acute IOP rise of 65 mmHg with the suction ring
- ? Will a glaucomatous optic nerve tolerate this
- Contraindicated in marked cupping and field loss
- Need to get baseline IOP before surgery because corneal thickness will change and throw out applanation readings
- No ablations in poorly controlled patients
- Ocular hypertension – more difficult to monitor post-op
- Suction ring cannot be placed on a filtering bleb
- Be careful with post-op steroids
- No IOP monitoring for at least 72 hours post-op because of flap

High myopia

- Symptomatic tears should be treated
- Asymptomatic lattice + atrophic holes – no treatment
- Asymptomatic tears and holes – no treatment
- No proven causal link between retinal detachment and ablation
- But IOP rise + acoustic shock waves from the laser may cause a PVD

13

Post-retinal surgery

- Myopia induced by a buckle or PPV
- Can be done, but less predictable

Amblyopia

- 2.5% in the general population
- Pre-op counselling is important because one eye will be less good
- Consider unilateral surgery only
- Although can cause a squint and diplopia
- Some people use LASIK to treat anisometropic amblyopia and accommodative esotropias not doing well with conventional treatments

HIV

- Potential post-op complications of low immunity
- But there are lots of healthy people on HAART who could do well

Diabetes

- Glucose must be stable for refraction
- Previous laser is a contraindicated to LASIK
- Corneal epithelium can be unhealthy
- Few long-term studies
- Complication rate is quite high and mostly due to epithelial problems
- Therefore, select patients well
- Minimise epithelial toxicity by not using too much local pre-op

Connective tissue disease

- Melts, corneal perforations + scarring
- Contraindicated

14

Systemic diseases

Acquired immune deficiency syndrome (AIDS) 397
Albinism 399
Chromosomal disorders 399
Haematological disorders and the eye 400
Leprosy 401
Liver disease and the eye 402
Metabolic disorders and the eye ... 402
Microphthalmos 403
Musculoskeletal disease and the eye 404
Myasthenia gravis 405
Phacomatoses 406
Rheumatoid arthritis 409
Skin diseases and the eye 410
Rubella 410
Syphilis 411

Acquired immune deficiency syndrome (AIDS)

Incidence in ophthalmology

- 10% of patients may first present with eye manifestations
- 75% of AIDS patients have eye involvement

Epidemiology

- North America and Europe – homosexual STD transmission + IV drug abusers
- Africa – heterosexual STD transmission
- Not spread through casual contact, only through contact with blood and other secretions

Virology

- Human immunodeficiency virus; types 1 and 2; retrovirus
- Strong propensity for genetic mutations with rapid emergence of new strains

Pathology

- Virus has selective tropism for CD4 receptors on T-helper cells in peripheral blood → destruction of T-helper cells → immune deficiency
- Penetrance is high, probably 100%

Laboratory tests

- Elisa test, to detect antibodies
  - If positive, then repeat
  - If repeat positive then →
- Western blot test; more specific test to detect antibodies to GP41 viral envelope protein
  - Will detect 99% of patients who are infected with HIV

Systemic manifestations of HIV

- Viral symptoms
  - Viral illness similar to glandular fever (fever, sore throat, headache, myalgia, rash, lymphadenopathy)
- Asymptomatic carrier state
  - Latent period; may last several years
- Neurologic syndrome

- AIDS-related complex
  - Generalised lymphadenopathy, fever, weight loss, chronic diarrhoea, malaise, oral thrush
- Slim disease – diarrhoea, wasting
- AIDS – weight loss, fever, lymphadenopathy, opportunistic infections, neoplasms
- Infections – pneumocystis carinii, cryptococcus, candidiasis, cytomegaloinclusion virus, toxoplasma, tuberculosis
- Neoplasms
  - Kaposi's sarcoma, non-Hodgkin's lymphoma
  - Occurs when CD4 T-lymphocyte count < 200 /Ul

Ocular manifestations of AIDS

- Retinal microangiopathy – cotton wool spots, haemorrhages, peripheral periphlebitis; ? due to immune complex deposition, ? due to HIV infection of vascular endothelium; seen in 50% of AIDS patients
- Kaposi's sarcoma of lids and conjunctiva – subconjunctival haemorrhage that does not clear, bluish discoloration of lid
- CMV retinitis – occurs in 20–45 % of AIDS patients; two forms are indolent form and fulminating form
  - Indolent from starts in periphery, mild granular opacification
  - Fulminating form shows dense white demarcated geographic area of confluent opacification, develops along vascular arcades, retinal haemorrhage within or overlying the leading edge, mild vitritis, brush fire like extension along course of blood vessels, complicated by retinal atrophy and retinal detachment; 33% bilateral on presentation; treat with intravitreal ganciclovir
- Herpes zoster ophthalmicus
- Herpes simplex keratitis – dendrites occur in corneal periphery
- Pneumocystis choroiditis – variable number of flat, yellow, round choroidal lesions, often bilateral, no vitritis, little visual impairment
- Other opportunistic infections – mycobacteria, toxoplasma, fungi (cryptococcus, candida), syphilis, TB
- Squamous cell carcinoma of conjunctiva
- Molluscum contagiosum – of lid skin + limbal conjunctiva

Ocular manifestations of HIV infection in Africa

- Herpes zoster ophthalmicus – marker for HIV with a high positive predictive value
- Molluscum contagiosum and verrucae of lids
- Kaposi's sarcoma of lids
- Stevens-Johnson syndrome – increased risk with HIV
- Squamous cell carcinoma conjunctiva – 75% of patients are HIV positive, human papilloma virus is causative, HIV plays a permissive role
- Syphilitic uveitis
- TB uveitis
- Retinopathy
- CMV retinitis – associated with CD4 count < 50
- Optic neuropathy (papillitis, optic atrophy) – due to neurosyphilis, cryptococcal meningitis, CNS toxoplasmosis, HIV encephalopathy, intracranial tumours

Treatment of ocular complications

- Retinal microangiopathy – no treatment required
- Kaposi's sarcoma – only treat if the size is a problem; chemotherapy, interferon, radiotherapy
- CMV retinitis
  Intravitreal ganciclovir 2–3 times a week to start, then weekly
- Zoster ophthalmicus – treat as usual, omit systemic steroids

- Pneumocystis carinii choroiditis – pentamidine

Albinism

Prevalence

- SA blacks – 1 in 3 000
- SA whites – 1 in 20 000

Classification

- Oculocutaneous (all autosomal recessive)
  - Tyrosinase positive (hair bulbs darken when incubated with tyrosine)
  - Tyrosinase negative (more severe form)
  - Yellow mutant
  - Hermansky-Pudlak syndrome (haemorrhagic diathesis due to platelet dysfunction)
- Ocular
  - Nettleship-Falls x-linked
  - Autosomal recessive
  - Chediak-Higashi syndrome (abnormal wbc → susceptibility to gram positive infection, develop lymphoma)
- Albinoidism
  - No significant visual impairment, no nystagmus
  - Autosomal dominant oculocutaneous
  - Punctate oculocutaneous
  - Apert's syndrome
  - Waardenburg-like syndrome

Ocular features

- Poor vision
- Photophobia
- Nystagmus; due to macular hypoplasia and visual pathway abnormality
- Strabismus
- Refractive errors
- Iris transillumination
- Visible choroidal vasculature
- Hypoplastic macula – absent pit, absent luteal pigment, absent hyperpigmentation of RPE; failure of retinal vasculature to wreathe fovea
- Visual pathway abnormality – abnormal cross-over of temporal fibres, therefore no stereopsis

Pathophysiology of visual imapairment

- Macular hypoplasia; RPE hyperpigmentation is necessary for normal foveal differentiation
- Congenital sensory nystagmus may contribute
- Temporal fibres cross at chiasm, therefore single binocular vision is not possible

Treatment

- Tinted lenses; no UV filter necessary
- Refraction; retinoscopy difficult, therefore test subjectively
- Low vision aids

Chromosomal disorders

Trisomy 21

Ocular features

- Lids
  - Mongoloid slant
  - Abnormal shaped palpebral fissures
  - Epicanthal folds
  - External hypertelorism
  - Narrowed interpupillary distance
  - Ectropion
  - Blepharitis
  - Nasolacrimal duct obstruction
- Cornea – keratoconus
- Anterior chamber angle – congenital glaucoma
- Iris
  - Peripheral hypoplasia
  - Brushfield spots (pale grey, in mid-periphery, local thickening of iris)
- Lens – cataracts (in 80%)
- Retina
  - Increased number of retinal vessels crossing disc margin, often in wheel spoke fashion
  - Retinal detachment

  - Retinitis pigmentosa
  - Retinoblastoma
- Refractive errors – high refractive errors
- Ocular motility
  - Esotropia (35%)
  - Nystagmus

Systemic features

- Appearance – low set ears, short stature, simian crease, rosebud mouth
- Mental retardation
- Cardiovascular anomalies

Trisomy 13

- Ocular features – microphthalmia, coloboma, retinal dysplasia, persistent hyperplastic primary vitreous, optic nerve hypoplasia, cataract, corneal opacity

Deletion of the long arm of chromosome 13

- Ocular features – retinoblastoma in 20–30%, hypertelorism, ptosis, uveal colobomas

Trisomy 18 (Edwards' syndrome)

- Ocular features similar to trisomy 13

Foetal alcohol syndrome

- Peters anomaly
- Lens opacities
- Ocular motility disorders
- Optic nerve hypoplasia

Haematological disorders and the eye

Anaemia

General

- Pallor of palpebral conjunctiva
- Retinopathy – haemorrhages including Roth's spots, soft exudates, distended veins, papilloedema

Specific

- Pernicous anaemia – retrobulbar neuritis
- Sickle cell anaemia – retinopathy
- Acute exsanguination – ischaemic neuropathy; low tension glaucoma

Leukaemia

- Ocular involvement in 50–90%
- If ocular involvement occurs in a treated patient, it indicates either bone marrow relapse or CNS involvement, and mortality is 100%
- Altered blood → anaemia, viscosity → retinopathy (background and proliferative)
- Leukaemic infiltrates
  - Eye – conjunctiva, episclera, sclera, iris → colour changes, hypopyon, elevated IOP, choroid → overlying serous retinal detachment, retina, disc, optic nerve
  - Orbit – chloroma in acute myeloid leukaemia (green due to myeloperoxidase), lymphosarcoma in acute lymphoblastic leukaemia
  - Cranial nerves – palsies, papilloedema
- Treat ocular infiltrates with irradiation, poor response to chemotherapy
- Opportunistic infections – CMV retinitis
- Drug toxicity
  - Busulphan → cataracts
  - Vincristine and vinblastine → motor nerve palsies
  - Cytosine → corneal epithelial toxicity
  - Methotrexate → blepharoconjunctivitis
  - Mustine → necrotising vasculitis

Hyperviscocity

- Polycythaemia, Waldenstrom's, multiple myeloma, lymphoma

- Retinopathy (venous engorgement, haemorrhages, exudates), vein occlusion

Multiple myeloma

- Hyperviscosity, eyelid necrobiotic xanthoma, corneal crystals (copper deposits in central cornea)

Septicaemia

- Retinopathy occurs in 25% cases
- Haemorrhages, soft exudates, Roth's spots

Leprosy

General

- Systemic disease with highest incidence of ocular complications
- World leprosy population 10–12 million; 5 million cases registered for treatment
- 30% suffer some form of disability
- 5% of people with leprosy are blind
- 21% of people with leprosy have potentially sight threatening lesions
- 24% people 'cured' of their leprosy and discharged from follow-up still have potentially sight-threatening lesions
- Paucibacillary/tuberculoid leprosy → lagophthalmos and corneal hypoaesthesia
- Multibacillary/lepromatous leprosy → uveitis with its sequelae, in addition
- Blindness in leprosy due to – corneal opacity, iridocyclitis, cataract
- Increased prevalence of ocular involvement if leprosy has been present for more than 15 years

Clinical features

- Madarosis
- Lepromatous nodules of skin, conjunctiva, sclera
- Lagophthalmos due to nerve damage affecting VII zygomatic and temporal branches; results in lower lid ectropion
- Dermatochalasis of upper lid; may result in entropion and trichiasis
- Keratitis
  - Opaque corneal nerves
  - Lepromatous nodules of cornea (usually limbal)
  - Interstitial keratitis
  - Avascular punctate keratitis – in upper outer quadrant; consists of clumps of bacilli-laden cells
  - Trophic keratopathy from corneal hypoaesthesia
  - Resultant corneal ulceration and scarring
- Uveitis
  - Acute – iris and ciliary body invaded by mycobacteria; all the features of acute iridocyclitis, but not painful
  - Chronic – mycobacteria lodge in iris and ciliary body, persist after skin smears are negative; results in autonomic paresis → decreased pupil reaction; decreased IOP; increased IOP postural response; decreased accommodation; end stage fixed miotic pupil
  - Sequelae of uveitis – cataract and glaucoma

Treatment

- Lower lid involvement
  - Acute stage – treat with systemic steroids, thalidomide, clofazamine; may recover
  - Chronic stage – treat with tarsorrhaphy or temporalis transfer
- Corneal involvement
  - Protect corneas at risk
  - Lid closure exercises + tear replacements
- Iris involvement
  - Treat acute iridocyclitis with steroids and mydriatics
  - Treat chronic iridocyclitis with 5% phenylephrine + atropine + steroids

Liver disease and the eye

Eyelids

- Xanthelasma in long standing cholestasis

Conjunctiva

- Jaundice in hyperbilirubinaemia
- Keratoconjunctivitis sicca in
  - Primary biliary cirrhosis
  - Chronic active hepatitis
- Pingueculae in Gaucher's disease

Cornea

- Wilson's disease → Kayser-Fleischer ring (copper deposit in region of Descemet's membrane in peripheral cornea)
- Chronic active hepatitis, primary biliary cirrhosis, any other severe jaundice → pigmented peripheral corneal ring
- Mucopolysaccharidoses and mucolipidoses → central corneal clouding and hepatomegally

Lens

- Developmental cataracts – galactosaemia, cerebrohepatorenal syndrome

Retina

- Mucopolysaccharidosis → pigmentary retinopathy
- Sphingolipidosis → cherry red spot
- Primary biliary cirrhosis → vitamin A deficiency

Optic nerve

- Mucopolysaccharidosis → optic atrophy

Cranial nerve palsies

- Wernicke's encephalopathy
- Parinaud's syndrome

Metabolic disorders and the eye

Mucopolysaccharidoses

- Eight types
- Corneal clouding in types 1, 4, 6
- RPE degeneration in types 1, 2, 3
- Optic atrophy in types 1, 2, 3, 4, 5

Glycogen storage diseases

- Eight types
- Glycogen accumulation in retinal ganglion cells in types 1 and 2 → yellow paramacular lesions

Sphingolipidoses

- Tay-Sach's – cherry red spot at macula, due to ganglioside accumulation in ganglion cells
- Later optic atrophy
- Niemann-Pick – cloudy cornea, macular cherry red spot
- Fabry's disease – whorl-like corneal epithelial opacity

Mucolipidoses

- Corneal clouding in some
- Cherry red spot in some

Neuronal lipofuscinosis (Batten-Mayou disease)

- Macular pigmentary retinopathy, optic atrophy

Aminoacidurias

- Homocystinuria – subluxed lens
- Cystinosis – crystals in cornea, conjunctiva, choroid; RPE degeneration
- Galactosaemia – cataracts

Lowe's oculocerebrorenal syndrome

- X-linked recessive
- Cataract
- Microphakia
- Congenital glaucoma

Refsum's disease

- Autosomal recessive; enzyme deficiency → increased phytanic acid
- Major features
  - Pigmentary retinopathy
  - Cerebellar ataxia
  - Peripheral neuropathy
  - Increased CSF protein
- Ocular features
  - Miosis
  - Posterior subcapsular lens opacities
  - Corneal clouding
  - Ophthalmoplegia

Microphthalmos

Definition

- Axial length less than normal
- < 19.2 mm at 1 year of age; < 20.9 mm in adulthood

Aetiology

- Genetic, usually; autosomal recessive, autosomal dominant, some x-linked recessive; autosomal dominant penetrance variable
- Teratogens, sometimes; irradiation, rubella, vitamin deficiency (A, E, folic acid, riboflavine)

Simple microphthalmos (nanophthalmos)

- Rare, unilateral or bilateral
- Small but otherwise normal eye; due to arrested development after embryonic fissure has closed
- Features include nystagmus and strabismus secondary to poor vision secondary to macular hypoplasia, hypermetropia, shallow anterior chamber, macular and retinal hypoplasia with attenuated and tortuous vessels, hypermetropic disc, late development of glaucoma

Colobomatous microphthalmos

- Unilateral or bilateral
- Due to involution of primary optic vesicle or failure of closure of embryonic cleft
- Associated with other colobomatous ocular features

Complex microphthalmos

- Unilateral or bilateral
- Clinical anophthalmos
- Associated ocular anomalies – corneal opacities, corneal staphylomata, cataract, aniridia, corectopia, persistent pupillary membrane, persistent tunica vasculosa lentis, persistent hyperplastic primary vitreous. thickening or ossification of choroid, retinal folds and gliosis, hypoplasia of visual pathways
- As part of systemic syndrome, systemic associations
  - Neurological abnormalities – oligophrenia, congenital spastic diplegia
  - Malformations of hands and feet – syndactyly, polydactyly
  - Cleft palate
  - Skeletal abnormalities
  - Dental abnormalities
  - Cardiovasular abnormalities
  - Urogenital abnormalities
  - 100 syndromes have been described, all modes of inheritance have been described

Clinical classification

- Unilateral or bilateral
- Anophthalmos
- Microphthalmos – remnant only, non-colobomatous, colobomatous

Aetiologic classification

- Associations
  - Sporadic, with unknown aetiology
- Genetic
  - Monogenic – autosomal dominant usually, sometimes autosomal recessive or x-linked recessive
  - Chromosomal anomalies
- Prenatal acquired – rubella is important

Systemic associations

- 50% have systemic associations
- May occur with the OAV spectrum (oculoauriculoverebral spectrum)

Musculoskeletal diseases and the eye

Mandibulofacial dysostosis (Treacher-Collins syndrome)

Ocular features

- Downward displacement of lateral canthi
- Notching of inferior lids, absent puncta
- Deficient lashes
- Astigmatism
- Iris coloboma
- Microphthalmia

Other features

- Maxillary hypoplasia

Craniofacial dysostosis (Crouzon's and Apert syndrome)

Ocular features

- Shallow orbits with prominent globes
- Hypertelorism
- Optic atrophy; secondary hydrocephalus, not due to bone encroachment
- V syndromes, squint (exotropia)

Other features

- Syndactyly in Apert syndrome

Oculoauriculovertabral dysplasia (Goldenhar syndrome)

Ocular features

- Limbal corneal dermoid (inferotemporal)
- Orbital lipodermoid (superotemporal limbus)
- Notching of the upper lid
- Also:
  - Duane's syndrome
  - Dacryocystitis
  - Microcornea
  - Iris coloboma
  - Anisocoria
  - Cataract

Other features

- Pre-auricular skin tag
- Pretragal fistula
- Vertebral anomalies

Marfan's syndrome

Ocular features

- Dislocated lenses
- Myopia
- Ptosis
- Megalocornea
- Blue scleras
- Strabismus
- Ciliary muscle hypoplasia
- Retinal degeneration

Muscular dystrophy

Ocular features

- Cataracts
- Ptosis
- External ophthalmoplegia
- Exophoria/tropia
- Keratoconjunctivitis sicca
- Decreased IOP
- RPE disturbance with diminished B-wave

Pierre Robin syndrome

Ocular features

- Occurs in 50%
- Esotropia
- Congenital glaucoma
- Retinal detachment
- High myopia

Other features

- Micrognathia
- Glossoptosis
- Cleft palate

Weill-Marchesani syndrome

Ocular features

- Myopia
- Microspherophakia
- Dislocated lenses
- Cataract
- Glaucoma

Myasthenia gravis

Definition

- Autoimmune disease; damage of acetylcholine receptors in striated muscle → weakness relieved by rest, with variability of muscle function and improvement with cholinergics

Incidence

- Rare, female > male, no racial predilection, 1 in 10 000

Pathophysiology

- Damage of postsynaptic acetylcholine receptors, ? on an autoimmune basis
- IgG against acetylcholine receptors demonstrable in 90% of patients
- Antibody against A, I and Z lines of skeletal muscle may be demonstrable
- Other autoimmune diseases are associated

Pathology

- Lymphocyte collections in muscle, end plate abnormalities, decreased number of acetylcholine receptors

Classification of myasthenia gravis

- Adult
  - Ocular (mild; 10% of cases)
  - Mild generalised
  - Moderate generalised
  - Acute fulminating (often associated thymoma)
- Paediatric
  - Neonatal (10 –30 % of babies of myasthenic mothers, lasts 6 weeks, due to placental transfer of anti-acetylcholine receptor antibodies)
  - Juvenile (good prognosis)

Features

- Ocular
  - Initial feature in 75%, eventually occurs in 90%
  - Diplopia and/or unilateral ptosis initially
  - Ptosis, unilateral or bilateral, asymmetric, may be apparent in upgaze (Simpson's sign)
  - Lid twitch, from looking down to straight ahead (Cogan's sign)
  - Weakness of orbicularis, 'afternoon ectropion'
  - Extraocular muscle pareses, variable patterns
  - Pupil and accommodation are never involved or very rarely involved
- Systemic
  - Face, tongue, masseter, neck, oropharyngeal, trunk, limbs
  - Characterised by weakness of muscles, relieved by rest, variable in severity, temporarily improved with cholinergics
- Thymoma
  - Occurs in 10%; severe, rapid progression
  - Also dysthyroidism in 5%

Tensilon test

- 1 ml tensilon (edrophonium – short acting anticholinesterase) IV → improvement of function within 3–4 mins

- 0.2 ml test dose, atropine on stand by; side effects are parasympathetic-like
- Paradoxic worsening, false positive or negative may occur
- May by used in conjunction with EMG, ocular tonography, oculography, red filter diplopia test
- Prostigmin should be used in children; response is seen after 10– 30 mins following IVI 1–2 mg

Ice Test

- Application of ice pack to ptotic lid for 2 mins
- 2 mm or more improvement of ptosis is positive for myasthenia gravis
- Decrease in temperature → decreased metabolism of acetyl choline

Differential diagnosis

- Myasthenia gravis should be suspected in any puzzling ocular motility disturbance, ± ptosis, with normal pupils
- Chronic progressive external ophthalmoplegia
- Dysthyroid ophthalmoplegia
- Neurogenic eye muscle palsies (combined III, IV, VI palsies)
- Lambert-Eaton syndrome (carcinoma bronchus → impaired acetylcholine release; ocular, facial and pharyngeal involvment is rare)
- Drugs – streptomycin, neomycin, kanamycin, polymyxin, bacitracin, colistein, penicillamine, vincristine, vinblastine

Special investigations

- Tensilon test
- Ice test
- Anti-acetylcholine receptor antibody
- Autostriated muscle antibody
- Chest x-ray and CT to demonstrate thymoma

Treatment

- Anticholinesterases – pyridostigmine 1–4 tablets 3–6 times daily; ?accelerate loss of acetylcholine receptors → long-term worsening
- Local eye treatment – prostigmine drops, phosphaline iodide drops
- Lid crutch
- Opaque lens for diplopia
- Steroids
    - Alternate day high dose, if unresponsive to anticholinesterases or thymectomy
    - Hospitalise initially, as there is initial exacerbation of the weakness
- Thymectomy – more effective response in patientrs without thymoma; eliminates abnormal clones of lymphocytes
- Azathioprine
- ± EOM surgery to achieve SBV if it is stable

Prognosis

- 90% of cases with ocular involvement develop systemic involvement, usually within 18 months
- Mortality rate 20–60%, due to respiratory paresis

Phacomatoses

Classification

- Von Hippel-Lindau disease
- Sturge-Weber syndrome (encephalofacial angiomatosis)
- Bourneville's disease (tuberous sclerosis)
- Von Recklinghausen's disease (neurofibromatosis)
- Naevus of Ota (oculodermal melanocytosis)
- Louis-Bar syndrome (ataxia telangiectasia)
- Wyburn-Mason syndrome
- Klippel-Trenaunay-Weber syndrome

Von Hippel-Lindau disease (angiomatosis retinae and cerebelli)

- 80% sporadic, 20% inherited – autosomal dominant, incomplete penetration + delayed expressivity
- Incidence: 1 in 36 000

Retinal capillary angiomatosis

- Early small red tumours with prominent afferent and efferent vessels; occurs in 60% of cases
- Histology shows endothelial cell proliferation
- Later opaque and white; histology shows sclerosis
- Bilateral in 50%, often multiple, occur in periphery
- May → haemorrhage, exudate, gliosis, retinal detachment, glaucoma, phthisis bulbi

CNS angiomatosis

- Of cerebellum, medulla, spinal cord

Systemic associations

- Renal cell carcinoma, hypernephroma, kidney cysts, pancreas cysts, ovarian cysts, anomalies of skull, epididymis cysts, phaeochromocytoma, meningioma

Sturge-Weber syndrome (encephalotrigeminal angiomatosis)

- No known inheritance
- Triad of
  - Cutaneous haemangioma/naevus flammeus (port wine stain)
  - Haemangioma of ipsilateral meninges + choroid
  - Glaucoma

Cutaneous haemangioma/naevus flammeus (port wine stain)

- Of Va (± Vb + Vc); nasal, buccal, conjunctival, episcleral hemangioma may also occur; iris telangiectasia → heterochromia may occur
- Vascular malformations may cross the midline

Haemangioma of ipsilateral meninges and choroid

- Meningeal haemangioma mainly in occipital region, → epilepsy, hemiplegia, and mental retardation; shows calficiation on x-ray
- Choroidal haemangioma yellow-grey, elevated, well-defined or poorly defined; may also occur in isolation; fluorescein → early lacy filling
- Differential diagnosis from malignant melanoma on ultrasound (high internal reflectivity cw poor internal reflectivity); overlying retina may degenerate, retinal detachment may occur

Glaucoma

- ? Due to increased episcleral venous pressure, occurs in 1/3rd of cases, onset
- Congenital → adult (especially if upper lid is involved)

Treatment

- Treat epilepsy, treat glaucoma, photocoagulate symptomatic choroidal haemangiomas

Bourneville's disease (tuberous sclerosis)

- Autosomal dominant, high penetrance + variable expressivity

Retinal lesion

- Astrocytic hamartomas (50%), occuring near disc; grey-white; may be calcified
- Grow very slowly, may break off and metastasise; may be associated nerve head drusen

CNS lesions

- Astrocytic hamartomas in cerebrum, basal ganglia, brainstem, cerebellum; → mental deficiency (60%), epilepsy, calcification on x-ray

Adenoma sebaceum

- Angiofibromas, appearing as yellow red papules in butterfly distribution
- Shagreen patch on the back, hypomelanotic macules on trunk or limbs, naevi, fibromas, café au lait spots

Systemic associations

- Rhabdomyosarcoma of heart, tumours of thyroid and kidney, spina bifida, ectopic testis, horseshoe kidney, renal tumours
- Treatment symptomatic

Neurofibromatosis Type 1

- Most common of all the phacomatoses, affects 1 in 4 000

Systemic features

- Neural tumours – of brain, spinal cord, and peripheral nerves
- Skeletal defects – acquired scoliosis, dysplasia of sphenoid bone, dysplasia of long bones, facial haemiatrophy, short stature, macrocephaly
- Skin lesions – café au lait spots, axillary freckles, fibroma molluscum, plexiform neurofibromas
- Miscellaneous – neurofibromas, leukaemia, lymphoma, hypertension, epilepsy, mental handicap

Ocular features

- Orbital involvement – optic nerve glioma, other neural tumours, spheno orbital encephalocoele
- Eyelid neurofibromas
- Iris lesions – Lisch nodules, ectropion uveae
- Prominent corneal nerves
- Glaucoma
- Fundus lesions – choroidal naevi, retinal astrocytomas

Neurofibromatosis Type 2

Systemic features

- Bilateral acoustic neuromas
- Central nervous system tumours – neurofibromas, meningiomas, gliomas, schwannomas

Ocular features

- Cataract
- Fundus lesions – combined hamartomas of RPE and retina
- Extraocular motor defects

Louis-Bar syndrome (ataxia telangiectasia)

- Autosomal recessive
- Progressive cerebellar ataxia, oculocutaneous telangiectasia, immunodeficiency, chromosomal instability, predisposition to malignancy (lymphoma + leukaemia)
- Mental retardation
- Progressive oculomotor apraxia, ophthalmoplegia

Wyburn-Mason syndrome

- Vascular hamartomatous lesions between the arterial + venous circulations
- Central nervous system arterovenous malformations → haemorrhage, epilepsy
- Racemose haemangiomas – usually asymptomatic
- Vision may reduce if they result in a vascular steal

Klippel-Trenaunay-Weber syndrome

- Autosomal dominant, variable expressivity
- Cutaneous vascular lesion affecting one or more limbs
- Ocular – uncommon, orbital varix, strabismus, iris heterochromia, coloboma, glaucoma, choroidal angiomas

Rheumatoid arthritis

Ocular manifestations

- Keratoconjunctivitis sicca
  - Most common
  - Occurs in 10–35% of patients, as part of Sjögren's syndrome
- Sclera and episclera
  - Episcleritis
  - Scleritis – anterior, posterior, diffuse, nodular, necrotising, scleromalacia perforans
- Cornea
  - Sclerosing keratitis, adjacent to limbal scleritis
  - Marginal ulcer – unilateral or bilateral, usually inferior, progressive → perforation, or non-progressive, ? due to immune complexes blocking limbal blood vessels, ? due to collagenase released from white blood cells, treat with bandage contact lens and cyclosporin 2% drops
  - Band-shaped keratopathy, secondary to uveitis
- Uveitis
  - In association with scleritis
- Cataract
  - Secondary to uveitis
- Choroid and retina
  - Secondary choroiditis and exudative retinal detachment overlying posterior scleritis
- Orbital myositis – episodic attacks, with proptosis, pain, paresis
- Superior oblique tendon sheath syndrome – ? due to rheumatoid nodule in region of trochlea
- Oculomotor palsies – due to central nervous system vasculitis

Ocular complications of treatment

- Corticosteroids
  - Cataract, glaucoma, herpes and fungal infections
  - Rebound phenomenon on steroid withdrawal → acute red eye
- Chloroqine
  - Cornea
    - Deposition in epithelium, reversible, occurs in 30–70% of patients
    - Decreased corneal sensation in 50% of patients
    - Accommodative weakness
  - Lens
    - Non-progressive flakes beneath posterior capsule
  - Retinopathy
    - 250 mg/day × 1 year is potentially retinopathic
    - Safe dose is < 3.5 mg/kg ideal body weight/day
    - Incidence 6–16%
    - May appear / progress after chloroquine is stopped
    - Chloroqine is bound to melanin and concentrated in RPE
    - Interferes with RPE metabolism and ability of melanin to protect surrounding tissues from action of free radicals
    - Results in RPE destruction with pigment dispersion and loss of rods and cones
    - Results in central or pericentral scotomata, pigmentary changes → bull's eye maculopathy (granular hyperpigmentation, surrounding hypopigmented ring, surrounding hyperpigmented ring), later more extensive retinal damage
    - Early detection is important; central red field loss, amsler grid, fluorescein → window defect, ERG and EOG normal early and decreased late, dark adaptation unaffected
    - Monitor central 12 degree red fields every 6 months
- Indomethacin
  - Cornea – deposition in epithelium and Descemet's membrane

    - Retinopathy – similar to chloroqine retinopathy
- Non-steroidal anti-inflammatories – toxic amblyopia, cortical visual hallucinations

Skin diseases and the eye

Pemphigus

- Conjunctivitis → entropion and trichiasis, cataract

Cicatricial pemphigoid

- Conjunctivitis → symblepharon formation, entropion, trichiasis, corneal scarring

Erythema multiforme

- Conjunctivitis → above, anterior uveitis

Toxic epidermal necrolysis

- Less severe form of erythema multiforme; limited to conjunctiva

Incontinentia pigmenti

- Retinal dysplasia, cataract, optic atrophy, strabismus, nystagmus

Xeroderma pigmentosum

- Progressive lower lid atrophy, lower lid tumours, chronic conjunctival congestion, conjunctivitis, symblepharon, pterygia, corneal ulceration, corneal scarring, limbal squamous cell carcinoma

Oculodermal melanocytosis

- Scleral pigmentation and skin pigmentation in the dermatomes of V – a, b and sometimes c, glaucoma, malignant change in < 25%
- Also Duane's, retinitis pigmentosa, congenital cataract

Psoriasis

- Lid involvement, conjunctival and corneal involvement, uveitis

Ehlers-Danlos

- Epicanthal folds, angioid streaks, blue sclera, keratoconus, ectopia lentis, myopia, strabismus, retinal detachment

Pseudoxanthoma elasticum

- Angioid streaks, drusen

Juvenile xanthogranuloma

- Tumours of iris and ciliary body, spontaneous hyphaema, glaucoma

Acne rosacea

- Blepharitis, recurrent chalazion, conjunctivitis, marginal corneal ulcers, rosacea keratitis of lower two-thirds

Ichthyosis

- Eyelid involvment, +/– ectropion and secondary corneal changes, deep corneal opacities in x-linked ichthyosis

Rubella

Congenital rubella

Ocular features

- Cataract (nuclear → total)
- Microphthalmos; associated with cataract
- Congenital or infantile glaucoma; in 10–20%
- Corneal haze; transient, ? due to endothelial dysfunction or keratitis
- Iris hypoplasia, iridocyclitis
- Speckled retinitis (salt and pepper retinopathy); visual acuity may be unaffected
- Viral dacryoadenitis
- Nasolacrimal duct obstruction
- Strabismus
- Nystagmus

Non-ocular features

- Congenital heart disease
- Neurosensory deafness
- Mental retardation

Acquired rubella

- Transient non-specific conjunctivitis

Syphilis

Congenital syphilis

Systemic early

- Coryza, hepatosplenomegally, etc.

Systemic late stigmata

- Saddle nose, frontal bossing, sabre tibia, Hutchinson's triad

Ocular early

- Thickening and redness of eyelids
- Conjunctivitis
- Chronic dacryocystitis
- Iridocyclitis
- Congenital cataract
- Chorioretinitis
  - Early multifocal exudates
  - Late salt and pepper fundus, peudoretinitis pigmentosa
- Optic neuritis and atrophy
- EOM paresis

Ocular late

- Interstitial keratitis
- Band keratopathy
- Corneal thinning and ectasia
- Iridocyclitis
- Secondary glaucoma
- Secondary cataract

Acquired syphilis

Systemic

- Primary – Chancre, lymphadenopathy
- Secondary – skin + mucous membrane lesions
- Tertiary – neuro, cardiovascular lesions, gummata

Ocular

- Primary – Chancre
- Secondary – uveitis, retinal vasculitis, optic neuritis
- Uveitis
  - Iritis roseola (small nests of capillaries)
  - Iritis papulosa (vascular papules)
  - Iritis nodosa (pinhead nodules)
  - Patchy iris hyperaemia
  - Retinal vasculitis
  - Optic neuritis
- Tertiary – features of secondary
  - Scleritis
  - Iris atrophy
  - Argyll-Robertson pupil
  - Ectopia lentis
  - Optic atrophy (vascular)
  - Disseminated chorioretinitis of Forster; acute and healed (with atrophy, gliosis, RPE clumping)
  - Neuroretinitis papulosa – periphlebitis, disseminated chorioretinitis, optic neuritis
  - Gummata – lids, extraocular muscles, optic nerve, orbit
  - Periostitis of orbit

15

Community eye health

Principles of prevention of blindness 412
Cataract 416
Refractive error 417
Childhood blindness 419
Glaucoma 422
Diabetic retinopathy 423

Principles of prevention of blindness

Definition of blindness and low vision

- The World Health Organisation classifies vision into four categories
- Based on the Snellen visual acuity
- The vision in the better eye with available correction
- The four categories are
  - 6/6–6/18 – normal
  - < 6/18–6/60 – visual impairment
  - < 6/60–3/60 – severe visual impairment
  - < 3/60–NPL – blind
- In addition blindness includes a visual field constricted to < 10 degrees around central fixation in the better eye
- Low vision includes a visual field constricted to < 20 degrees around central fixation in the better eye

Magnitude of global blindness – prevalence (existing cases)

Category of vision	Number	Visual acuity
Blind	36.9 million people	< 3/60
Low vision	124.3 million people	< 6/18–3/60
Visual impairment	161.2 million people	< 6/18
Normal	6 052.7 million people	6/6–6/18

Correlation of prevalence of blindness in different countries and in different regions with the economy and level of health care

Economy/health care	% Blind	Number blind per million
Good	0.25	2 500
OK	0.50	5 000
Poor	0.75	7 500
Very poor	1.00+	10 000+

The prevalence of blindness increases with increasing age	
Age (years)	**Prevalence of blindness (number per million)**
0–14	800
15–44	1 000
45–59	19 000
60+	44 000

Exponential increase in number of blind people in the world since 1975	
Year	**Number blind (millions)**
1975	28
1980	30
1984	31
1990	38
1995	45
2000	50

- If present trends and present blindness prevention activities continue, the exponential increase is set to grow to 75 million by the year 2020
- The global Vision 2020 programme is an initiative of the World Health Organisation and the International Agency For The Prevention Of Blindness to reverse this increase

Magnitude of global blindness – incidence (current estimate of new cases)

- Incidence – 6 million per year
- Treatment – 1 million per year
- Mortality – 4 million per year
- Therefore, net increase in prevalence (backlog) – 1 million per year

Causes of global blindness		
Disease	**Number blind (millions)**	**%**
Cataract	17.6	47.8%
Glaucoma	4.5	12.3%
Age-related macular degeneration	3.2	8.7%
Corneal scar	1.9	5.1%
Diabetic retinopathy	1.8	4.8%
Childhood blindness	1.4	3.9%
Trachoma	1.3	3.6%
Onchocerciasis	0.3	0.8%
Other	4.8	13

Major causes of blindness throughout the world	
■ Africa and Asia	□ Cataract □ Glaucoma □ Trachoma □ Other corneal opacity □ Onchocerciasis (Africa)
■ Latin America	□ Cataract □ Glaucoma □ Diabetic retinopathy
■ North America and Europe	□ Age-related macular degeneration □ Diabetic retinopathy □ Glaucoma

Prevalence of blindness

- Up to 75% of all blindness is avoidable
- Only about 50% of childhood blindness is avoidable
- The numbers and proportions of the different causes vary in different countries and regions, depending on their economies and levels of health care

Causes of blindness in relation to economy

Cause of blindness	Very poor economy (number blind per million)	Poor economy (number blind per million)	Fair economy (number blind per million)	Good economy (number blind per million)
Cataract	5 000	4 000	2 000	–
Corneal scar	3 000	1 500	–	–
Glaucoma	1 000	1 000	1 000	500
Diabetic retinopathy	–	–	1 000	500
Other retinal disease	–	–	–	1 000
Other	1 000	1 000	1 000	500
Total adult blind	10 000+	7 500	5 000	2 500
Blind children	250	200	150	100

Blind person years

- Blind person years is a measure of disability over time
- Blind person years = number blind × average number of years a person lives blind with this disease
- When blind person years is considered, childhood blindness ranks second in importance after cataract

15

Summary of blinding eye diseases	
Cataract	**Trachoma**
Glaucoma	**Onchocerciasis**
Diabetic retinopathy	**Vitamin A deficiency**
■ Occur everywhere	■ Focal diseases
■ Affect individuals	■ Affect communities
■ Affect mainly adults	■ Start in children
■ Require surgery/laser	■ Require medicine
■ Need an eye doctor	■ Do not need an eye doctor
■ Hospital-based	■ Community-based

- Both hospital based services and community based services are essential for the provision of comprehensive services in a Vision 2020 programme

Primary, secondary and tertiary prevention of blindness

Primary prevention

- Prevent the disease ever occurring

Examples

- Vitamin A deficiency
  - Good nutrition
- Trachoma
  - Good water and sanitation
- Rubella and measles
  - Immunisation

Secondary prevention

- Prevent loss of vision from established disease

Examples

- Cataract
  - Surgery when vision is down but better than 3/60
- Glaucoma
  - Sight preservation from surgical or medical treatment
- Diabetic retinopathy
  - Sight preserving laser treatment
- Vitamin A deficiency
  - If keratomalacia, saving the sight of the other eye
- Onchocerciasis
  - Treatment with ivermectin

Tertiary prevention

- Restore vision to a blind patient

Examples

- Cataract
  - Surgery when vision is < 3/60
- Corneal scarring
  - Keratoplasty
- Low vision
  - Low vision aids

Cataract

Prevalence and incidence of age related cataract

Planning estimates per million population				
	Good economy	**Fair economy**	**Poor economy**	**Very poor economy**
Prevalence of blindness	–	2 000	4 000	5 000
Prevalence of visual impairment and severe visual impairment	–	8 000	16 000	20 000
Total backlog needing surgery	–	10 000	20 000	25 000
Annual incidence of blindness	1 000	1 000	1 000	1 000
Annual incidence of visual impairment and severe visual impairment	4 000	4 000	4 000	4 000
Total new cases each year needing surgery	5 000	5 000	5 000	5 000

Cataract surgery rate

- Cataract surgery rate (CSR) = number of cataract operations per million population per year
- CSR allows comparison between different districts and different countries with differing population sizes
- In order to eliminate blindness due to cataract, the CSR needs to equal the incidence (new cases) of cataract blindness
- Because not all the surgery that is done is on people who are blind due to cataract, it needs to be somewhere between 1 000–5 000
- If the proportion of surgeries that are done on blind people is around 30–50%, the CSR that is required to equal the incidence is 2 000–3 000 cataract operations per million population per year
- If the CSR is less than 2 000, the surgery rate will not keep up with the incidence (new cases), people who become blind due to cataract will remain untreated and will remain blind until they die and the backlog will continue to increase
- If the CSR is 3 000 or more, the CSR will keep up with the incidence, people who become blind due to cataract will be treated and will be cured of their blindness, and the backlog will be abolished over a period of 5 years

Barriers to the uptake of cataract surgery	
■ Sub-Saharan Africa	□ Only 1 out of 10 people who are blind due to cataract attend for surgery □ Only 1 out of 20 people with cataract who are not blind but who should have surgery attend for surgery

15

- Summary of barriers precluding attendance for surgery
  - Awareness (lack of)
  - Bad service
  - Cost
  - Distance
  - Expectation (lack of)
  - Fear
- Strategies to overcome the barriers
  - Publicity campaigns (radio, newspapers)
  - Outreach clinics
  - Networking with other organisations and agencies
  - Use of pseudophakic motivators
  - Employment of cataract case finders

Cataract surgery capacity

- In order to implement Vision 2020 and to eliminate blindness due to cataract, it is necessary to achieve a cataract surgery rate of 2 000–3 000 per million population per year
- The capacity of a Vision 2020 surgery centre for a district with a population of 1 million should be 2 000–3 000 cataract surgeries per year, which is 40–60 cataract surgeries per week

Monitoring of cataract services

- Monitoring of output (quantity)
  - Number of cataract operations per year
  - Number of cataract operations on blind people
  - Cataract surgery rate
- Monitoring of outcome (quality)
  - Success rate – % eyes achieving 6/18 or better
  - Failure rate – % eyes achieving less than 6/60
- Monitoring of outlay (cost)
  - Number of cataract operations per surgeon per year
  - Number of cataract operations per bed per year
  - Cost of consumables per surgery

Improving cataract services

Improving output

- Is there a waiting list?
- No → increase demand
  - Consider barriers to uptake
  - Consider cataract case finding
- Yes → Increase capacity
  - Consider volume of surgery
  - Consider efficiency of surgery

Improving outcome

- Ensure each surgeon does a minimum of 500 surgeries per year
- Monitor outcome

Reducing cost

- Cost containment – increase productivity; improve efficiency
  - Increase volume
  - Purchase cheap consumables
- Cost recovery + cost sharing – use a multitier system, with cross subsidisation

Refractive error

Definition of significant refractive error	
Adults	**Children**
< 6/18 binocularly	< 6/12 binocularly

15

Myopia of −1.00DS or more in both eyes	Myopia of −0.50DS or more in both eyes
Astigmatism of 1.50DC or more in both eyes	Astigmatism of 1.00DC or more in both eyes
Hypermetropia of +3.00DS or more in both eyes	Hypermetropia of +3.00DS or more in both eyes

Magnitude of significant refractive error in children

From population bases prevalence surveys				
Country	**Myopia −1.00DS or more (% of children) (number per million population)**	**Hypermetropia + 3.00DS or more (% of children) (number per million population)**	**Astigmatism 1.50DC or more (% of children) (number per million population)**	**Total significant refractive error (% of children) (number per million population)**
Nepal (5–15 years)	0.7% 3 000	0.4% 1 500	1.0% 4 000	2.1% 8 500
Chile (5–15 years)	4.6% 18 500	5.6% 22 500	14.9% 59 500	25,1% 100 500
China (5–15 years)	13.6% 54 000	1.3% 5 000	2.0% 8 000	16.9% 67 000
Urban India (5–15 years)	4.2% 17 000	1.9% 7 500	3.8% 15 000	9.9% 39 500
Rural India (7–15 years)	2.8% 11 000	0.3% 1 000	1.8% 7000	4.9% 19 000
South Africa	0.5% 2 000	10% 4 000	1.0% 4 000	2.5% 10 000

Strategy for school screening for refractive error

- Screen all children once between ages 5 and 9 years (25 000 children per million population) and screen all children again once between ages 11–15 years (25 000 children per million population) (50 000 children screened each year)
- Use a binocular vision of less than 6/12 to screen for significant refractive errors, but test monocular
- Screening should be done by trained teachers, trained health care workers or school nurses, using a 6/12 E chart with 4 letters
- Refer identified cases to an optometrist, refractionist or eye nurse
- Refract (retinoscopy + subjective, with cycloplegia when necessary)
- Spectacles should be prescribed and dispensed for
  - Myopia – 1.0 dioptre sphere or more both eyes

- Astigmatism 1.5 dioptre cylinder or more both eyes
- Hypermetropia + 3.0 dioptre sphere or more both eyes

- The prevalence in individual countries correlates with the level of economic development of the country and the under 5 mortality rate

Childhood blindness

Prevalence

- The global prevalence is estimated to be 1.4 million (7.5 per 10 000 children)

Childhood blindness related to economic development		
Level of economic Development	**Under 5 mortality rate (per 1 000 children)**	**Estimated childhood blindness (per 1000 children)**
Industrialised	20	0.3
Middle developing	100	0.6
Poor developing	200	0.9
Very poor	300	1.2

Incidence

- The incidence is unknown
- The global incidence is estimated to be 500 000 new cases per year
- This is 1 new case each minute
- Over 50% die within 1–2 years of becoming blind
- The prevalence underestimates the magnitude of the problem, as this only takes account of the children who survive

Causes

- The causes of childhood blindness can be classified in two ways: Anatomically and aetiologically
- Anatomically – according to the anatomical site of the lesion in the eye
  - Cornea
  - Lens
  - Uvea
  - Retina
  - Optic nerve
  - Glaucoma
  - Globe
  - CNS
- Aetiologically – relating to when the insult occurred which resulted in blindness
  - Hereditary
  - Intrauterine
  - Perinatal
  - childhood
- Data from surveys at schools for the blind
  - Globe is an important cause in Asia, but not in Africa
  - Cornea is an important cause in all the poor regions
  - Retina is an important cause everywhere
  - Optic nerve is an important cause in rich countries
- Hereditary causes are important everywhere
- Perinatal causes are important in richer regions
- Childhood causes are important in poorer regions

Summary of the main causes of childhood blindness in different socio-economic groups

Affluent communities

- For every 1 million population
  - 20% 0–15 years = 0.2 million
  - Prevalence = 0.3 per 1 000 = 60 blind
  - Corneal scar – 0%
  - Cataract + glaucoma – 10% – 6
  - Retinopathy of prematurity – 10% – 6
  - Other – 80% – 48

Middle income communities

- For every 1 million population
  - 30% 0–15 years = 0.3 million
  - Prevalence = 0.6 per 1 000 = 180 blind
  - Scar – 0%
  - Cataract + glaucoma – 20% – 36 blind
  - Retinopathy of prematurity – 25% – 45 blind
  - Other – 55% – 95 blind

Poor communities

- For every 1 million population
  - 40% 0–15 years = 0.4 million
  - Prevalence = 0.9 per 1 000 = 360 blind
  - Scar – 20% – 72
  - Cataract + glaucoma – 20% – 72
  - Retinopathy of prematurity – 0%
  - Other – 60% – 216

Very poor communities

- For every 1 million population
  - 50% 0–15 years = 0.5 million
  - Prevalence = 1.2 per 1 000 = 600 blind
  - Scar – 50% – 300 blind
  - Cataract + glaucoma – 15% – 90 blind
  - Retinopathy of prematurity – 0%
  - Other – 35% – 210 blind

Management of cataract in children

Primary prevention

- Genetic counselling
- Rubella immunisation

Secondary prevention

- Nil

Tertiary prevention

- Surgery + refractive correction
- Low vision services
- The management of these patients (surgery, refractive correction and follow-up) should be done by a paediatric ophthalmology team (ophthalmologist, refractionist and contact lens practitioner, orthoptist, anaesthetist, etc.) working in a paediatric ophthalmology unit with appropriate instruments and equipment
- One quaternary paediatric ophthalmology unit is recommended for every 10 million population

Management of corneal scarring in children

Primary prevention

- Ophthalmia neonatorum prophylaxis
- Measles immunisation
- Nutrition education
- Vitamin A supplementation
- Health education about the harmful effects of traditional eye medicines

Secondary prevention

- Treatment of ophthalmia neonatorum
- Treatment of vitamin A deficiency
- Treatment of measles keratitis

Tertiary prevention

- Optical iridectomy
- Keratoplasty
- The emphasis of the control of corneal scarring is on primary and secondary prevention, which are largely community-based strategies

Management of glaucoma in children

Primary prevention

- Rubella immunisation
- Genetic counselling

Secondary prevention

- Early diagnosis and surgery
- Treat amblyopia + refractive errors

Tertiary prevention

- Low vision services
- As for paediatric cataract, paediatric glaucoma should be managed in a quaternary paediatric ophthalmology unit

Management of retinopathy of prematurity

Primary prevention

- Retinopathy of prematurity can be prevented by adequate monitoring of oxygen therapy in neonatal units

Secondary prevention

- Consider screening if retinopathy of prematurity accounts for more than 10% of new admissions/ registrations of blind children
- Or if there is a neonatal unit where, each year, 100 babies or more with birth weights of less than 1 500 gms are surviving to 6 weeks of age
- Which neonates should be screened?
  - < 1 500 gm birth weight
  - And/or < 32 weeks gestation
- When should they be examined?
  - The first examination should be 6 weeks after birth or 33 to 34 weeks gestation
- How should they be examined?
  - By indirect ophthalmoscopy
  - With dilated pupils
  - By a skilled ophthalmologist
- For how long should they be checked?
  - Until there is either regression or vascularisation

Tertiary prevention

- Stage 3 plus threshold disease should be treated as soon as possible after diagnosis and within 1 week at the latest
- The time window available for treatment and re-treatment, if necessary, is short (about 2–3 weeks)
- Treatment is usually around 36–44 weeks post-conceptual age (mean 37.7 weeks)
- Cryotherapy or laser is applied to the whole of the area of avascular retina
- Treatment for stage 3 plus disease reduces the progression to stage 4 and 5 disease from approximately 50% to 25%

Summary of control of childhood blindness

- Why are children blind?
- Examine 200 blind children
- Which causes are avoidable?
- Which can be prevented?
- Which can be treated?
- How can we prevent these diseases?
- Primary prevention – prevent disease occurring
- Secondary prevention – prevent visual loss from disease
- Tertiary prevention – restore vision
- Methods of control
  - Integration in health care system
  - Or specific disease control
- The principal strategies for prevention of blindness due to corneal scar are based in the community and include
  - Ophthalmia neonatorum prophylaxis
  - Measles immunisation
  - Nutrition education
  - Health education about harmful effects of traditional eye medicines
  - Prompt treatment of infection
- The principal strategies for prevention of blindness due to cataract, glaucoma and retinopathy of prematurity are based in a quaternary paediatric ophthalmology unit and include
  - Screening for retinopathy of prematurity
  - Treatment of retinopathy of prematurity
  - Surgery for cataract
  - Surgery for glaucoma
  - Refractive correction of aphakia after cataract surgery

- Refractive correction for glaucoma
- Low vision treatment as necessary
- The team in the paediatric unit comprises
  - Paediatric ophthalmologist
  - Paediatric anaesthetist
  - Refractionist and contact lens practitioner
  - Orthoptist
  - Low vision therapist

Glaucoma

Global prevalence of chronic glaucoma		
Type	**Number of cases**	**Number blind**
Open angle	33 million	3.3 million
Closed angle	17 million	1.7 million
Total	50 million	5.0 million (10% global blind)

Prevalence of chronic glaucoma in Africa					
Country	**South Africa (Western Cape)**	**Tanzania**	**South Africa (KwaZulu-Natal)**	**South Africa (North West)**	**Ghana**
Age group surveyed	40 years and older	Over 40 years	40 years and older	40 years and older	40 years and older
All glaucoma		4.16	4.5	5.3	
Primary open angle glaucoma	1.5	3.1	2.7	2.9	8.5
Primary closed angle glaucoma	2.3	0.59	0.1	0.5	
Secondary glaucoma		0.47	1.7	2.0	

For planning purposes – conservative estimate of prevalence of chronic glaucoma

- 4% in the age group 40 years and older
- 1% in the total population
- Up to 50% of cases are already blind in one eye
- Up to 90% of cases are not diagnosed

Case detection of glaucoma in the community

- Glaucoma does not meet the criteria for a community-based screening programme
- Opportunistic case detection may be considered if it is prioritised for a Vision 2020 programme
- Testing the pinhole visual acuity and using a cut point of 6/18 in one or

both eyes has a sensitivity > 90% and a specificity > 90% for detection of cataract and glaucoma

- This test would be suitable for use by nurses working in a primary care clinic
- Examining the optic disc with a direct ophthalmoscope and using a cut point of 0.7 vertical cup : disc ratio has a sensitivity > 90% and a specificity > 90% in those eyes in which the disc can be seen for detection of glaucoma
- Combining this test with testing for an afferent pupil defect has a sensitivity > 90% and a specificity > 90% in all eyes, including those in which disc examination is not possible
- This combination of tests would be suitable for use by ophthalmic nurses working in secondary level eye clinics

Treatment of glaucoma in Vision 2020 programmes in Africa

- Primary trabeculectomy with antifibrosis adjunct should be the treatment of choice
- Medical treatment should be added if there is inadequate intraocular pressure control

Glaucoma surgery rate

- For an African population of 1 million people
  - Population at risk (those aged over 40 years) = 25% = 250 000
  - Prevalence rate in this group = 4% = 10 000 cases
  - Of the 10 000 cases – 5 000 early; 4 000 intermediate/moderate/ detectable/ treatable; 1 000 late
  - 50% (5 000) have early glaucoma
  - 10% (1 000) are already blind
  - 40% (5 000) have moderate, detectable, treatable glaucoma
- This is the priority target group for case detection and treatment
- Assuming a rate of progression of 10 years from onset of moderate disease to blindness, and an incidence of 400 new cases per year, the glaucoma surgery rate should be trabeculectomies for 400 patients per million population per year

Recommendations for including glaucoma in Vision 2020 programmes in Africa

- All people aged 40 years and over seen in primary care clinics should have their visual acuity screened once every 2 years
- If the visual acuity is less than 6/18 in one or both eyes, they should be referred to the eye nurse
- The eye nurse should examine the cases referred, and use the optic cup : disc vertical ratio (> or = 0.7) and pupil response (afferent pupil defect) to categorise patients as – normal or suspicious
- Suspicious cases should be referred to the eye doctor, who should use visual field testing to confirm the diagnosis
- Trabeculectomy with antifibrosis adjunct should be the first line of treatment
- Medical treatment should be added if there is inadequate intraocular pressure control following trabeculectomy
- Follow-up of cases should be done by the eye nurse, using the intraocular pressure to decide if there is adequate control. A register of diagnosed cases should be kept, so that persons who default on follow up can be traced

Diabetic retinopathy

Magnitude

General

- There is an increase in diabetes mellitus throughout the world

- Diabetic retinopathy is the fifth most common cause of global blindness (1.8 million people)
- It accounts for 5–10% of all blindness in economically intermediate countries
- It is the main cause of blindness in the economically active age group in developed countries
- It is becoming increasingly important in developing countries

Prevalence

- Diabetic retinopathy is associated with increased mortality
- 50% of diabetic retinopathy is undiagnosed
- Prevalence of diabetes mellitus (types 1 and 2) = 3–5% (= 30 000–50 000 diabetics per million population)
- Prevalence of any retinopathy in diabetics = 20% (= 6 000–10 000 with diabetic retinopathy per million population)
- Prevalence of blindness amongst these = 5% (= 300–500 blind per million population i.e. 5% of all blindness)

Incidence

- 0.05% of the population develop sight threatening retinopathy per year (= 500 people per million population per year)

Recommendations for including diabetic retinopathy in Vision 2020 programmes in Africa

Screening

- This can be done by eye nurses, optometrists, general doctors, physicians or ophthalmologists
- It might be done by fundoscopy or by fundus photograpghy
- Juvenile onset diabetics should be screened at puberty and then annually
- Adult onset diabetics should be screened at diagnosis and then annually
- For each 1 million population, the number of people needing screening each year can be conservatively estimated to be 30 000

Referral to ophthalmologist

- All patients with retinopathy should be referred to the ophthalmologist for assessment

Laser

- For each 1 million population, the number of patients requiring laser each year can be conservatively estimated to be 500
- Posterior pole laser should be done by an ophthalmologist
- Peripheral laser could be done by a general doctor

Index

A patterns 292
abducens nerve palsy *see* palsy sixth nerve
abduction deficit, causes of 17
abetalipoproteinemia 197
acanthamoeba keratitis52–53
accommodating IOL 394
accommodation
  abnormalities of 377
  fatigue of 377
  paralysis of 377
  pupil disorders of 356
  spasm of 377–378
  theories of 393–394
accommodative convergence strabismus 283
accommodative esotropia 287–288
acne rosacea 410
acquired immune deficiency syndrome (AIDS) 397–399
acute multifocal posterior placoid pigment epitheliopathy 177
acute retinal necrosis (ARN) 170
adenoviral
  keratoconjunctivitis 33–34
  corneal disease 58
Adie's tonic pupil 8
adult vitelliform dystrophy 222
Advanced Glaucoma Intervention Study (AGIS) 126–127
afferent pupil defect 8, 354
after image test 302
age related macular degeneration (ARMD) 203–207
  dry/atrophic 204–205
  wet/exudative 205–206
albinism 200, 221, 399
alkaptonuria 71
allergic
  conjunctivitis 35
  eyelid disorders 23–24
  rhinoconjunctivitis 35
alpha agonists 122
Alport syndrome 223–224
amblyopia 298–299
  ametropic 299
  anisometropic 299
  meridional 299–300
  preschool screening for 283
  refractive surgery 396
  strabismic 298–299
  tobacco-alcohol 320
  visual deprivation 299
amino acid metabolism, disorders of 69, 70–72
aminoacidurias 402
amniotic membrane 86
Amsler grid 11
amyloidosis 71–72, 253
anaesthesia, cataract surgery 136
angioid streaks 199–200
angiomatosis retinae and cerebelli 407
aniridia 119, 129, 145–146
aniseikonia 376
anisocoria
  causes of 16
  physiologic 353
anisometropia 376
anisophoria 376–377
ankylosing spondylitis 149, 151
anophthalmos 260
anterior ischaemic optic neuropathy 313–315
anterior segment ischaemia 303–304
anterior chamber cleavage syndromes 44–46
anterior chamber IOLs 114
antifibrotic agents 124
antiphospholipid syndromes 211
Anton's syndrome 326
Apert syndrome 260–261
aphakia
  congenital 128
  correction of 141
  spectacle correction of 380–381
arcus juveniles 45
Argyll-Robertson pupil 9, 354
arthritis
  and uveitis 149–150
  psoriatic 150
aspergillosis 270
asteroid hyalosis 252
asthenopia 379–380
astigmatism 373
  post-operative 139
  surgery 382
atopic
  dermatitis 23
  keratoconjunctivitis 35
Avellino dystrophy 46, 49–50

Axenfeld-Rieger syndrome 45, 117

Bagolini striated lens 302
Balint's syndrome 326
basal cell
carcinoma 26
cell papilloma 25
Bassen-Kornzweig syndrome 197
Batten-Mayou disease 402
Behçet's disease 150–151
Bell's palsy 345
benign acquired
melanosis 41
familial fleck retina 224
hamartoma of childhood 321
raised intracranial pressure 310
Bergmeister's papilla 186
Best disease 222
beta-adrenergic antagonists 122
beta-blockers 122
bevacizumab 207
Bietti's crystalline corneoretinal dystrophy 70, 223
biometry 133–134
bioptics, refractive surgery 390
birdshot choroidopathy 178
blepharitis 23
blepharochalasis 24
blepharophimosis syndrome 20–22
blepharospasm 24, 306
blindness
causes of 413–414
childhood, community eye health 419–4222
definition of 412
global magnitude of 412, 413
prevalence of 412
prevention of 415
principles of prevention of 412–415
blindsight 325–326
blowout fractures 277–279, 366–367
blunt trauma 363
retinal 258–259
Botulinum toxin (Botox) 306
Bourneville's disease 407–408
branch retinal vein occlusion 209–211
Brown's superior oblique tendon sheath syndrome 297
burns
acid 81, 362
alkaline 80–81, 361–362
chemical 361–362
butterfly dystrophy 223

CMV retinitis 169–170
central retinal vein occlusion 208–209
carbohydrate metabolism, disorders of 69
carbonic anhydrase inhibitors 123
carcinoma
adenocyctic 268
basal cell 26
conjunctiva squamous cell 40
mucoepidermoid 40
sebaceous gland 26
squamous cell 26
carotid artery occlusion and stenosis 211–212
carotid cavernous fistula 280–281, 347
cat scratch disease 35
cataract surgery
and diabetic retinopathy 137
surgery, community eye health 416–417
surgical complications 136–137
in special situations 141–142
in uveitis 142–144 182–183
post-operative astigmatism 139
pre-operative evaluation 132–133
pre-operative examination 9–10
cataracts
classification of 128
community eye health 416–417
developmental 139–141
drug-induced 132
examination technique 9
prevalence and incidence of 416
secondary 131–132
senile 131
traumatic 132
unilateral 140,
unilateral, diplopia following 336
uveitic 143
cavernous sinus syndrome 347
central areolar choroidal dystrophy 250
central serous choroidopathy 217–218
chalazion 22
chlamydial conjunctivitis 34–35
chloroquinemaculopathy 218
cholinergic agonists 122–123
choristoma, epibulbar 39–40
choroidal

dystrophies 220–221, 249–251
folds 251
haemangioma 173
melanoma 174–177
naevus 173, 175–176
neovascularisation 207–208
osteoma 173
choroideraemia 249–250
chronic progressive conjunctival cicatrisation 37–39
chronic progressive external ophthalmoplegia 298, 329
cicatricial pemphigoid 37–38, 410
climate droplet keratopathy 68
clinically significant macular oedema 228–229
Coat's disease 234–235
Coat's white ring 77
Cockayne's syndrome 197
Cogan's microcystic dystrophy 46, 47
Cogan's syndrome 73
Collaborative Initial Glaucoma Treatment Study (CIGTS) 126
coloboma 25, 129
Fuchs' typical 308
ocular 309
coma, spherical aberration 379
combined oculomotor palsies 346–347
commotio retinae 371
computer vision syndrome 380
conductive keratoplasty 392, 394
congenital
cloudy cornea 44
corneal guttata 43
disc anomalies 307–309
disc crescent 308
hereditary endothelial dystrophy 46, 48
hereditary stromal dystrophy 45
hypertrophy of the RPE (CHRPE) 185–186
monochromatism 222
nasolacrimal duct obstruction 27
ocular melanocytosis 41
ocular motor apraxia 350
retinal pigment epithelium and vascular abnormalities 185–186
stationary night blindness 221
conjunctival
cicatrisation, chronic progressive 37–39
degenerations 31–32
epithelial melanosis 41
intraepithelial neoplasia 40
malignant melanoma 41
naevus 41
papilloma 39
pigmentation sources of 39
conjunctivitis 32–39
allergic 35
chlamydial 34–35
giant papillary 36–37
herpes simplex 34
ligneous 36
molluscum contagiosum 34
neonatal bacterial 33
Parinaud's oculoglandular 34–35
simple bacterial 32–33
toxic 36
viral 33–34
contact lenses 385–387
convergence
insufficiency 284, 292
retraction nystagmus 334
spasm 288–289
cornea 42–89
congenital abnormalities 42–44
congenital, cloudy 44
examination technique 5–6
guttata 48
plana 43
pre-operative examination 9
corneal
arcus 77
astigmatism post-operative control of 84
autograft procedures 84
crystal deposits, causes of 75–76
deposits, differential diagnosis of 70–71
corneal dystrophies 46–50
farinata 77
grafts 118
guttata 43
inlays 394
keloids 77
nerves 73
oedema 77
optics 387
reconstruction 86
refractive surgery 389
scrape 54–58
topography 385
cortical blindness 325–326
corticosteroids 161–162
cranial nerve palsies 402
craniopharyngioma 336
craniosynostoses 260–261

Criswick-Schepens syndrome 224
crocodile shagreen 78
crocodile tears 345
Crouzon syndrome 260
cutis marmarata telangiectasia congenital 203
cyclodialysis 108
cysticercosis 171, 270
cystinosis 70
cystoid macular oedema 216–217

dacryoadenitis 268
dacryocystitis 28
dacryops 261
dark adaptometry 11
deep anterior lamellar keratoplasty 85
deep lamellar endothelial keratoplasty 85
dermatochalasis 24
dermoid cysts 261
Devic's disease 319
diabetic retinopathy 227–232, 423–424
  cataract surgery and 137
  clinical classification of 230
  factors aggravating 229
  factors reducing severity of 229–230
  management of 230–232
diktyoma 174
diplopia 16, 18, 336–337
disc
  abnormalities 307
  anomalies congenital 307–309
  changes in glaucoma 95–97
  crescent congenital 308
  drusen 307
  swollen 309
dissociated
  nystagmus 333
  vertical deviation (DVD) 293
distichiasis 23–24
divergence paralysis 288
dominant
  neovascular inflammatory vitreo-choroidopathy 225
  vitreoretinochoroidopathy 225
dorsal midbrain syndrome 351
double depressor palsy 298
  elevator palsy 296, 298
drusen 204–205
  disc 307
  familial dominant 223
dry eye syndrome 29–30
Duane's retraction syndrome 296–297
duochrome test 378
dysthyroid eye disease 262–265

Eale's disease 233–234
ectopia lentis 129–131
ectropion 20
Edwards' syndrome 72, 400
Ehlers-Danlos syndrome 200
electrodiagnostics 256–257
empty sella syndrome 336
encephalocoele 262
encephalotrigeminal angiomatosis 202–203, 407
endophthalmitis 138–138, 364–365
  aseptic, post-op 166
  bacterial 164–166
  fungal 166–167
entropion 20
epiblepharon 25
epibulbar
  choristoma 39–40
  dermoid 43
epicanthic folds 24
epicanthus inversus 21, 22
epidermoid cysts 261
epiphora 26, 27
epiretinal membrane 214–215
episcleritis 86, 87–88
erosions, recurrent 74–75
erosive vitreoretinopathy 224
erythema multiforme 410
esotropia 285–290
  accommodative 287–288
  acute acquired comitant 289–290
  congenital 285–286
  consecutive 289
  cyclic 289
  stress induced 289
exophoria 290
exotropia 290–292
  congenital 292
  constant 291
  intermittent 290–291
  secondary comitant 291–292
  vertical deviations 292
eyelid retraction, causes of 4
eyelashes, disorders of 23–24
eyelids 13, 20–26, 172

FDT (Frequency Doubling Technology) perimetry 121
facial nerve palsy *see* palsy seventh nerve
familial
  dominant drusen 223
  exudative vitreo-retinopathy 224, 252

fat adherence syndrome 296
Favre-Goldmann syndrome 224
fibrosis syndromes, strabismus 297–298
fleck dystrophy 46, 50
floppy eyelid syndrome 24
fluorescein angiography 11, 254–255
foetal alcohol syndrome 400
foreign bodies, intraocular 364, 367–369
fourth nerve (IV) palsy see palsy fourth nerve
Fuchs'
  endothelial dystrophy 46, 48
  heterochromic iridocyclitis 157–158
  superficial marginal keratitis 63
  typical coloboma 308
functional visual loss 19
fungal
  endophthalmitis 166–167
  infections of the orbit 270
  keratitis 55
  uveitis 168–169

gelatinous drop-like dystrophy 46, 50
giant cell arteritis 212–213
giant papillary conjunctivitis 36–37
giant tears 246
Gillespie's syndrome 145
glaucoma 90–127, 407
  acute neovascular 110–111
  angle closure 90–91
  aniridia 146
  aphakic 114
  cataract surgery in 142
  ciliary block 116–117
  community eye health 422–423
  congenital 92, 104–106, 119
  disc changes 95–97
  drainage devices 109
  drugs 122–123
  ghost cell 107
  imaging 124–125
  inflammatory 113–114
  lens induced 107, 114, 144
  management 110–111
  neovascular 108–111
  normal pressure 100–101
  open angle 91–92
  phacolytic 114
  phacomorphic 114
  pigmentary 111–112
  primary angle closure 102–104
  red cell 108
  secondary 106–108
  studies 125–127
  surgical management 105–106
  uveitic 113–114
glaucomatocyclitic crisis 107
glaukomflecken 144
glycogen storage diseases 402
Goldenhar syndrome 43, 404
gonioscopy 6, 97
goniotomy 108–109
gonococcal keratoconjunctivitis 33
graft vs host disease 38–39
granular dystrophy 46, 49
Graves disease 296
gyrate dystrophy 250
haemangioma
  choroidal 173
  capillary 279–280
  cavernous 280
Harada-Ito procedure 304
Hassall-Henle bodies 77
headache 326–327
helicoidal parapapillary choroidal degeneration 251
Helmholtz's theory 393
hepatolenticular degeneration 72
hereditary
  fundal dystrophies 220–225
  vitreoretinal degenerations 221, 224–225
herpes simplex
  conjunctivitis 34
  keratitis 56
herpes zoster
  iritis 170
  ophthalmicus (HZO) 51–52
histiocytosis 275
HIV 396, 397–399
Holmes-Adie pupil 354
homocystinuria 130
hordeolum 22–23
Horner's syndrome 8, 17, 354–355
Humphrey perimetry 119–120
hut eye 78
Hutchinson's pupil 356
hyaloid artery, persistent 186
hydatid cyst 270
hypermetropia 372, 373–374
hypertelorism 20
hypertensive retinopathy 236–237
hyperviscocity 400–401

hyphaema 369–370
hypopyon, causes of 151

IOLs (intraocular lenses) 134–135, 183
accommodating 394
anterior chamber 114
calculation formulae 134–134
materials 134
multifocal 390
phakic 389
power calculation after refractive surgery 393
toric 390
ice test 406
ichthyosis 410
idiopathic
juxtafoveolar retinal telangiectasia 234
orbital inflammatory disease 265
polypoidal choroidal vasculopathy 219–220
immunosuppressives, classification of 161
incontinentia pigmenti 410
indocyanine green (ICG) angiography 255–256
inferior oblique overaction 292, 293–294
internuclear
gaze palsies 348–349
ophthalmoplegia 333, 350–351
interstitial keratitis 73
intrastromal corneal ring segments 392–393
intravitreal antibiotics 166
iridocorneal dysgenesis 117
iridocorneal endothelial (ICE) syndrome 46, 117, 146–147
iridoschisis 147
iris
degenerations and atrophies 146–147
heterochromia causes of 158
melanoma 173
naevus 173
non-pigmented tumours of 174

Jones dye testing 4
juvenile idiopathic (JIA) arthritis and uveitis 162–164
American Academy of Pediatrics screening schedule 163–164
juvenile xanthogranuloma 25, 173–174, 410

Kaposi sarcoma 26, 41
Kearns-Sayre-Daroff syndrome 197
keratitis 52–63
acanthamoeba 52–53
autosomal dominant 119
disciform 74
Fuchs' superficial marginal 63
fungal 55
herpes simplex 56
in measles 58
in ocular leprosy 172
in polyarteritis nodosa 63
in rheumatoid arthritis 62
in SLE 62
interstitial 73
in Wegener's granulomatosis 63
peripheral ulcerative 60–63
rosacea 63
stromal 57
suppurative bacterial 53–54, 55
Thygeson's superficial punctuate 74
keratoacanthoma 25
keratoconjunctivitis
adenoviral 33–34
adult gonococcal 33
atopic 35
neonatal chlamydial 34
neonatal gonococcal 33
sicca 29, 142
superior limbic 35–36
vernal 35
keratoconus 65–67
keratoglobus 43, 67
keratopathies
miscellaneous 73–76
metabolic 69–73
keratopathy
calcific band-shaped 78
climate droplet 68
exposure 74
neurotrophic 58, 74
keratoplasty 67, 82–85
Kleppel-Trenaunay-Weber syndrome 203, 408
Kohner's disease 209

LASEK (laser-assisted subepithelial keratomileusis) 387, 390
LASIK (laser-assisted in situ keratomileusis) 94, 387, 391–392
LOCS (Lens Opacification Classification System) score 9
lacrimal gland
adenocyctic carcinoma 268
enlargement 267
infections 268
inflammations 268–269
lymphoma 268–269
sialadenosis 269

tumours 267–268
lamellar keratoplasty 84–85, 389
lattice degeneration 244–245
lattice dystrophy 46, 50
Lawrence-Moon-Biedl syndrome 197
Leber's
congenital amaurosis 196, 221–222
hereditary optic atrophy 313
military aneurysms 234
lenticonus 128
lentiglobus 128
leprosy 401, 171–172
leukaemia 274, 400
leukoria 189
light-near dissociation 17, 354, 356
ligneous conjunctivitis 36
limbal stem cell transplants 85–86
Linkoff's rules 11
Louis-Bar syndrome 203, 408
Lowe's oculocerebrorenal syndrome 402
Lyme disease 150
lymphangiectasia 40
lymphangioma 40, 280
lymphoma 40–41
lacrimal gland 268–269
orbital 269

macroaneurysm 237
macular
dystrophy 46, 50
dystrophy, juvenile 222
dystrophy, North Carolina 223
dystrophy, Sorsby pseudo inflammatory 223
function tests 10
hole, idiopathic 225–226
hole, traumatic 371
oedema, cystoid 216–217
pucker 215
maculopathy
chloroquine 219
drug-induced 218–219
optic disc pit 220
solar 220
valsalva 220
Maddox rod 383
mandibulofacial dysostosis 404
Marcus Gunn
jaw winking phenomenon 298
pupil 8
Marfan's syndrome 72, 130, 404
masquerade syndromes 159, 172–173
medulloepithelioma 174
Meesman's dystrophy 46, 47–48
megalocornea 42–43
meibomian cyst 22
meibomianitis 23
melanocytoma 323
melanocytosis congenital ocular 41
melanoma 26
choroidal 174–177
conjunctival malignant 41
iris 173
melanosis
benign acquired 41
conjunctival epithelial 41
primary acquired 41
Melkersson-Rosenthal syndrome 345
meningiomas 322
orbital 273
parasellar 336
microcornea 43
microcystoid degeneration 244
microphakia 129
microphthalmos 403–404
microspherophakia 114, 129
migraine 327–32
Miller's syndrome 145
Mittendorf's dot 129
Möbius syndrome 297
molluscum contagiosum 22, 34, 58
monochromatism congenital 222
monofixation syndrome 300–301
Mooren's ulcer 61
Moorfields-Florida (MorFlo) protocol 124
morning glory disc 308
mosaic degeneration 78
Mourits score 14, 265
mucocoele 262
mucoepidermoid carcinoma 40
mucolipidoses 70, 402
mucopolysaccaridoses 69, 197, 402
mucormycosis 270
mucous fishing syndrome 36
mucous membrane pemphigoid, benign 37–38
multiple evanescent white dot syndrome (MEWDS) 177
multiple myeloma 401
multiple sclerosis 317–319
Murphree classification 193–194
muscular dystrophy 404
myasthenia gravis 328–329, 405

myopia 248–249, 373, 374–37, 395
myotonic dystrophy 329

naevus 25
 choroidal 173, 175–176
 conjunctival 41
 flammeus 25–26, 407
 iris 173
nanopthalmos 142, 403–404
nasolacrimal duct obstruction 27, 287
neurilemmoma 273
neurofibroma 40, 273
neurofibromatosis 201–203, 408
neuromyelitis optica 319
neuroprotection 124
neuroretinitis, causes of 15
neurotrophic keratopathy 58, 74
Niemann-Pick disease 225
North Carolina macular dystrophy 223
nystagmus 329–335
 acquired primary position 332
 adult neurological 332
 blockage syndrome 289
 classification of 330
 congenital 331
 convergence retraction 334
 dissociated 333
 downbeat 333
 drug induced 333
 elliptical 333
 gaze evoked 332–333
 induced 331
 latent 331–332
 management of 334–335
 monocular of childhood 332
 periodic alternating 333
 rebound 333
 seesaw 332
 upbeat 332

ocular hypertension 101–102, 126
Ocular Hypertension Treatment Study 125–126
ocular ischaemic syndrome 211–212
oculoauriculovertebral dysplasi 43, 404
oculodermal melanocytosis 410
oculogyric crisis 351
oculomotor palsies, combined 346–347
oculomotor palsy *see* palsy third nerve (III)
oculopalatal myoclonus 333
ophthalmoplegia
 chronic progressive external 329
 internuclear 333, 350–351
 painful causes of 346
optic
 chiasm syndrome 335–336
 disc pit 308
 disc tumours 253–254
optic nerve
 glioma 272
 sheath meningioma 273
 tumours 321–323
optic neuritis 15, 315–317, 318
optic neurophathies
 optic neuropathy
 anterior ischaemic 313–315
 nutritional 320–321
 posterior ischaemic 315
 traumatic 319–320
 toxic 320–321
optical coherence tomography (OCT) 125, 256
orbital
 abscess 269–270
 apex fractures 277, 364
 apex syndrome 347
 cellulitis, bacterial 269–270
 decompression 272
 floor fracture 296, 366–367
 infections 269–270
 lymphoma 269
 pseudotumour 266–267
 roof fractures 277, 365–366
 trauma 276–279
 tumours 269, 272
orbitotomy 271–272
orthokeratology 393
osteoma, choroidal 173

Paget's disease 200
 supranuclear gaze 348–352
palsy
 Bell's 345
 combined oculomotor 346–347
 fourth nerve (IV) 18, 340–341
 internuclear gaze 348–349
 pontine conjugate gaze 350
 progressive supranuclear gaze 351
 saccadic 349–350
 seventh nerve (VII) 344–346
 supranuclear gaze 348–352
 sixth nerve (VI) 295, 342–344

smooth pursuit 350
third nerve (III) 338–340
pannus, causes of 75
panretinal photocoagulation 109, 118
papillitis 315, 316
papilloedema 307, 309–310
papilloma
basal cell 25
conjunctival 39
squamous cell 25
paralysis of
accommodation 377
parasellar
meningiomas 336
tumours 191
parasympathomimetics/miotics 122–123
Parinaud's
oculoglandular conjunctivitis 34–35
syndrome 351
Parkinson's disease 352
pars plana vitrectomy 118, 241
pars planitis 155
pattern dystrophy 223
pavingstone degeneration 244
pegaptanib sodium 207
pellucid degeneration 62, 67
pemphigoid, cicatricial 37–38
pemphigus 410
penetrating
eye injuries 363–365
keratoplasty 82–84
perimetry 8, 119–122
periodic alternating nystagmus 333
peripheral ulcerative keratitis 60–63
persistent
foetal vasculature 251–252
hyaloid artery 186
primary hyperplastic vitreous 251–252
Peter's anomaly 45117, 119, 129
phakomatoses 406–409
phlyctenular keratoconjunctivitis 63
photodynamic therapy 206–207
photoreceptor dystrophies 220, 221–222
Pierre Robin syndrome 404
pigment dispersion syndrome 111–112, 119
pigmentary retinopathy, systemic disease associated with 209–210
pigmented
paravenous retinochoroidal atrophy 251
tumours of the conjunctiva 39
pinealoblastoma 191
pingueculum 31–32, 78
pituitary adenoma 335–336
pleomorphic adenoma 267–268
porphyria 72
port wine stain 25–26, 407
Posner-Schlossmann syndrome 107
post chiasmal lesions 359–360
posterior
capsule opacification 183
corneal dystrophies 46, 48–49
embryotoxon 45
ischaemic optic neuropathy 315
polymorphous dystrophy 45, 46, 49
vitreous detachment 252
presbyopia 377, 393–394
presumed ocular histoplasmosis syndrome 168–169
primary acquired melanosis 41
progressive
cone dystrophy 221
outer retinal necrosis (PORN) 170
rod-cone dystrophy 221
supranuclear gaze palsy 351
proliferative
retinopathy 232–233, 236
vitreoretinopathy 243
proptosis
causes of 274–275
differential diagnosis 13
examination technique 12–13
thyroid eye disease 13
prostaglandin analogs 123
pseudocapsular exfoliation 112–113
pseudoproptosis 13
pseudoretinitis pigmentosa 198
pseudoxanthoma elasticum 200, 410
psoriasis 410
psoriatic arthritis 150
pterygium 32, 79
ptosis 3–4, 20-22
punctuate inner choroidopathy 178
pupil
block 115
disorders 8–9
disorders of accommodation 356
examination technique 8
Purtscher's retinopathy 371

radial keratotomy 392
radiation retinopathy 371

Raeder's syndrome 355
Ramsay-Hunt syndrome 345
Reese-Ellsworth classification 193
refractive surgery 385–396
  aberrations 385–386
  basic principles of 385
  biomechanics of 386–387
  corneal 389
  ocular and systemic disease 395–396
  intraocular 389–390
  IOL power calculation after 393
  pre-operative examination 18–19
Refsum's disease 197, 403
Reis-Buckler's dystrophy 46, 47
Reiter's syndrome 149, 151
retinal
  arterial occlusive disease 211–214
  artery occlusion 213–214
  breaks 245–246, 258
  cavernous haemangioma 201
  degenerations, peripheral 244–245
  detachment 238–242
  hole (trophic) 244
  necrosis progressive outer (PORN) 170
  pigment epithelium congenital and vascular abnormalities 185–186
  pigment epithelium detachment 247
  ischaemia 109
retinitis pigmentosa 196–198
  sclopeteria 371
retinoblastoma 190–195
  classification and staging 193–195
  differential diagnosis of 192
  management 195
  metastases 191
  surgical staging 194
  treatment protocol South African Children's Cancer Study Group 195
  trilateral 191
retinopathies 109
  diabetic *see* diabetic retinopathy
  hypertensive 236–237
  of prematurity (ROP) 186–190, 421
  proliferative 36, 232–233
  radiation 371
  Sickle Cell 235–236
  traumatic 371
retinoschisis 224, 244, 247–248
retrobulbar optic neuritis 316–317
rhabdomyosarcoma 276
rheumatoid arthritis 62, 409–410
Richardson-Steele-Olszewski syndrome 351
Riddoch's phenomenon 326
Rieger's syndrome 119
Roth-Bielschowsky syndrome 350
Ranibuzumab 207
rubella congenital 58, 170
rubeosis iridis 108, 109–110

saccadic intrusions 333–334
saccadic palsy 349–350
Salzman's hyaline degeneration 78
Sandhoff disease 225
sarcoidosis 152–155
Schachar's theory 393–394
Schaffer grading angle width 7
Schiötz tonometry 94
Schnyder's dystrophy 46, 48
schwannoma 273
Schwartz syndrome 108
scleritis 58, 86–87
sclerocornea 43, 45
sebaceous gland carcinoma 26
seborrhoeic
  anterior blepharitis 23
  keratosis 25
serpiginous choroidopathy 177–178
seventh nerve (VII) palsy *see* palsy seventh nerve (VII)
short wavelength automated perimetry (SWAP) 121
sialidosis 225
sickle cell retinopathy 235–236
siderosis 259
simultanagnosia 326
sixth nerve (VI) palsy *see* palsy sixth nerve (VI)
Sjögren's syndrome 29–30
skew deviation 351–352
smooth pursuit palsy 350
solar
  keratosis 25
  maculopathy 220
Sorsby pseudo inflammatory macular dystrophy 223
South African Children's Cancer Study Group retinoblastoma treatment protocol 195
spasm of accommodation 377–378
spasm of the near reflex 289

spasmus nutans 332
spherical aberration 378
sphingolipidoses 70, 225, 402
squamous cell
  carcinoma 26, 40
  papilloma 25
stabbed orbit 365
Stargardt disease 222
steroids 178–182
Stevens-Johnson syndrome 38
Stickler syndrome 224
strabismus 282–306
  abnormal head postures 301
  abnormal retinal correspondence 302
  accommodative convergence 283
  classification of 282–283
  convergence insufficiency 284
  examination technique 11–12
  fibrosis syndromes 297–298
  fusional vergence 284–285
  motor adaptations 301
  paralytic 295–296, 306
  preschool screening for 283
  prevalence of 282
  restrictive 295–296
  sensory adaptations 301
  surgery 303–304
  surgical complications 305
  syndromes 296–298
Sturge-Weber syndrome 202–203, 407
sulphite oxidase deficiency 131
superior
  limbic kerato-conjunctiviti 35–36
  oblique myokemia 334, 341–342
  oblique overaction 292, 294
  oblique palsy 294–295
  orbital fissure syndrome 347
supranuclear gaze palsies 348–352
Swedish interactive threshold algorithm (SITA) 121
Sylvian aqueduct syndrome 351
sympathomimetics 122
synchisis scintillans 252–253
syphilis 73, 168, 411

tamoxifen 219
tapetochoroidal degeneration 244
Tay-Sachs disease 225
telangiectasias 234–235
telecanthus 20, 24–25
temporal arteritis 212–213, 313
tensilon test 405–406
Terrien's marginal degeneration 61, 78–79
Terson syndrome 253
thermokeratoplasty 389, 392
third nerve (III) palsy *see* palsy third nerve (III)
thrombophilia 211
thrombophlebitis 281
Thygeson's superficial punctuate keratitis 74
thyroid eye diseases 13–14, 265
tobacco-alcohol amblyopia 320
Tolosa-Hunt syndrome 347
toxic
  epidermal necrolysis 410
  optic neurophathies 320–321
toxocariasis 171
toxoplasmosis 158–159
trabeculotomy 108
trabulectomy 109
trachoma 34
trauma 110, 361–371
  blunt 363
  glaucoma secondary to 108
  orbital 276–279
  retinal 258–259
  uveal 369–370
traumatic
  cataracts 132
  hyphaema 369–370
  macular hole 371
  optic neuropathy 279, 319–320
  proptosis 13
  retinal breaks 246–247, 258
  retinopathy 371
Treacher-Collins syndrome 404
trichiasis 23–24
triple procedure 142
trochlear nerve palsy see palsy fourth nerve (IV)
tuberculosis (TB) ocular 167–168
tuberous sclerosis 202, 407–408
tubulointerstitial uveitis 150
tumours
  lacrimal gland 267–268
  optic disc 253–254
  optic nerve 321–323
  orbital 269, 272
  parasellar 191
  secondary 191

uveal 173–174
tunica vasculosa lentis 252
tyrosinaemia 71

Usher's syndrome 197
uveitis
acute anterior 48, 148
arthritis and 149–150
cataract surgery in 142–144, 182–183
causes of 151
childhood 159–162
chronic anterior 48
classification 147–148
clinical features of 148
fungal 168–169
GIT diseases associated with 150
glaucoma secondary to 106
intermediate 148
JIA and 162–164
lens-induced 144
masquerade syndromes 159, 172–173
ocular leprosy 172
parasitic 170–171
phacoantigenic 144
posterior 148
renal diseases associated with 150
sympathetic 156–157
tubulointerstitial 150
viral 169–170

valsalva maculopathy 220
vasculitis 237–238, 281
viscoelastics 135–136
vernal keratoconjunctivitis 35
visual fields 356–360
vitreomacular traction syndrome 227
vitreoretinal
degenerations hereditary 221, 224–225
interface abnormalities 225–227
vitreoretinochoroidopathy, dominant 225
vitreoretinopathy
erosive 224
familial exudative 224, 252
proliferative 243
vitreous
detachment posterior 252
haemorrhage 253, 258
Vogt-Koyanagi-Harada (VKH) syndrome 155–156
Von Hippel-Lindau disease 200–201, 254, 407
von Recklinghausen's disease 201–202

WEBINO syndrome 351
wavefront
analysis 387
guided PRK + LASIK 391–392
Wegener's granulomatosis keratitis in 63
Weill-Marchesani syndrome 130, 405
Wernicke's encephalopathy 351
white without pressure 245
Wilson's disease 72
Worth 4-dot test 302
Wyburn-Mason syndrome 201, 408

X-linked juvenile retinoschisis 248
X patterns 292
xanthelesma 22
xanthogranuloma juvenile 25, 410, 173–174
xeroderma pigmentosum 410
xerophthalmia 30–31